Type 2 Diabetes
in Adults
of All Ages

How to become an expert
on your own diabetes

Reviews of the first edition of
Type 2 Diabetes in Adults of All Ages

I purchased this book for my Diabetes Diploma. Although there are numerous titles available I was attracted to this one, and it has proven an excellent choice. If you want to understand diabetes, why it occurs, how it progresses, and what you can to do slow down the process whilst continuing to lead a normal life then I strongly recommend it to you.

Martin Gray, (From the Amazon website)

This is a very informative book. I have recently been diagnosed with Type 2 diabetes and had loads of questions that I didn't want to bother my doctor with so I thought it better to buy a book that can answer everything, which this one does. It also covers insulin treatment which doesn't apply to me but it is interesting to read it all the same. I would recommend this book if you are confused about diabetes as it is very helpful.

JC, (From the Amazon website)

I bought this book for my mother. She's a medical expert, being an officionado of Holby City and Casualty. She doesn't want to know less than her doctor. If you've got Type 2 diabetes and you want to understand the scientific reasons for how your condition is managed, and why certain treatments are picked for you, then this is for you. Become an expert.

Dr Phil, (From the Amazon website)

Reviews of
Type 2 Diabetes: Answers at Your Fingertips
(by the same authors)

'I can pass on much more information now after this marathon read!'

Clare Mehmet, Diabetes UK Newham Voluntary Group

'… an invaluable guide to the subject: authoritative, nicely written and packed with facts.'

P L, Acton

'This book will go a long way in helping anyone diagnosed with diabetes – or their relatives – understand what lies ahead. It explains everything you need to know about what causes diabetes and how to manage it.'

Jimmy Tarbuck, Honorary Vice-President Diabetes UK

Type 2 Diabetes in Adults of All Ages

How to become an expert on your own diabetes

Second edition

Charles Fox BM, FRCP

Consultant Physician with Special Interest in Diabetes,
Northampton General Hospital

Anne Kilvert MD, FRCP

Consultant Physician with Special Interest in Diabetes,
Northampton General Hospital

Class Publishing

NOTICE
For dosages and applications mentioned in this book, the reader can be
assured that the authors have gone to great lengths to ensure that the
indications reflect the standard of knowledge at the time this work was
completed. However, diabetes treatment must be individually tailored for
each and every person with diabetes. Treatment methods and dosages
may change. Advice and recommendations in this book cannot be
expected to be generally applicable in all situations and always need to
be supplemented with individual assessment by a diabetes team. The
author and the publishers do not accept any legal responsibility or
liability for any errors or omissions, or the use of the material contained
herein and the decisions based on such use.

Neither the authors nor the publishers will be liable for direct, indirect or
consequential damages arising out of the use, or inability to use, the
contents of this book.

Printing history
First edition 2008
Second edition 2014, reprinted 2017

The authors and publishers welcome feedback from the users of this
book. Please contact the publishers.

Class Health, The Exchange, Express Park, Bristol Road, Bridgwater, TA6 4RR, UK
Telephone: 44(0)1278 427800
Fax: 44(0)1278 421077 [International +4420]
email: post@class.co.uk Website: www.classhealth.co.uk
Class Health is an imprint of Class Publishing Ltd

A CIP catalogue for this book is available from the British Library
ISBN 978 1 85959 374 5 (Paperback)
ISBN 978 1 85959 375 2 (E-book)

10 9 8 7 6 5 4 3 2

Edited by Richenda Milton-Daws
Designed and typeset by Typematter, Basingstoke
Additional artwork by David Woodroffe
Printed in the UK by Bell & Bain Ltd, Glasgow

Contents

Contents

Contents

Contents

Contents

Preface

The first edition of this book on Type 2 diabetes was inspired by Dr Ragnar Hanas's book on *Type 1 Diabetes in Children, Adolescents and Young Adults*, which contains a wealth of detail and wisdom. The aim, in both the Type 1 book and this book, is to enable readers to become the experts on their own diabetes.

Diabetes is a condition which forces people to make unwelcome changes in their lives. This is true of both Type 1 and Type 2 diabetes. The more information available to you, the more motivated you are likely to be when it comes to making choices.

There is no such thing as 'mild diabetes', but that it is not to say it needs to rule your life. Type 2 diabetes is a progressive condition and people move inevitably through different stages of treatment starting with diet, through increasing numbers of tablets and eventually to insulin. Each new stage leads to anxiety and a feeling of failure and loss of control. This book aims to provide you with the information you need to understand what it happening to you at each stage, and why. Once you are armed with this information, you will begin to be able to take back control of your life.

We hope that, in its new edition, this book will continue to be a valuable source of information for people with Type 2 diabetes, and for everyone with whom they share their lives. The style is informal and friendly and we have tried to avoid jargon. More detailed information about physiology or research findings can be found in boxes so it is readily available for reference but does not interfere with the readability of the text itself. We write for the reader who wants to be fully informed so that they can make the choices necessary for staying healthy. Wherever possible, we provide evidence to support our views.

We want this book to be as good as it can be, and to remain so. In order to achieve this, we welcome feedback from our readers. If you feel there are errors or gaps, please contact Class Publishing at The Exchange, Express Park, Bristol Road, Bridgwater, TA6 4RR, UK, or via info@class.co.uk.

Enjoy the book, explore the information, and live your life to the full!

Dr Charles Fox, Northampton, UK

Dr Anne Kilvert, Northampton, UK

1

Introduction

If you want something done properly, do it yourself. This is all very well, but of course you need to know how to do it first. If you are to manage your diabetes, you will need a thorough understanding of the condition and how it may affect you. As anyone living with diabetes knows, it is with you 24 hours of every day.

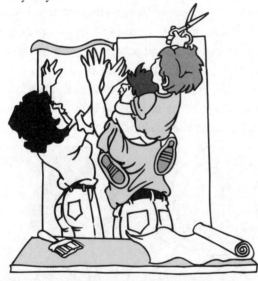

The underlying theme of this book is: 'If you want something done properly, do it yourself'. You are the only person who will be involved with your diabetes 24 hours every day so it won't be long before you are the greatest expert on it.

This book helps you take control of your own life with Type 2 diabetes. The only person you can rely upon to be there 24 hours a day is yourself. So after a while you will become the best authority on your own diabetes. Learning to care for your diabetes from scratch, like learning anything else, is a matter of trial and error. During the process you are bound to make some mistakes – but you can learn from each one of these. Indeed you will learn more from your own mistakes than from the mistakes other people have made. Taking an active part in lifestyle management and having an understanding of your drug treatments and why they are important is crucial to preserving your health over the longer term. It is rapidly becoming clear that consultations in which treatment is truly a partnership between the healthcare professional and the patient achieve far better long-term results.

If you want something done properly, do it yourself. This is all very well, but of course you need to know how to do it first.

Once you have come to terms with your diagnosis of diabetes, you will probably find it takes about a year to experience most of the day-to-day situations that are likely to be affected. These may include holidays, birthdays, parties, heavy exercise and periods of sickness. As you become more confident, you will begin to draw upon your own experiences and discover things about your condition that your diabetes team will find it helpful to know about. This sort of free exchange of information not only helps us to help you. It also enables the practice nurse to function as an information centre, passing on suggestions and knowledge from one person to another. You are not alone, and you can be sure that whatever problem you've had, someone attending your surgery will already have encountered it.

Knowledge changes over time. What was advisable 10 or 15 years ago may not necessarily apply today. At one time, health professionals would tell a person about some new development only to hear, 'Actually, I have been doing it that way for years, I just didn't dare tell anyone'. Nowadays, we share knowledge and learning with each other instead. Ask your practice nurse or doctor about your local Diabetes UK group. Most groups hold regular meetings which encourage sharing of experiences and usually have a speaker who is an expert in some aspect of diabetes – maybe your local diabetes specialist, a dietitian or an exercise coach. Even if you can't attend the meetings, you may at least be able to acquire some telephone numbers so you can 'phone a friend' for advice.

This book deals with Type 2 diabetes in adults of all ages, including the specific problems of Type 2 diabetes encountered by older people. It does not address the treatment of Type 1 diabetes, except in the briefest of ways. This is dealt with in the companion book *Type 1 Diabetes in Children, Adolescents and Young Adults*, by Dr Ragnar Hanas. This book describes methods of treating diabetes that are common in much of Europe as well as in

North America and elsewhere in the world. However, the methods used may vary from one centre to another. The goal is to find a way of managing your diabetes effectively, and there may be more than one way of reaching this goal.

Don't try to read the book from cover to cover or memorise it. Rather, use it as a reference book. A number of medical jargon terms are included, but their meaning should be obvious from the context so you don't necessarily need to learn them. If you find some parts of the book difficult to understand, especially on the first reading, please don't be discouraged. When you come back and read it a second time, and when you have more experience of living with diabetes, it will all begin to fit together. More detailed information, aimed at those who want to learn a little bit more, can be found in the boxes in the text. Key references that have been used in the writing of each chapter can be found at the back of the book.

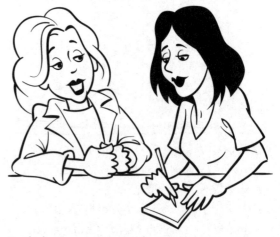

Body language can make more impact than words, and many people find that if it comes to a choice between remembering official information or informal information, they usually find it easier to remember informal information.

Remember that you can learn things in many different ways. Many places offer group education programmes (for example DESMOND or X-PERT). You will be encouraged to attend with a partner or friend who will help you to take in everything you're told. Generally, people learn better in a relaxed atmosphere where they are encouraged to participate. While you will be given official information during a formal consultation, you will also hear unofficial views and additional information from health professionals, other people with diabetes and their family members.

Your previous experience of diabetes from a relative or colleague may give you a false picture of what living with diabetes will be like for you. In particular, perhaps, your treatment immediately after diagnosis is likely to be very different from that taken by someone who has been living with diabetes for a number of years.

It will be quite natural after diagnosis to be preoccupied by concerns about your future and the difficulties that may lie ahead.

Your diabetes team will give you straightforward information about possible complications, and how to avoid or reduce the risks. During the first few weeks, you may find it hard to come to terms with the diagnosis, particularly if it was discovered by chance rather than because you felt unwell. You may question whether you really have the condition or feel angry that this has happened to you. Alternatively, you may have been worrying about a number of unexplained symptoms, in which case you may be relieved that you now know the reason and glad that you can do something to make you feel better To begin with, you may feel overwhelmed at the prospect of having to make changes to your life. This book aims to provide you with the knowledge to deal with your diabetes with confidence and to help you make the adjustments needed to lead a healthy life with diabetes.

2

Getting to grips with diabetes

Managing Type 2 diabetes involves a journey of therapy, which begins with changes to your diet and pattern of exercise. In time, this should become a way of life. In due course you will probably need to start taking tablets, moving on to combine different treatments, and possibly eventually to taking insulin injections. Good diabetes care includes both medical treatment and education. Everyone with Type 2 diabetes, and their relatives, should feel that they can assume responsibility for their own treatment and take charge of their own life. You can control your diabetes rather than letting your diabetes control you.

When you first find out you have diabetes

In the UK and many other countries, newly diagnosed Type 2 diabetes is usually looked after in general practice, where patients have an initial consultation with their GP, and later with the practice nurse. If you have Type 2 diabetes it is usual to receive advice about changes to your diet and lifestyle at the time of diagnosis, but this should be reinforced a

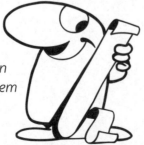

Keep a list of your questions so you can remember to ask them at your next review.

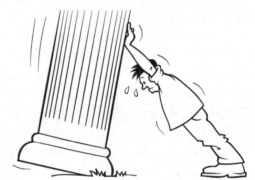

When a problem is too large and seems to have no solution, don't feel you have to cope with it all at once, by yourself.

few days later by a longer consultation with the practice nurse. In many areas you will be offered a structured education session which will tell you what you need to know to help you manage your diabetes. A few months later, you should have a follow-up appointment to look at whether the changes you have made to your lifestyle have brought your blood glucose levels under control. Long-term glucose control is measured by a test called HbA_{1c} which gives you an estimate of how much sugar is being carried in your red blood cells. This can improve substantially in people who are able to change the way they eat and the amount of exercise they take. It is essential to ask questions about your diet in the early stages and you should try to work out the best way of changing your pattern of eating. Changes made early on can set you up for better glucose control throughout your life with Type 2 diabetes.

Structured patient education programmes

People living with diabetes have a crucial role in managing their condition on a day-to-day basis so supporting self-care should be an integral component of any local diabetes service. Patient education is a vital part of this support package. There is a considerable amount of excellent work already being done to ensure that quality-assured training and education are available to all those who need it. For more information, consider contacting your local Diabetes UK group for advice on courses available in your area.

DESMOND

DESMOND is an acronym for Diabetes Education and Self Management for Ongoing and Newly Diagnosed. Still in development, this is a structured education programme based on recognized principles of adult learning and is promoted by the Department of Health. People are invited to DESMOND sessions in groups of eight, accompanied by partners if they wish. The sessions are run by two nurses or dietitians who have been specially trained to deliver patient education. Ideally, patients should have access to a DESMOND session within 4 weeks of their diagnosis. After this, they should be able to identify their own health risks and set their own specific goals.

To date, only people with newly diagnosed Type 2 diabetes are able to take part in DESMOND sessions, and a research project to test its effectiveness has been published. However, individuals who take part in these groups describe how their attitude towards diabetes has been altered completely by the programme. They have been able to tell their own story and listen to the accounts of diabetes from several other people in the same situation.

The results of the research study looking at 824 people showed a numerically greater reduction in HbA_{1c} for individuals enrolled in a DESMOND group compared with those receiving normal care, but this wasn't statistically different from the normal care group.

It is important to note though that the DESMOND group had significantly greater rates of smoking cessation and weight loss, and much stronger beliefs that they could have an impact on their own illness.

The Desmond course is run either as a one-day (6 hour) session, or as two half-day (3 hour) sessions.

DESMOND topics covered at the newly diagnosed patients' session

DESMOND:
Newly-diagnosed curriculum

Housekeeping

The patient story

What diabetes is

Main ways to manage diabetes

Consequences/personal risk

Monitoring and taking action

Food choices

Physical activity

Stress and emotion

Annual screening and clinics

X-PERT

X-PERT is a 6-week structured patient education programme developed by Dr Trudi Deakin, which was trialled initially in the North of England but has been rolled out throughout the UK and Ireland. It consists of six sessions, leading to goal setting for a healthier lifestyle. Visit the X-PERT website for a selection of materials for self-learning, including books and patient packs with interactive DVDs.

X-PERT programme: content

Week 1	What is diabetes?
Week 2	Weight management
Week 3	Carbohydrate awareness
Week 4	Supermarket tour
Week 5	Complications of diabetes
Week 6	Questions and evaluation
Lifestyle experiment	Goal setting

Coming to terms with the diagnosis

The first weeks may seem strange as you come to terms with the diagnosis of diabetes. You may have felt quite well at the time diabetes was diagnosed, but suddenly you are being given a number of depressing facts about long-term problems associated with diabetes. You may also be given one or more new medicines which you will be advised to take to protect you from future problems.

However, these drugs are not designed to make you feel better and simply act as a reminder of this condition you now have to live with. Many people may experience a feeling of resentment, disappointment and thoughts of 'Why me?' If you are in this situation, you may not accept that you actually have diabetes. You will need time to examine your feelings and adjust gradually to this new situation which affects you and the rest of your family. You will begin to understand how making careful choices about what you eat and drink can make a big difference to your blood sugar.

What happens next?

In the first few months, you should expect to meet a specialist dietitian. There is only so much that you can learn about healthy eating from books; a face-to-face meeting helps to put the information about food into context.

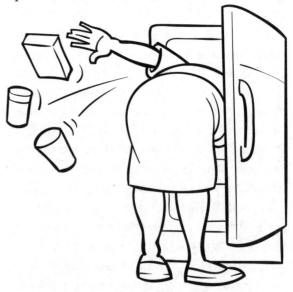

As you discover how taking control of what you eat can help your symptoms, you may find yourself clearing out most of the contents of the fridge.

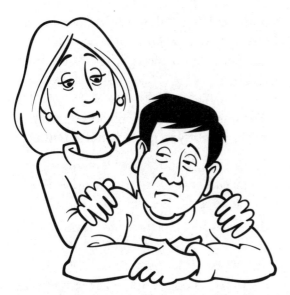

As you begin to come to terms with your diagnosis, it's worth having the courage to talk about it with close colleagues and friends. This will help them understand why you have to make changes in your lifestyle.

Older people

Older people are being diagnosed with Type 2 diabetes in ever greater numbers as GPs are now actively looking to make the diagnosis. Unfortunately, as you get older it may be more difficult to make the necessary lifestyle changes. With help and support from relatives and carers, people often find the motivation to accept the diagnosis and alter their eating habits and take the medication. If you're on your own, there will be a skilled practice nurse to offer advice and support.

More information about diabetes and older people can be found in Chapter 34.

Teenagers and young adults

Unfortunately, more and more young people are now being affected by Type 2 diabetes. This is due, in part, to the increasing burden of weight gain affecting our society in general. If you are in your teens or 20s and have just been diagnosed with Type 2 diabetes, it can be depressing and frightening. You should be referred to a specialist clinic, where staff will have experience of working with young people in your situation. They will be able to offer you the help and support you need. Specific strategies around weight loss and the management of Type 2 diabetes in teenagers and young adults will be discussed in Chapter 22.

Self-help groups

You may encounter people who have strong beliefs about diabetes and how to treat it and they may give you advice which differs from the education you have received. Knowledge and self-confidence are your best defence in this situation. This will help you to recognize and deal with the prejudice and out-of-date views. It is important for patients and health professionals to help increase knowledge and understanding about diabetes.

Our goal is for everyone with Type 2 diabetes, however young or old, to feel empowered to manage their own condition. You don't suddenly have to get up every morning and run a marathon. Simple changes like getting off the bus one stop early, or forgoing that mid-morning snack, can make a real difference to your long-term health with diabetes.

Routine check-ups

After the initial phase, you are likely to see the nurse or doctor at the surgery for a check-up every third month or so. At these check-ups, you can discuss your health over the last few months, and the nurse or doctor will measure your long-term blood sugar control using an HbA$_{1c}$ measurement. You will also be weighed, and the healthcare professional leading the clinic will ask about changes to your diet or routine. You may not achieve perfect results straight away, but as long as there is a steady improvement, that in itself is enough. Because raised blood pressure and cholesterol go hand in hand with Type 2 diabetes, you will also have these checked at regular intervals. There is good evidence that keeping these other risk factors under control has a positive effect on your long-term health.

If you are in a steady relationship, it is important that you feel able to bring your partner with you when you visit your diabetes healthcare team.

Once a year, you should have a more thorough check-up, including weight and blood pressure measurement, examination of your feet and photographs of your eyes. Your practice nurse will need to ensure that you have all nine annual checks required to make sure that you are keeping healthy. This will include blood tests to check on your diabetes control, cholesterol and kidney function.

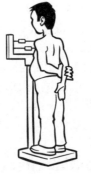

It is important that you continue to maintain a healthy weight. We check your weight at every visit to monitor and encourage your efforts with respect to weight loss.

Diabetes UK and NICE (National Institute for Health and Care Excellence) have both produced recommendations for a number of checks that need to be carried out on people with diabetes. These are known as the NICE 9

and the D UK 15. Both can be found in the Diabetes UK *State of the Nation* www.diabetes.org.uk/documents/reports/State-of-the-Nation -2012.pdf

The nine vital health checks you need every year if you have diabetes (NICE)

1. Get your blood glucose levels measured at least once a year – including an HbA$_{1c}$ blood test.

2. Have your blood pressure measured and set a personal target (of less than 140/80) that is right for you. Discuss with your doctor how you might achieve this target.

3. Have your cholesterol measured every year.

4. Have your eyes screened once a year, for retinopathy and other problems.

5. Have your legs and feet checked annually and discuss with your doctor whether you should be referred to a foot clinic.

6. Have a urine test for protein (a sign of possible kidney problems) every year.

7. Have an anuual blood test for creatinine to check your kidney function.

8. Have your weight checked and your waist measured to see if you need to lose weight. Your dietitian will advise you if you do.

8. Get support if you are a smoker, including advice and support on how to quit.

The Diabetes UK 15 standards of care include NICE health checks but recommend additional standards of good care.

Diabetes UK's 15 Healthcare Essentials

1. **HbA₁c**   Get your blood glucose levels (HbA_{1c}) measured at least once a year.
2. **Blood pressure**   Have your blood pressure measured and recorded at least once a year.
3. **Cholesterol**   Have your blood fats (cholesterol) measured every year.
4. **Retinopathy**   Have your eyes screened for signs of retinopathy every year.
5. **Foot checks**   Have your legs and feet checked – the skin, circulation and nerve supply in your legs and feet should be examined annually.
6. **Kidney function**   Have your kidney function monitored annually.
7. **Weight**   Have your weight checked, and your waist measured, to see if you need to lost weight.
8. **Smoking**   Get support if you are a smoker, including advice and support on how to quit.
9. **Care planning**   Receive care planning to meet your individual needs.
10. **Education**   Attend an education course to help you understand and manage your diabetes.
11. **Paediatric care**   Receive paediatric care if you are a child or young person.
12. **Inpatient care planning**   Receive high-quality care if you are admitted to hospital.
13. **Pregnancy care**   Get information and specialist care if you are planning to have a baby.
14. **Specialist care**   See specialist diabetes healthcare professionals to help you manage your diabetes.
15. **Emotional support**   Get emotional and psychological support.

Living the life you choose

Diabetes is a long-term condition that will affect you every day for the rest of your life. If you are able to accept your diabetes and incorporate the necessary changes into your daily routine you will find it easier to manage. Although it is important to adapt your lifestyle to support your treatment goals, you can still be flexible in your day-to-day work and leisure activities. You should try from the beginning to carry on with your life in a manner that suits you. Some people find themselves thinking: 'I can't do such and such any more, now that I have diabetes … but I used to enjoy it so much before my diagnosis'. However, most activities are perfectly compatible with diabetes. You should try to work with your practice nurse and doctor to agree a treatment regime which fits in with your lifestyle. If your diabetes progresses with time and you need insulin, this could have an impact on certain occupations (Chapter 27, Social and employment issues).

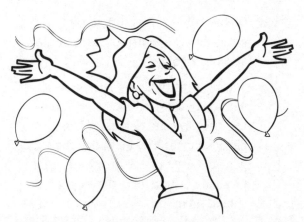

Whether it is a birthday, an anniversary or a new job, some days call for a celebration. Once in a while you can be a bit more relaxed about routines and rules.

3

Caring for your own diabetes

Goals for managing diabetes

International, North American, European and national bodies have all put together detailed guidelines for the management of Type 2 diabetes. However, the most relevant to England and Wales have been produced by NICE and should be followed by healthcare professionals working with diabetes. The NICE guidelines acknowledge that diabetes is a complex condition and that treatment and care should take account of the patients' individual needs and preferences. NICE recommend the following priorities:

- Patient education. This should be at diagnosis and ongoing and should include carers.

- Dietary advice. This should be given by an expert in nutrition and should also be ongoing.

- Setting a target HbA$_{1c}$. The person with diabetes should be involved in this decision and depending on circumstances may be above the general target of 6.5%. If there are problems with hypos, the target should be raised.

- Self-monitoring. At diagnosis, this may be a valuable educational tool but should only be used when the patient knows how to react to the results.

- Starting insulin therapy. This requires education especially about hypos, telephone support, frequent self-monitoring, insulin dose titration, understanding of diet, support from an experienced professional.

The following goals of treatment are recommended:

- No symptoms or discomfort in everyday life.

- Good general health and wellbeing.

- Normal social relationships.

- Normal professional life.

- Normal family life including the possibility of pregnancy.

- Prevention of long-term complications.

An important goal of diabetes management is to reduce the number and severity of the symptoms and side effects you may experience. During the early stages after diagnosis you may suffer tiredness, frequency of passing urine and thirst. It is important for your own personal wellbeing to protect yourself from these as much as possible. For this reason we regularly review control of blood sugar and ensure it is the best it can possibly be.

Diabetes should not disrupt your work patterns. It is difficult to apply yourself if your blood glucose is too high or too low, as this disturbs concentration. During times of stress, there may be a temptation to relax your pattern of eating. But of course, it may be even more important to keep yourself feeling well when there are extra pressures in your life. You should aim to lead an enjoyable and full life but maintain good control in order to reduce the long-term risks of diabetes.

How can you achieve these goals?

Traditionally, exercise and lifestyle changes have been the cornerstone of good Type 2 diabetes management – and this is still the case. Lifestyle changes underpin the way most of our treatments for diabetes work and improve their effectiveness. In the past, clinicians have started their first choice treatment to lower blood sugar but have not added a second medication unless control cannot be achieved on the maximum dose of the first – a stepwise approach. Many doctors and health professionals are starting to question this now, and believe that earlier combination of two drugs may be more effective at lowering blood sugar, with fewer side effects. Managing Type 2 diabetes isn't just about blood sugar: studies have shown that changing what you eat in order to reduce your fat intake can be combined with drugs to reduce fats in the blood. Along with exercise and tablets to help reduce your blood pressure, these can be important in helping you avoid problems later. See also Chapter 8, Nutrition, and Chapter 9, Control Weight.

Doctors' understanding of Type 2 diabetes, and the different treatments they can prescribe to help you manage it, have both increased with time. Unfortunately, those aspects of your lifestyle that put you at risk of developing Type 2 diabetes tend to be with you for a very long time. So health professionals have learned that they must work with people to help them change habits and behaviour patterns which are particularly damaging. Drug combinations, not just for sugar but for blood pressure and blood fats as well, allow you to avoid or reduce the chance of complications later in life. But the key factor in all of this is you, and your own level of motivation. If you have the knowledge and commitment to be fully involved in managing your own diabetes care, this will be lead to the best possible outcomes.

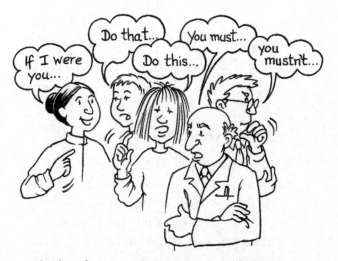

The key factor in managing your diabetes is you.

Traditional approach

- Diet and exercise.
- Stepwise addition of tablets when blood glucose control is lost.
- Insulin – eventually.

Diabetes today – cornerstones of management

- Education and knowledge.
- Diet and exercise.

- Earlier combinations of drugs to lower sugar to improve effectiveness and reduce side effects.

- Avoidance of complications by managing a range of problems, not just sugar.

If you want to manage well with diabetes you must:

1. Become your own expert on diabetes.

2. Be motivated to take responsibility for your own diabetes.

3. Have more knowledge about diabetes than the average doctor.

4. Accept your diabetes and learn to live with it.

'It is no fun getting diabetes, but you must be able to have fun even if you have diabetes.'

Professor JOHNNY LUDVIGSSON, Sweden

Becoming your own expert

The more motivated you are, the better you will be able to manage your own diabetes. It is important to realize that the treatment is for your benefit, not for your family, and certainly not for your doctor or nurse. Your motivation for the best possible self-treatment might be:

- to participate in the same activities as you did before diabetes was diagnosed;

- to achieve a good performance at work while keeping good control of your blood sugar levels;

- to be able to enjoy an active retirement and look after your grandchildren.

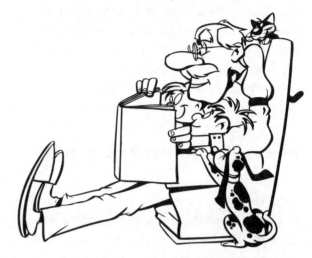

No matter how good our health or our fortune, we all need to feel loved and needed.

The treatment of diabetes has changed a great deal in recent years, but public awareness has not necessarily caught up. So you are likely to come across a lot of people with out-of-date or fixed ideas, who think they know a great deal more than they actually do. You need to be able to rely on your own knowledge. Indeed, in order to live your life in the way you want, you may need to know even more about diabetes than the average doctor. To gain this knowledge you will have to ask questions and clarify your own thoughts about diabetes. Be sure to contact a member of your diabetes team whenever you have questions about your medication or anything else. If you save the question until your next visit, which might be months away, you may simply forget all about it.

Becoming fully engaged with your diabetes and your own care is vitally important. Because you have to live with diabetes 24 hours a day, it is crucial to decide as early as possible whether you are going to adjust your life around your diabetes, or whether you prefer to adopt a particular lifestyle and adjust your diabetes treatment to enable you to achieve it. We encourage all people both young and old to be as active as possible in the management of their own diabetes from the start.

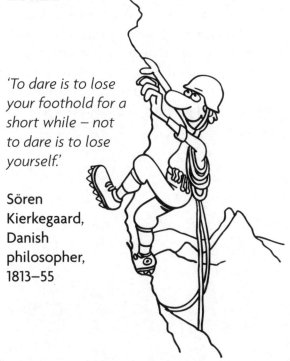

'To dare is to lose your foothold for a short while – not to dare is to lose yourself.'

Sören Kierkegaard, Danish philosopher, 1813–55

Can you take time off from diabetes?

This really isn't possible since your diabetes is with you 24 hours a day. But you can make a distinction between everyday life and having a good time on special occasions. Most people (with or without diabetes) will allow themselves something extra once in a while, even if they know that this little extra is not necessarily terribly healthy. If your usual lifestyle is appropriate for diabetes, you too can allow yourself to be a bit more relaxed

with food, if you are celebrating for example (see also 'Party-time' on page 52).

If you go on holiday or a business trip, your routine is bound to differ from the one you have at home. The goal on these occasions should not be to have perfect control over your blood glucose. The important thing is that you feel well enough to participate in all activities. This may mean you have to accept having a slightly higher than usual blood glucose level, but of course you shouldn't let it get so high that it affects your wellbeing.

Alternative and complementary therapies

Sometimes we encounter questions about complementary or alternative treatment methods. Unfortunately, some stories from the world of Type 1 diabetes, where insulin is required in all patients, make disturbing reading – particularly where choosing an 'alternative' has resulted in the death of a child.

In Type 2 diabetes, many herbalists claim to have products which promote weight loss or improve blood glucose levels. Although some may be genuine and well-meaning practitioners, others may prey on vulnerable individuals who have had trouble losing weight or maintaining a diet in the past.

Unlike an alternative therapy, which is used instead of a conventional one, complementary therapy means exactly what its name implies. It should be used in addition to medical treatment, to complement rather than replace it. So, while a complementary therapy cannot be a substitute for prescription medicines, you may benefit from it in other ways. For example, an aromatherapy massage may help you to relax, or a reflexology treatment may make it easier for you to cope with the anger you feel at having to organize your life rather differently from the way you did before.

Three issues are especially important when thinking about complementary or alternative treatments:

1. If you want to try an alternative or complementary treatment for your diabetes despite recommendations not to, it is better that you do this openly and tell your doctor and diabetes nurse about it.

2. Adolescents and adults with diabetes must continue taking their medical treatments as prescribed by the doctor, otherwise their health may be in serious danger.

3. The alternative or complementary treatment must not be in any way dangerous or harmful to the person with diabetes.

Bitter gourd or bitter melon

These are alternative names for the same fruit/vegetable, which is in common use in India. It is used to treat Type 1 and Type 2 diabetes and some patients find it has an effect on lowering the blood glucose. However, it is never given in a standardized dose and if you want to try it out, be sure to continue the normal treatment you take for diabetes. Apparently the taste is very off-putting.

4

Diabetes: some background

Diabetes mellitus, usually referred to simply as 'diabetes', has been known to mankind since ancient times. Diabetes means 'flowing through' and mellitus means 'sweet as honey', referring of course to the high volume of urine laden with sugar found in uncontrolled diabetes. Diabetes used to be described as either 'insulin-dependent' (IDDM) (now known as Type 1 diabetes or 'non-insulin dependent' (NIDDM) (now known as Type 2 diabetes).

Egyptian hieroglyphic findings from 1550 BC illustrate the symptoms of diabetes. In the past, diabetes was diagnosed by tasting the urine. No effective treatment was available. Before insulin was discovered, Type 1 diabetes always resulted in death, usually quite quickly.

Insulin history

■ The first human to be treated with insulin was a 14-year-old boy, Leonard Thomson, in Canada in the year 1922.

■ James Havens was the first American to be treated with insulin, in 1922.

■ In the UK, insulin was first given as part of a research trial later the same year.

■ In Sweden, the first insulin injections were given in 1923 to, among others, a 5-year-old boy who subsequently lived almost 70 years with his diabetes.

■ In the early days, insulin was distributed as a powder or tablets which were mixed with water before being injected.

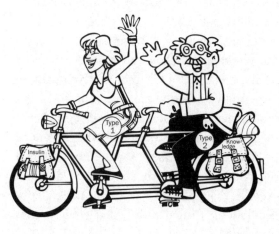

Type 1 diabetes

Most people who get Type 1 diabetes develop it before their 40th birthday, but having said this, it can happen at any age. In the past, if diabetes was diagnosed in childhood or the teenage years it was always Type 1 diabetes, but now there is an alarming increase in Type 2 diabetes in young people.

Type 1 diabetes is treated with insulin from the time it is first diagnosed. The insulin-producing cells of the pancreas are destroyed by a process in the body known as 'autoimmunity' (i.e. the body's cells attack each other). This leads eventually to a total loss of insulin production. In the absence of insulin, the blood glucose level continues to rise resulting in severe illness and eventually in death.

Type 2 diabetes

Type 2 diabetes used to be called adult-onset diabetes as it usually occurred after the age of 40. Unfortunately, due to lifestyle changes over the last few decades, it is no longer rare for children and young people to develop Type 2 diabetes. Nowadays, many more people are overweight and this leads to 'insulin resistance'– meaning that insulin is less effective so more and more insulin has to be produced to control the blood sugar. (You can read more about insulin resistance in Chapter 9.) Eventually, in some individuals, the pancreas can no longer produce enough insulin and blood sugars begin to rise. This is the point at which Type 2 diabetes occurs. The best way to improve blood sugar levels in the early stages is by diet and exercise, though there is a case to be made for people to be treated with tablets straight after diagnosis.

A minority of people who develop Type 2 diabetes are not overweight and the reason for their diabetes is that their pancreas is unable to produce sufficient insulin, even for someone of normal weight. People in this situation are very likely to need tablets immediately and sometimes need insulin within a year of diagnosis. After 5–10 years of diabetes the body's ability to produce insulin tails off and the majority of people require insulin injections eventually.

Risk factors for Type 2 diabetes

- Overweight, particularly around the middle: (a waist measurement of 37 inches in men and 33 inches in women puts you at greater risk).
- Genetics (i.e. having a parent or other close relative with Type 2 diabetes).
- Poor nutrition.
- A history of high levels of cholesterol and other fats in your blood.
- A history of heart problems.

Non-insulin treatments for Type 2 diabetes

The mainstay of Type 2 diabetes drug treatment in patients both young and old is metformin. This drug reduces the amount of glucose produced by the liver in the period between meals and has been shown in a very large study called the United Kingdom Prospective Diabetes Study (UKPDS) to reduce the risk of heart attacks and strokes in people with Type 2 diabetes.

A number of different types of drug are available if metformin alone is insufficient to control the blood sugar. The longest established, the sulphonylureas, act by increasing the amount of insulin released by the beta cells in the pancreas. They are good at bringing blood sugars down quickly and are useful in thinner patients with Type 2 diabetes or those with many symptoms of high blood sugar. Patients taking sulphonylureas must be careful about their blood sugars falling too low (hypoglycaemia).

Since the year 2000, a class of drugs, called the glitazones or insulin sensitizers have been available. Glitazones act by improving the action of insulin and making it more effective, so that muscle and fat can take up and use the sugar from the bloodstream. Originally there were two glitazones, rosiglitazone and pioglitazone, but rosiglitazone has been withdrawn because of worries that it may lead to a small increase in the risk of heart attack. Pioglitazone remains available and there are no concerns about heart attacks although evidence has recently emerged to suggest that there may be a possible association with bladder cancer. This is being closely monitored. Pioglitazone also increases the risk of fractures and the reason for this is not clear. Glitazones also cause fluid retention and should not be used in people with heart failure.

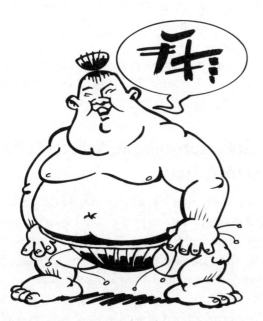

Being overweight will make you more vulnerable to Type 2 diabetes as, in the long run, your body will not be able to produce the large amounts of insulin necessary to keep your blood sugar normal. Japanese sumo wrestlers with a body weight of 200–260 kg (31–41 stones) have an increased risk of Type 2 diabetes when they stop their intensive training.

More recently, two new types of drug have been introduced to widen the choice of treatment for Type 2 diabetes; the GLP-1 agonists and the gliptins. The GLP-1 agonists, exenatide and liraglutide, are available for people who are overweight. Both are taken by injection and act by reducing appetite, leading to weight loss. They also stimulate insulin production to lower blood glucose. Their use is strictly regulated and NICE has stipulated that they can only be continued beyond six months of treatment if specified weight and blood glucose targets are met. The gliptins are related to the GLP-1 agonists but do not lead to weight loss and can be taken in tablet form.

Your doctor will advise which of the available treatments will best suit your circumstances; if necessary several different types can be used in combination. Most tablets and injections for diabetes can be used in combination but GLP-1 agonists and gliptins should not be used at the same time. More information about non-insulin treatments for lowering blood sugar is given in Chapter 13.

Young people with Type 2 diabetes

An increasing number of reports from North America, Japan, the UK and other parts of the world indicate that overweight teenagers are now developing Type 2 diabetes. This appears to be more common in girls than in boys. In North America, Type 2 diabetes and heart disease among young and middle-aged members of the native American population is reaching epidemic proportions.

In certain groups, the number of people with Type 2 diabetes is so high that all newly diagnosed children have Type 2 rather Type 1 diabetes. Type 2 diabetes is often diagnosed in African Americans after they become ill with the symptoms of ketoacidosis (see page 35).

Other risk factors for Type 2 diabetes in children and young people are low birth weight, Type 2 diabetes in the family, ethnic origin, high-fat and low-fibre diet, lack of exercise, and signs of insulin resistance such as high blood pressure and dark velvety discoloration of the skin (known as acanthosis nigricans).

A possible reason for the increase in Type 2 diabetes in young people may be that some people were 'programmed' thousands of years ago to survive famine by conserving energy during periods when there was better access to food. Today, when we have easy access to food, these 'survival capacities' may lead to obesity. For example, the number of young people with Type 2 diabetes is much higher in African Americans than among Africans still living in their home continent, although the genetic make-up of these two groups is very similar. This suggests that lifestyle and diet are important in reducing the risk of diabetes.

Principles of treatment for Type 2 diabetes

- Change what you eat to include smaller portions with less fat and carbohydrate.

- Take up a form of regular exercise that involves your friends too.

- Walking, jogging or team sports can all be fun in groups.

- Metformin can generally be used across all age groups, young and old, as long as they don't have kidney trouble. It is the mainstay of drug treatment for high blood sugar levels in Type 2 diabetes, and other drugs are added around it.

- Newer drugs such as the glitazones can't be used in children but offer promise for the future.

Maturity-onset diabetes of the young (MODY)

Some young adults, and even adolescents and children, have a rare form of genetic diabetes (MODY, maturity-onset diabetes of the young). This is associated with a definite family history of diabetes, and people with this condition are usually slim at time of diagnosis.

More information about MODY can be found in Chapter 22, Type 2 diabetes and young people.

Latent autoimmune diabetes in the adult (LADA)

This is a form of Type 1 diabetes that appears in adults and is caused by the body's own immune mechanisms. People with LADA are relatively thin and are very insulin-sensitive. They usually produce insulin of their own for many years, much longer than the typical remission or 'honeymoon' period seen in most young people with Type 1 diabetes. Because of their age on presentation, many people with LADA are initially diagnosed wrongly as having Type 2 diabetes, but this can sometimes be determined by measuring the level of certain antibodies that are specific for Type 1 diabetes.

How common is diabetes?

It is not just the absolute number of people in the UK with Type 2 diabetes which is frightening healthcare planners but the relentless increase in frequency. Thus the

Diabetes UK website tells us that an extra 130,000 people were diagnosed in 2011. By 2012, there was a total of 2.9 million people with diabetes in the UK which is a 50% rise since this information first became available in 2005. The average for the country is just below 5% but in some areas where there is a concentration of older people or racial minorities from the Indian subcontinent, this percentage already reaches 8%. Large areas of the UK are predicted to have a prevalence of 10% of diabetes by 2030.

Can you catch diabetes?

Diabetes is not infectious. This may be obvious to adults but young children may be less confident. It is very important to get the message across to all friends – and children and grandchildren – that they cannot 'catch' diabetes off you or anyone else.

Does eating too much sweet food cause diabetes?

Eating sweet food will not influence your risk of getting Type 1 diabetes at any stage of life. You can fall into the trap of thinking: 'If only I had done this or that differently, perhaps I wouldn't have diabetes'. Generally speaking, there is nothing you can do to change your chance of getting Type 1 diabetes.

Type 2 diabetes is rather different, however. While sweet foods do not in themselves cause Type 2 diabetes, excess calories of any kind (sweets, cake, potatoes, sugary drinks, alcohol), or just insufficient physical exercise coupled with eating too much, is clearly related to obesity. And if you have a genetic susceptibility to Type 2 diabetes, obesity and lack of exercise will make it much more likely that you will actually develop it. Nutritional issues relating to diabetes are discussed more fully in Chapter 8.

5

How your body works

It is important to understand how your body works in order to understand what goes wrong when you have diabetes. The three most important components of the food we eat are carbohydrates (sugar and starch), fat and protein. When we eat, the digestion of starch (long chains of sugar joined together) begins immediately in the mouth with the help of a special enzyme known as salivary amylase. (An enzyme is a substance that breaks down the bonds holding chemicals together.) The food collects in the stomach, where it is mixed and broken down by the acidic gastric juice. The stomach then empties this mixture, a little at a time, into the small intestine through the lower opening of the stomach (see illustration below).

Once the food is in the small intestine, it will be broken down further by digestive enzymes from the pancreas. Sugar cannot be absorbed directly from the mouth or stomach and can only reach the bloodstream once it has passed through the stomach into the small intestine. The emptying rate of the stomach varies for different foods and has an impact on the rate at which glucose is absorbed into the blood. Thus if you have a hypo (see Chapter 18) and need to increase your` blood glucose as quickly as possible, fluids containing concentrated glucose (e.g. Lucozade™, orange juice) are most effective as they pass through the stomach rapidly.

Phases in glucose metabolism

1. **Storage after meals:**
   During a meal and for the following 2–3 hours, glucose from the meal will be used as fuel by the cells. At the same time the stores of glycogen (glucose in long chains; see illustration 42), fat and protein are rebuilt.

2. **Fasting between meals:**
   After 3–5 hours, the carbohydrate content of the meal is used up and the blood glucose level starts to decrease. The glycogen stores in the liver will then be broken down to maintain a constant blood glucose level. The glucose produced in this way will be used by the brain while the body uses free fatty acids from fat tissue for its fuel.

The carbohydrates we eat are broken down into simple sugars known as glucose (dextrose, grape-sugar), fructose (fruit sugar) and galactose. Fructose must first be transformed into glucose in the liver before it can affect your blood glucose level. The two other components of food, protein and fat, are important for building muscles and bones (protein) and for storing energy (fat) but when you eat them they have no effect on your blood sugar. When you eat starch or sugar it is broken down into glucose, which is carried via the bloodstream from the stomach and intestines to the liver, to be stored as a form of starch (glycogen). Glycogen stores can be converted back to glucose as necessary between meals, during the night, and when a person is starving. Insulin is needed to take up glucose and transform it into glycogen (see illustration overleaf). If insulin is not available, glucose cannot be converted into glycogen and stores of glycogen in the liver will be broken down to form glucose. All this contributes to a high blood glucose level and insufficient insulin is the cause of diabetes. The body's ability to store glucose is very limited. The glycogen stores are only sufficient for 24 hours without food for an adult and 12 hours for a child.

The glucose content of the blood remains surprisingly constant during both day and night in a person without diabetes (approximately 4–7 mmol/L, 70–120 mg/dl). In adults, this blood glucose level corresponds to only about two lumps of sugar. If you think about it this way, you won't find it surprising that even a small amount of sugar, a few sweets for example, can disturb the balance of glucose in the body of a person with diabetes.

The smallest building blocks in your body are called cells. All the cells in your body need glucose to function well. With the help of oxygen, glucose is broken down into the vital energy to make cells work throughout the body.

How insulin works

1. Insulin switches off glucose production by the liver.
2. It stimulates the storage of glucose as glycogen.
3. It opens the door for glucose to enter the cells.
4. It stimulates the development of fat from excess carbohydrates.
5. It stimulates the production of protein compounds in the body.

Insulin

Insulin is one of a number of hormones, which act throughout the body, travelling in the bloodstream to work like keys, 'opening doors' to different functions in the body. Insulin is produced in the pancreas in special types of cells called beta cells. The beta cells are found in a part of the pancreas known as 'the islets of Langerhans' which also contain alpha cells

Pancreas

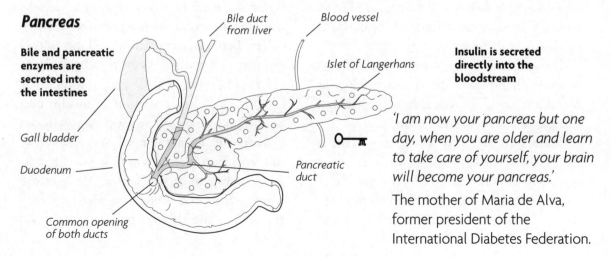

Bile duct from liver

Blood vessel

Bile and pancreatic enzymes are secreted into the intestines

Islet of Langerhans

Insulin is secreted directly into the bloodstream

Gall bladder

Duodenum

Pancreatic duct

Common opening of both ducts

'I am now your pancreas but one day, when you are older and learn to take care of yourself, your brain will become your pancreas.'

The mother of Maria de Alva, former president of the International Diabetes Federation.

Insulin and blood glucose

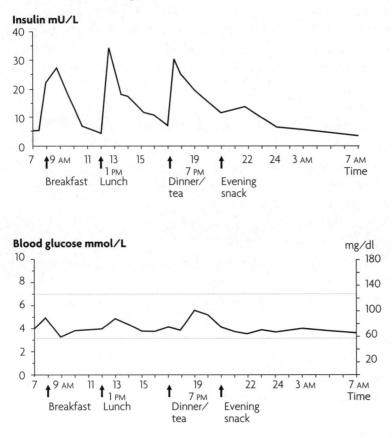

Insulin mU/L

Blood glucose mmol/L

A person without diabetes

If an individual doesn't have diabetes, the insulin concentration in the blood will increase rapidly after a meal. When the glucose in the food is absorbed from the intestine, and the blood glucose has returned to normal levels, the insulin level will drop back to baseline once again. However, the insulin level will never go right down to zero, as a low level of basal insulin is needed to take account of the gluose coming from the reserve stores in the liver between meals and during the night. The resulting blood glucose level will be very stable in a person without diabetes as this graph illustrates.

The normal blood glucose level is between about 4 and 7 mmol/L (70–120 mg/dl).

producing the hormone glucagon (see illustration on previous page). All the islets together contain approximately 200 units of insulin in an adult. The volume of them all combined is no larger than a fingertip.

The pancreas has another very important function. It produces enzymes to help you digest your food. In someone with diabetes, this part generally works normally.

The reason that insulin is so important is that it acts as the key that 'opens the door' for glucose to enter the cells. As soon as you see or smell food, signals are delivered to the beta cells to increase insulin production. Once the

food has gone into your stomach and intestine, other hormones, such as glucagon like peptide (GLP-1), send signals to the beta cells to continue increasing their insulin production.

The beta cells contain an inbuilt 'blood glucose meter' that measures the level of glucose in your blood and responds by sending the correct amount of insulin into your bloodstream. When a person without diabetes eats food, the insulin concentration in their blood increases rapidly (see illustration above) to make use of the glucose coming from the food, transporting it into the cells. The blood glucose level will

Insulin and blood glucose

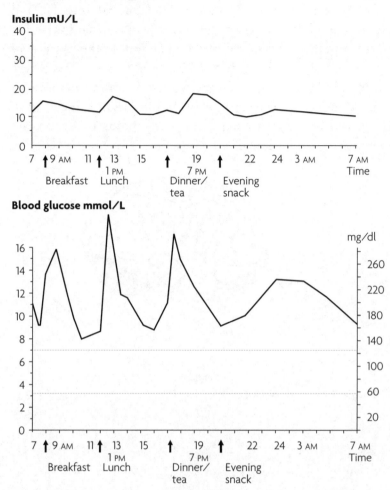

Insulin mU/L

7 ↑9 AM 11 ↑ 13 15 ↑ 19 ↑ 22 24 3 AM 7 AM
   1 PM   7 PM   Time
Breakfast Lunch   Dinner/ Evening
                   tea   snack

Blood glucose mmol/L

mg/dl

7 ↑ 9 AM 11 ↑ 13 15 ↑ 19 ↑ 22 24 3 AM 7 AM
   1 PM   7 PM   Time
Breakfast Lunch   Dinner/ Evening
                   tea   snack

A person with diabetes

In newly diagnosed Type 2 diabetes, because of insulin resistance, the basal levels of insulin may be high, but the pancreas loses the capacity to respond to a meal. Thus, fasting blood glucose may be only slightly raised, but the blood sugar rises to high levels after food, particularly if high in carbohydrate.

The resulting blood glucose level will be very unstable and only occasionally within normal levels. Every time the blood glucose level is higher than the renal threshold (see Chapter 7, High blood glucose levels), glucose will be passed out into the urine.

normally not rise more than 1–2 mmol/L (20–25 mg/dl) after a meal in a person without diabetes.

Insulin travels in the bloodstream to the different cells of the body, where it sticks onto special insulin receptors on the surface of the cell. The receptors allow the glucose to pass into the cell. As glucose enters the cell the blood glucose level falls. In this way, insulin regulates the blood glucose level. If the glucose level starts to fall, insulin will be switched off and cells will be unable to take up glucose, leaving it in the bloodstream, available for the essential body organs.

Certain cells can absorb glucose without insulin. If there is not enough glucose in the body, insulin production will be stopped, thus keeping the glucose in reserve for the most important organs such as the brain. If you have diabetes and your blood glucose level is high, the cells that can absorb glucose without the need for insulin will absorb large amounts of glucose. This includes the retina, nerves and kidneys. In the long run, this will poison the cells, putting those organs at risk of long-term damage.

The body needs a small amount of insulin, even between meals and during the night, to prevent the liver from breaking down glycogen stores to form glucose. This is often referred to as 'background' or 'basal' insulin to distinguish it from the 'boluses' of insulin needed to control the blood glucose after food. Around 40–50% of the total amount of insulin produced by a person without diabetes, over any 24-hour period, will be secreted as basal insulin between meals.

If you eat more than you need, the excess carbohydrate is transformed into fat and stored in the fat tissue. Excess fat in the diet is stored in the same way so the capacity of the body to form fat from excess food is very high. However, there is no mechanism for storing protein, and if insulin is deficient in the long term, body proteins are broken down.

What happens to the carbohydrates in the food?

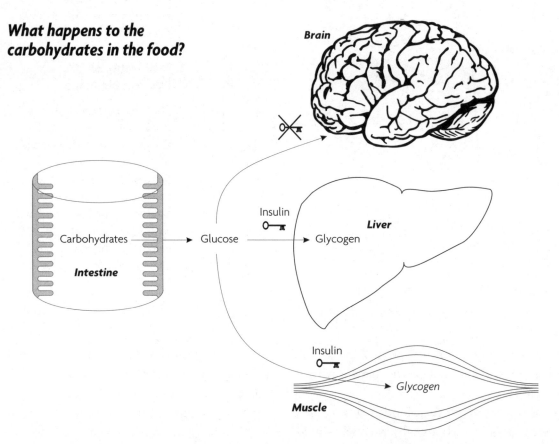

The complex carbohydrates in food are broken down to simple sugars in the intestine. Glucose is absorbed into the bloodstream and stored as glycogen in the liver and muscles. The key hormone insulin is needed to transport glucose into the cells of these organs. The brain cannot store glucose, so it has to depend upon a regular supply if it is to function well. The nervous system and some other cells (for example, those in the eyes and kidneys) can take up glucose without the help of insulin. There are advantages to this in the short term as the nervous system will not experience a lack of glucose, even if no insulin is present. However, in the long term, there are disadvantages for a person with diabetes, as the nervous system will be exposed to high levels of glucose inside the cells when the blood glucose level is high.

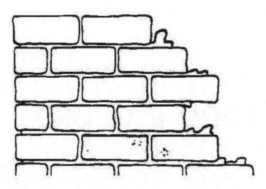

All the organs in your body are built of cells which are like the bricks in a house. Each organ contains specialized cells to enable it to perform its function, so there are identifiable kidney cells, liver cells and muscle cells.

Your body doesn't realise it has diabetes

When you read about how your body functions if you have diabetes, remember that it always 'thinks' and reacts as if it does not have diabetes, that is to say, as if insulin were being produced and working normally. Your body doesn't understand why things go wrong when you are short of insulin, because it doesn't realize what has happened. You will need to use your brain to work out what you need to do to compensate for lack of insulin – this may mean eating less carbohydrate or taking more exercise, but could mean taking insulin injections. It is very important therefore that you remember to stop and think about how your body reacts in particular situations, why it reacts like this, and how you can influence these reactions.

If you are taking insulin, the doses will vary as a result of changes in diet or exercise. If you did not have diabetes, your beta cells would adjust to any changes automatically. It is now up to you to notice how your body reacts on different days, and how much insulin you need in different situations.

Diabetes, insulin deficiency and insulin resistance

Type 2 diabetes is a condition which results from increased requirements of insulin at a time when the beta cells are no longer able to produce adequate supplies of this hormone. Thus, Type 2 diabetes is caused by insulin deficiency in the face of insulin resistance. This makes the insulin that is available less effective, and puts extra demands on the pancreas at a time when it is failing. This lack of insulin leads to an increase in the fasting glucose. However, the insulin resistance is usually more obvious when insulin is required to cover a meal. The pancreas is unable to produce enough insulin and the blood glucose levels rise after food, taking many hours to return to baseline levels.

So, while Type 1 diabetes is a 'deficiency disease' in which the hormone insulin is missing, people with Type 2 diabetes often have reasonable levels of insulin, but not enough to overcome the insulin resistance. In Type 1 diabetes, lack of insulin leads to breakdown of fat, with the formation of ketone bodies. This can lead to a very serious condition called ketoacidosis. In Type 2 diabetes complete insulin lack is unusual and ketone bodies rarely appear in large amounts. This means that ketoacidosis hardly ever occurs in Type 2 diabetes.

6

Regulation of blood glucose

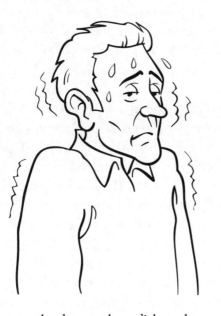

remaining glucose to the brain, which in general terms can only operate when enough glucose is available as fuel. Cells outside the brain attempt to use as little glucose as possible. The brain is unable to store glucose, so it depends on an uninterrupted supply of glucose from the blood. However, if no food has been eaten for several days, the brain can adapt to use other types of fuel, such as ketones, which are a produced when fat stores are broken down.

Where does the glucose in your blood come from?

1. From your food, via the liver.

2. From the breakdown of glucose stored as glycogen in the liver (called glycogenolysis).

3. From protein and fat, converted in the liver to form glucose (called gluconeogenesis).

Someone who does not have diabetes has a very small amount of glucose in their blood. The glucose content of their entire bloodstream in the fasting state amounts to only 5 g (1/5 ounce) of glucose – barely two lumps of sugar. However, the liver, which produces glucose, needs to provide 10 g of glucose every hour as fuel to the organs of the body. Thus if the supply of glucose dries up, the level of blood glucose will fall rapidly.

In someone who does not have diabetes, the body is able to regulate its own blood glucose levels within narrow boundaries, normally between 4 and 7 mmol/L (70–120 mg/dl). When your blood glucose falls below 3.5–4.0 mmol/L (65–70 mg/dl) you will feel unwell. A reduction in blood glucose level affects all bodily reactions, as the body struggles to channel all

While the hormone insulin lowers your blood glucose level, there are a number of hormones in your body which can raise it. The body reacts to low blood glucose (hypoglycaemia) with a defensive reaction known as counter-regulation. In this process, the brain and nerves work with a number of different hormones to raise the blood glucose level. This defence against hypoglycaemia is extremely important. The symptoms associated with hypoglycaemia are caused by the brain's response to a lack of glucose as well as by the direct effects of the counter-regulatory hormones.

Counter-regulatory hormones that increase blood glucose levels

1. Adrenaline.
2. Glucagon.
3. Cortisol.
4. Growth hormone.

In Type 2 diabetes, insulin is less effective due to insulin resistance, in particular with respect to blood glucose and blood fats. This leads to increased glucose production in the liver, and reduced uptake of glucose into the cells. The level of fats in the blood is also increased.

Effects of insulin

- Insulin is produced in the beta cells of the pancreas.
1. Insulin decreases blood glucose by:
   - Decreasing the production of glucose from the liver.
   - Increasing the uptake of glucose into the cells.
   - Increasing the body's ability to store glucose as glycogen in the liver and muscle.
2. Insulin prevents the production of ketones from the liver. It stimulates utilization of ketones in the cells.
3. Insulin also increases the production of muscle protein.
4. It increases the production and decreases the breakdown of body fat.

The liver

The liver functions as a bank for glucose. When times are good (after feeding) glucose is laid down in the liver and when times are bad (starvation) glucose is released. Excess glucose following a meal is stored in the 'reservoir' of the liver and muscle cells in the form of glycogen (see illustration on page 24). Insulin is needed to transport the glucose into both liver and muscle cells.

Body reserves during fasting and hypoglycaemia

- The store of glycogen in the liver is broken down to glucose.
- Fat is broken down to free fatty acids that can be used as fuel. Fatty acids can be transformed into ketones in the liver. Ketones can also be used as fuel, mainly by the brain.
- Proteins from the muscles are broken down to be used in the liver in order to produce glucose.

The liver can also produce glucose from fat and proteins to raise the blood glucose level (by a process called gluconeogenesis). The adult liver produces about 6 g (1/5 ounce) of glucose per hour in between meals. The majority of this glucose will be consumed by the brain which can make use of glucose without the help of insulin. After a longer period without food, the kidneys can produce glucose in the same way as the liver does. Recent research suggests that the kidneys can contribute as much as 20% of the body's total glucose production after a night without food.

People use the stores of glycogen in their liver to produce glucose if their blood glucose is low. This is the body's way of reversing hypoglycaemia.

A healthy pancreas produces insulin. Since the blood from the pancreas goes directly to the liver, this organ will be the first in line to receive a high concentration of insulin. When people with diabetes inject insulin subcutaneously, it has to pass through the general circulation and the heart before it reaches the liver. Because the insulin has been diluted on its passage through the circulation, the concentration reaching the liver is much lower than when insulin is provided naturally.

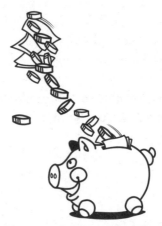

The liver acts like a bank for the glucose in your body. When times are good, i.e. during the hours after a meal, glucose is deposited in the 'liver bank' to be stored as glycogen.

Liver and muscle stores

- Liver cells can release glucose into the blood from the store of glycogen.

- Muscle cells can only use the glucose released from the glycogen stores as fuel inside the cell.

- An adult has about 100–120 g (3.5–4.2 ounces) of glucose stored in the liver.

- The glycogen store can be broken down to glucose when the blood glucose is low (glycogenolysis) and can compensate for about 24 hours without food in an adult.

- Children have smaller glycogen stores and can compensate for a shorter time without food.

- A pre-school child has enough glucose for about 12 hours without food, a smaller child even less.

- A child will use up glucose faster than an adult will, even when not very active. This is because a child's brain is larger in relation to body mass than an adult's brain.

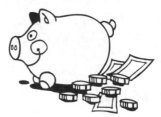

When times are bad, i.e. a couple of hours after the meal, glucose is withdrawn from the 'liver bank' to keep the blood glucose level adequate.

Glucagon

During the day you tend to feel hungry at intervals of about 4 hours, whereas during the night you can do without food for up to 8 or even 10 hours. This is because glycogen from the liver is broken down into glucose during the night, with the help of the hormones glucagon and adrenaline.

Glucagon is produced by the alpha cells in the pancreas and has the opposite effect to insulin, namely it leads to glucose production by the liver. In Type 1 diabetes, glucagon production is normal at the time of diagnosis but becomes blunted after about a year and by 5 years is absent. The cause for this failure of alpha cells is not well understood but may be related to the nervous system control of glucagon release. People with Type 2 diabetes do not lose the ability to produce glucagon as long as they are able to produce some insulin themselves. However, if they reach the stage of being completely devoid of their own insulin, they also lose the ability to produce glucagon and this will affect the body's ability to respond to a low blood sugar.

Glucagon injections

If a person with diabetes is unconscious or unable to eat or drink, an injection of glucagon will stimulate the breakdown of glycogen in the liver and raise the blood glucose level. Glucagon injections are not difficult to administer. If you take insulin and are prone to severe hypos, a partner or family member could learn how to give glucagon so they are able to help in the unlikely event of you being unable to deal with a hypo yourself. In practice, very few people with Type 2 diabetes have hypos which are serious enough to need glucagon.

The effects of glucagon

Glucagon is produced by the alpha cells in the pancreas.

1. Glucagon raises blood glucose by:

    – release of glucose from the glycogen stores in the liver

    – activation of production of glucose from proteins

2. Glucagon stimulates the production of ketones in the liver.

Adrenaline

Adrenaline is a stress hormone secreted by the adrenal glands. It raises the blood glucose primarily by breaking down the glycogen stores in the liver. The concentration of adrenaline rises when the body is exposed to any stress, such as fever or danger. One of the greatest stresses the body can experience is a low blood glucose, which immediately puts the brain at risk. For this reason, hypoglycaemia causes a brisk release of adrenaline.

Adrenaline also reduces the amount of glucose taken up by the cells of the body. This is in order to allow as much glucose as possible to go to the brain, which can only operate if glucose is available.

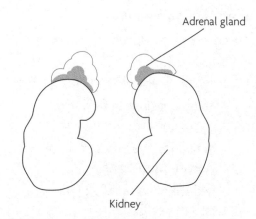

Adrenal gland

Kidney

Adrenaline and cortisol are produced in the adrenal glands.

The human body was originally designed for living in the Stone Age. If a person ran into a polar bear or a mammoth, the only alternatives were to fight or take flight. In both situations extra fuel, in the form of glucose, was needed by the body. The problem with our present way of life is that adrenaline is still secreted when we get excited or fearful, though this is more likely to be caused by a frightening TV programme than by an activity which actually calls for extra strength. A person whose insulin production is working as it should will not find this causes a problem. However, a person with diabetes will find that their blood glucose level rises if they are anxious or stressed (see Chapter 20 on Stress).

When a person with diabetes becomes hypoglycaemic, secretion of adrenaline can raise the blood glucose by stimulating the breakdown of the glycogen stores in the liver and at the same time causing shakiness, anxiety, and a pounding heart. Adrenaline also stimulates the breakdown of body fat to fatty acids which can be converted into ketones in the liver.

Effects of adrenaline

Adrenaline is produced in the adrenal glands.

1. Adrenaline raises blood glucose by:
   - Releasing glucose from the glycogen stores in the liver.
   - Activating the production of glucose from proteins.
   - Reducing the uptake of glucose into the cells.
   - Reducing insulin production in people who don't have diabetes.
2. Adrenaline causes symptoms of hypoglycaemia, such as shakiness, rapid heartbeat and sweating.
3. It also stimulates the breakdown of body fat.

Cortisol

Cortisol is another important hormone which is secreted by the adrenal glands in response to stress and affects the body's metabolism in many ways. It increases the amount of glucose in the blood by producing glucose from proteins (called gluconeo genesis) and by decreasing the amount of glucose that is absorbed and used by the cells. Cortisol also promotes the breakdown of body fat into fatty acids that can be converted into ketones.

Effects of cortisol

Cortisol is produced in the adrenal glands.

1. Cortisol raises blood glucose by:
   - Reducing the cellular uptake of glucose.
   - Breaking down proteins that can be used to produce glucose in the liver.
2. It also stimulates the breakdown of body fat.

Growth hormone

Growth hormone is produced in the pituitary gland, which is found just below the brain. Some of the body's most important hormones are produced in this gland. The most important effect of growth hormone is to stimulate growth. It has the effect of raising blood glucose by counteracting insulin on the cell surface, thereby reducing the uptake of glucose into the cells. Growth hormone not only stimulates growth during childhood and adolescence; it also increases muscle tissue and stimulates the breakdown of body fat.

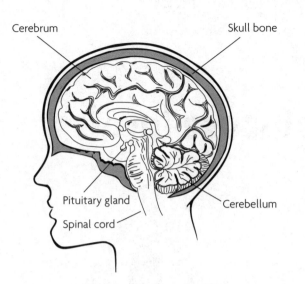

Cerebrum

Skull bone

Pituitary gland

Spinal cord

Cerebellum

Diagram of the brain. Growth hormone is produced in the pituitary gland.

The effects of growth hormone

Growth hormone is produced in the pituitary gland:

1. It stimulates growth.

2. It raises blood glucose by reducing the cellular uptake of glucose.

3. Growth hormone breaks down body fat.

4. It increases muscle mass.

7

High blood glucose levels

When your blood glucose level is high, the only way the body can eliminate the excess sugar is via the urine. Because there are large amounts of glucose to be removed, the body has to provide a lot of fluid to dilute the glucose. Thus anyone with a high glucose level and normal kidneys will pass a copious volume of sugary urine. This in turn leads to dehydration, a potentially serious condition. In order to correct this problem, you will become very thirsty and will need to drink abnormally large quantities of fluid. If you choose to slake your thirst with high sugar drinks, such as Coca Cola or lemonade, you will add fuel to the flames and cause a further rise in your blood glucose level. This then leads to the vicious circle of even greater thirst and urine output. When your sugars are high, your skin and mucous membranes can become dry and uncomfortable as a result of dehydration. High blood glucose levels also leave you prone to infection, particularly with candida, which in men may cause balanitis (infection of the penis), or in women, vulvovaginitis (infection, inflammation and itching around the vagina). In addition, your immune system is less effective at fighting off infections once your blood sugar goes above 14 mmol/L (250 mg/dl).

If your blood glucose level rises temporarily (e.g. following a large meal), you may not even notice. Many people feel fine, even with a blood glucose level of 16–18 mmol/L (290–325 mg/dl). You may be a bit more tired

Infection can often precipitate an increase in symptoms of Type 2 diabetes and may be associated with a rapid loss of control over blood sugar levels.

and thirsty than usual, but the symptoms are not nearly as obvious as when your blood glucose level is low. One study of adults found no difference in neuro-psychological function (simple motor abilities, attention, reaction time, learning and memory) when comparing blood glucose levels of 8.9 and 21.1 mmol/L (160 and 380 mg/dl).

Insulin resistance – not enough insulin to do the job?

In Type 2 diabetes, insulin is less effective (insulin resistance), and although the actual amount of insulin produced by the pancreas can be high, it is still not sufficient to keep the blood sugar in the normal range. A moderate increase in sugar levels will cause the usual symptoms of thirst, tiredness and frequent visits to the bathroom. However, if there is another medical problem, such as a chest infection or even a heart attack, blood sugar levels may rise above 25 mmol/L (450 mg/dl). Very high blood sugar levels can also result from trying to quench the thirst with sugary drinks such as lemonade or cola. Confusion, profound drowsiness and lethargy and even coma (loss of consciousness) may follow, and patients can rapidly become very unwell. This condition is called HHS (hyperglycaemic hyperosmolar state) and was previously known as HONK (hyperosmolar non-ketotic coma). More information about HHS is given on page 34. (See Chapter 21, Coping with sickness, for further information about what to do in an acute illness.)

Remember that your blood glucose level may rise during an acute illness even if you don't eat anything. This is caused by an increased level of hormones stimulating the liver to release more glucose (see Chapter 6, Regulation of blood glucose).

Early need for insulin in Type 2 diabetes

Some people who apparently have Type 2 diabetes do not respond to the normal early treatment with diet and tablets. They continue to have the symptoms of thirst and especially weight loss despite large doses of tablets and careful diet. In such cases, the only treatment is insulin. It is sometimes difficult to know whether such people actually have Type 1 diabetes at an older age, or whether they have simply progressed rapidly through the stages of Type 2 diabetes.

What to do about a high blood glucose level

If your blood glucose levels are higher than usual for more than a few days, you will have to take action. If you are feeling unwell, you should contact your doctor, who may identify an underlying cause such as an infection. If you do not feel unwell, your response will depend on the treatment you normally have for your diabetes.

Diet alone

If there is no obvious reason for the high glucose levels, it is likely that your diabetes has just moved into a different phase – this often happens quite suddenly. If so, you will need tablets and metformin is the usual first-line treatment.

Anti-diabetes tablets

If you take metformin and your sugars are high, you could try taking an extra one or two tablets each day to a maximum of 4 tablets. Unfortunately, higher doses of metformin are more likely to cause the recognized side effects of nausea and diarrhoea. If you take a sulphonylurea (such as gliclazide or glimepiride), you could try increasing the dose. These drugs normally have a fairly fast response but if you are already taking 4 of these tablets a day, increasing the dose will not have any effect.

Pioglitazone is a very slow acting drug so increasing the dose in the short term will not have an effect on the blood sugar levels for several weeks. There is no scope for altering the dose of the gliptins or GLP-1 agonists.

Sometimes the rise in blood glucose may be caused by your diabetes reaching the stage where you either need to add in a new type of tablet or to move to insulin treatment. The nurse or doctor who normally sees you about your diabetes will be able to advise you about this.

Symptoms of persistently high blood glucose

1. Glucose in the urine:
   - Needing to go to the toilet more frequently, including at night.
   - Passing a lot of urine at a time.
   - Fluid loss:
     Very thirsty, dry mouth.
     Dry skin, dry mucous membranes.
   - Lack of energy.
2. Weight loss, weakness.
3. Blurred eyesight.
4. Difficulty in concentrating, irritable behaviour.

Insulin treatment

This is the only heading in this section where the advice is simple. If you are taking insulin and, for whatever reason, your glucose levels suddenly run high, you need to increase the dose of insulin. How you do this will depend on the type of insulin you are taking. If your blood glucose is high first thing in the morning, an increase in the evening insulin should help. If, on the other hand, your sugar level rises during the day, you should take larger doses of morning or mealtime insulin.

Hyperglycaemic hyperosmolar state (HHS)

Hyperglycaemic hyperosmolar state was previously known as 'hyperosmolar non-ketotic coma' or 'HONK'.

The onset of HHS usually occurs slowly with several days of ill health and severe dehydration before people ask for medical help. Unfortunately, the dehydration (which may amount to 9–10 litres of fluid) leads to confusion, which may prevent people from realizing how unwell they are, especially if they live alone. Eventually, drowsiness, coma and, sometimes, even fits occur.

People with HHS have enough residual insulin to prevent the formation of ketones (see section on ketoacidosis below) but not enough to prevent very high blood glucose levels, which may reach 30–60 mmol/L (540–1000 mg/dl) or more. The high blood glucose causes very large volumes of urine to be passed with consequent severe dehydration. This dehydration, in combination with high blood glucose levels, causes increased thickness (viscosity) of the blood leading to a risk of heart attack or stroke. For this reason, people with HHS are treated with heparin to thin the blood and prevent the formation of clots.

Up to two thirds of cases of HHS occur in people who have not previously been known to have Type 2 diabetes. Because they don't know they have diabetes, they tend to quench their thirst with drinks containing sugar, such as squash or lemonade. This leads to very high blood sugar levels and makes the situation rapidly worse.

HHS is a very serious condition and always requires urgent hospital treatment with fluids and insulin. Although people with HHS always require treatment with insulin initially, it is unusual for insulin to be needed long term. Once things are stable the pancreas will probably be able to produce enough insulin to allow the blood glucose to be controlled with tablets.

If you have already experienced HHS, the best way to avoid problems in the future is to be aware of the symptoms of high blood glucose and dehydration, to recognize early when things are running out of control, and to consult your doctor or diabetes nurse at an early stage.

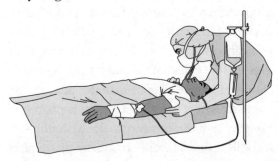

Hyperglycaemic hyperosmolar state (HHS) can rapidly develop into a life-threatening condition. This must be treated adequately in hospital with intravenous fluid and insulin.

Ketoacidosis

This is a condition which can develop in Type 1 diabetes as a result of a severe lack of insulin. People with Type 1 diabetes usually have no insulin production of their own and are dependent on injected insulin. If this is omitted, or if it is insufficient because of another condition, such as infection, keto-acidosis may develop. This is a serious condition which usually develops over the space of several hours or even days. Because of insulin lack, the body breaks down fat stores, which leads to the production of ketones as an alternative fuel to glucose. Since ketones themselves can only be utilized if insulin is present, they accumulate in the bloodstream. Because they are very acidic, they unbalance the body chemistry, cause the blood to become too acid and lead to

vomiting. At this stage people are already dehydrated from the raised glucose levels, and vomiting tips the balance into an emergency situation. Ketoacidosis requires urgent admission to hospital for therapy with fluids and insulin and can be life threatening.

Most people with Type 2 diabetes can produce enough insulin to avoid ketoacidosis, although it can occur in situations of extreme stress such as heart attack or severe infection. However, high blood sugar levels may lead to severe dehydration without ketones (see HHS above), and people may not feel well enough to drink to replace all the fluid they have lost in the form of urine. They may then end up being admitted to hospital as an 'emergency' in a very unwell state. This is particularly likely to affect teenagers.

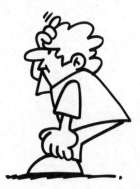

Symptoms of a low blood glucose level are usually fairly easy to recognize. However, when the blood glucose level is high many people won't have any symptoms at all. Thirst and the need to pass a lot of urine both occur when your blood glucose level goes above the renal threshold, but remember that this level can vary from one person to another. Other common symptoms are apathy and a sense that everything is 'slowing down'. What signs do you notice when your own blood glucose level is high?

Blurred eyesight and diabetes

Blurred eyesight can be a symptom of a high blood glucose level. This is caused by a mismatch between the glucose content of the lens and that of the blood. The lens contains no blood vessels (if it did, they would block the passage of light into the eye). Glucose from the blood must therefore be transported into the lens through the surrounding fluid (aqueous humour; see illustration on page 224). So when the glucose content of the blood is changing rapidly, the glucose content of the lens is bound to be different. If the glucose level of the lens is higher than the blood glucose, fluid enters the lens and interferes with focusing. This may last for several weeks after diagnosis. It can be corrected by glasses but as the changes are only temporary, it is important not to buy a new pair of glasses until your vision has stabilised.

The eye itself will not be damaged by short-term high blood sugar levels, and vision often returns to normal within a few hours. It is like borrowing somebody else's glasses – you can still focus, but it is tiresome for your eyes. This type of visual disturbance is common at the onset of diabetes and usually happens when the glucose level is changing rapidly. It has nothing to do with the eye complications that can occur after many years of diabetes. See Chapter 31, Microvascular complications.

Nutrition

The eatwell plate

Use the eatwell plate to help you get the balance right. It shows how much of what you eat should come from each food group

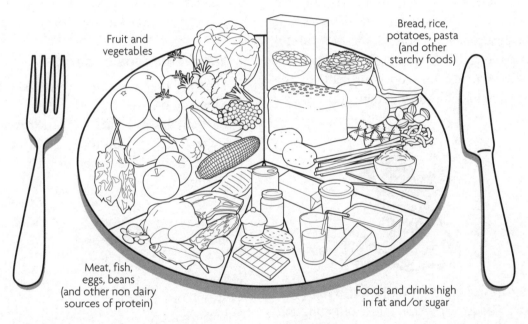

Fruit and vegetables

Bread, rice, potatoes, pasta (and other starchy foods)

Meat, fish, eggs, beans (and other non dairy sources of protein)

Foods and drinks high in fat and/or sugar

The food we eat is made up of three main categories: carbohydrate, fat and protein. While all three types of food are required for a balanced diet, it is important to understand that only carbohydrate can cause a rise in the blood sugar. Consequently, people tend to assume that once someone has been diagnosed with Type 2 diabetes, they should severely restrict the carbohydrate in their diet. However, while it is important to avoid refined carbohydrate (sugar), it is equally important to maintain a balanced diet

containing adequate amounts of carbohydrate in the form of starch. This chapter will explain how the type of carbohydrate you choose, and the foods you eat with it, can affect the blood sugar level. Understanding this will help you to keep your diabetes well controlled.

It is not necessary to stick to a rigid pattern of mealtimes and selected food unless you are taking a sulphonylurea or insulin – both of which are more likely to cause hypoglycaemia if meals are delayed. If you are on multiple injections of insulin, you should tailor your insulin dose to the size or type of meal that you are eating. The more you know about the composition of the food you are eating, the better you will be able to control your diabetes.

This chapter will give you many details about blood glucose and different foods.

Everyone with newly diagnosed diabetes has lots of questions about what they should or should not eat, and you can obtain advice from many different sources but you should insist on seeing a dietitian for personal advice. Many dietitians offer group sessions for people with newly diagnosed diabetes and the group can generate some very useful discussion. It helps if the person who normally prepares the food is present for the consultation with the dietitian.

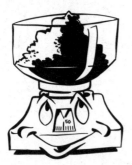

Kitchen scales can be useful for weighing food. Reducing portion size is difficult, and actually being able to visualize the weight of food being eaten is important. If you are estimating calories, then weighing portions of foods like meat or cheese can also help make your estimates more accurate.

Most people who develop Type 2 diabetes are overweight and this leads to insulin resistance. The best way to tackle this, and to reduce blood glucose levels, is to lose weight. This means reducing your total calorie intake, so the dietary advice should focus on portion sizes and a balance of carbohydrate, protein and fat. If you are able to increase the amount of exercise you do, this will help to burn off the calories and help you to lose weight.

An alternative to weighing food is to buy a book which provides photographs of foods with a guide to the carbohydrate content, for example *Carbs and Cals* by Chris Cheyette and Yello Balolia (available via Amazon). For those with a smartphone, apps which serve the same purpose are available for downloading.

What is our food made of?

The food that we eat is mainly made up of a mixture of:

Carbohydrates	Fat	Protein
Sugar	Butter	Meat
Bread/flour	Margarine	Fish
Biscuits	Oil	Egg
Potatoes	Cream	Cheese
Pasta	Milk	Milk
Rice	Yoghurt	Yoghurt
Fruit	Cheese	
Cereals		
Sweetcorn, taro		
Milk, yoghurt		

Aims of nutritional management

- To provide appropriate energy and nutrients for optimal health.
- To maintain or achieve an ideal body weight.
- To achieve the best possible control of your blood glucose, by balancing food intake with oral medication or insulin, energy requirements and physical activity.

- To prevent and treat acute complications of insulin or sulphonylurea therapy, for example hypoglycaemia, crises with high blood glucose, illness and exercise-related problems.

- To reduce the risk of long-term complications through optimal glucose control.

- To reduce the risk of heart complications and blood vessel disease.

- To preserve your quality of life and your social and psychological wellbeing.

How can this be achieved?

- Healthy eating principles should involve partners and other family members too.

- Your total calorie intake should allow you to maintain an ideal weight which, in turn, reduces insulin resistance.

- Cut down the amount of saturated fat.

- Eat more fruit and vegetables on a regular basis (the Department of Health recommends 5 portions a day of fruit or vegetables).

Absorption of carbohydrates

Glucose from food can only be absorbed into the bloodstream after it has passed into the intestines. Carbohydrates can be simple – as in sugar (sucrose) or fruits (fructose) or they can be complex, made up of long chains to form starch, which is found in foods such as bread, potatoes, pasta and rice. Complex carbohydrates must first be broken down to simple sugars so they can be absorbed into the bloodstream. The length of the carbohydrate chain does not seem to affect absorption, since 'cleavage' (breaking into smaller sections) is a fairly rapid process. Simple carbohydrates are broken down by enzymes in the intestinal lining while more complex carbohydrates are first prepared for digestion by amylase, an enzyme found in the saliva and pancreas, before moving on to the intestine for further digestion.

The term 'glycaemic index' (GI) is used to describe how the blood glucose level is affected by different foods. Dietary fibre content and particle size seem to be particularly important. The starch in vegetables is broken down more slowly than the starch in bread. The starch in potatoes is quick to break down to glucose. The starch from pasta products is broken down much more slowly, even though it is made from white flour, which is low in fibre.

How much you chew the food and the size of the food particles swallowed also influence the blood glucose response. Industrially manufactured mashed potatoes contain a fine powder that is mixed with fluid. The glucose in mashed potatoes is absorbed just as quickly as a glucose solution. Pasta and rice are swallowed in larger bites and must be digested before they can be absorbed. Likewise, a whole apple will give a slower rise in blood glucose than apple juice which contains smaller particles and is in a liquid form.

Heating decomposes starch, making sugar more accessible and faster to digest. Industrial food processing usually involves higher temperatures, which give food a quicker blood glucose raising effect compared with home-cooked meals. Indigestible carbohydrates (dietary fibre) cannot be broken down in the intestines and will therefore not give a blood

Structure of different foods

Slow
absorption

Quick
absorption

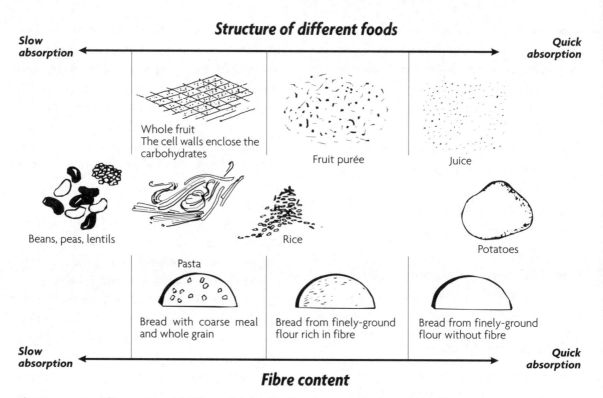

Whole fruit
The cell walls enclose the
carbohydrates

Fruit purée

Juice

Beans, peas, lentils

Rice

Potatoes

Pasta

Bread with coarse meal
and whole grain

Bread from finely-ground
flour rich in fibre

Bread from finely-ground
flour without fibre

Slow
absorption

Quick
absorption

Fibre content

The structure and fibre content of different foodstuffs affect how quickly the carbohydrate content is absorbed. The illustration is from the book *Food and Diabetes* by the Swedish Diabetes Association, printed with permission.

glucose response. The amount of carbohydrate listed on a food label can be misleading as no distinction is made between digestible and indigestible carbohydrates. Do ask your dietitian for more information about this.

Glycaemic index

The glycaemic index (GI) is an attempt to describe the blood glucose-raising effect of different foods. Glucose is used to give a baseline GI index of 100. The GI of a mixed meal can be predicted from the GI of single foods. It may be difficult to estimate the GI for some combined meals from the GI of the single ingredients since the fat content also affects the speed with which carbohydrates are absorbed. A foodstuff with a low but easily accessible sugar content (e.g. carrots)

has a high glycaemic index but you would need to eat a very large portion of carrots to have any effect on your blood glucose.

Although the use of low-GI food may reduce blood glucose levels after meals, more research is required before GI can be used as a general tool in diabetes care. The Diabetes and Nutrition Study Group of the European Association for the Study of Diabetes recommends the substitution of high-GI with low-GI foods to improve glycaemic control. A summary of many studies (called a meta-analysis) found that a low-GI diet reduced HbA_{1c} by 0.43% compared with conventional or high-GI diets. In Australia, the GI concept is much more accepted and widely used than, for example, in the US or the UK.

Potatoes (GI 74) give a faster blood glucose response than pasta (GI 46–52). Adding a small amount of oil or margarine to mashed potatoes (GI 85) will delay the glucose peak. If you replace one item in a meal with another (e.g. potatoes with pasta), the GI of the individual foods will help you determine the likely effect on the blood glucose. GI is very useful when you are looking at eating between meals (single items of food often, such as yoghurt, an apple, a bun, ice cream, crisps, etc.). Glucose tablets have a GI of 100 and can be used for treating hypoglycaemia if a rapid response is required.

Factors that raise the blood glucose level more quickly (increase the glycaemic index)

1. **Cooking:**
   Boiling and other types of cooking will break down the starch in food.

2. **Preparing food:**
   Prepared food, e.g. polished rice, will give a quicker rise in blood glucose than unpolished, mashed potatoes quicker than whole potatoes and grated carrots quicker than sliced. Wheat flour gives a higher blood glucose response when baked in bread than when used for pasta.

3. **Fluids with food:**
   Drinking fluids with a meal causes the stomach to empty more quickly.

4. **Glucose content:**
   Extra sugar as part of a meal can cause the blood glucose level to rise. Particle size and cell structure in different food compounds give them different blood glucose responses in spite of their containing the same amount of carbohydrate.

5. **Salt content:**
   Salt in the food increases the absorption of glucose into the bloodsteam.

Factors that raise the blood glucose level more slowly (decrease the glycaemic index)

1. **Starch structure:**
   Rice and pasta give a slower blood glucose response, while boiled and mashed potatoes give a blood sugar response which can be as fast as ordinary sugar.

2. **Gel-forming dietary fibre:**
   A high fibre content (as in rye bread) gives a slower rise in blood glucose by slowing down the emptying rate of the stomach and binding glucose in the intestine.

3. **Fat content:**
   Fat in the food will delay the emptying of the stomach.

4. **Cell structure:**
   Beans, peas and lentils retain their cell structure even after cooking. Whole fruits affect the blood glucose level more slowly than peeled fruits and juice.

5. **Size of bites:**
   Larger pieces of food take longer to digest in the stomach and intestine. Larger pieces also cause the stomach to empty more slowly.

Carbohydrates

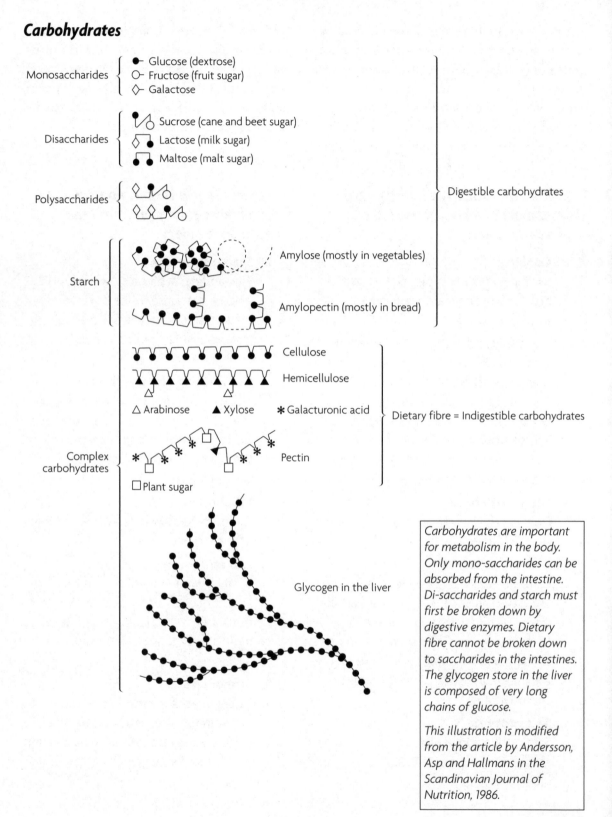

Monosaccharides
- Glucose (dextrose)
- Fructose (fruit sugar)
- Galactose

Disaccharides
- Sucrose (cane and beet sugar)
- Lactose (milk sugar)
- Maltose (malt sugar)

Polysaccharides

Digestible carbohydrates

Starch

Amylose (mostly in vegetables)

Amylopectin (mostly in bread)

Cellulose

Hemicellulose

△ Arabinose   ▲ Xylose   ✻ Galacturonic acid

Dietary fibre = Indigestible carbohydrates

Complex carbohydrates

Pectin

☐ Plant sugar

Glycogen in the liver

Carbohydrates are important for metabolism in the body. Only mono-saccharides can be absorbed from the intestine. Di-saccharides and starch must first be broken down by digestive enzymes. Dietary fibre cannot be broken down to saccharides in the intestines. The glycogen store in the liver is composed of very long chains of glucose.

This illustration is modified from the article by Andersson, Asp and Hallmans in the Scandinavian Journal of Nutrition, 1986.

Glycaemic index

High glycaemic index	GI
Glucose 100	
Instant mashed potatoes	85
Potato, baked	85
Corn flakes	81
Jelly sweets	78
White bread (gluten free)	76
Waffles	76
French fries	75
Weetabix	75
Oatmeal porridge	74
Rice, puffed	74
Potato, boiled	74
Watermelon	72
Popcorn	72
White bread	70
Sucrose (sugar)	68
Pineapple	66
Rice, white	64

Low glycaemic index	GI
Orange	44
Milk chocolate	43
Nectarine	43
Banana, yellow and green	42
Peach	42
All Bran	42
Prunes	40
Apple	38
Pear	38
Ice cream	37–61
Yoghurt	36
Lentils, green	30
Kidney beans	28
Strawberries	28
Milk, 3% fat	21
Fructose (fruit sugar)	19
Soya beans (dried)	18
Peanuts	14

Average glycaemic index	GI
Rye bread (wholemeal)	58
Rice, long grain	56
Gluten-free pasta	56
Honey	55
Banana, all yellow	51
Pasta	46–52
Lactose (milk sugar)	46
Grapes, green	46
Rye bread (whole grain)	46

See also www.mendosa.com/gilists.htm for an extensive list of foods.

Emptying the stomach

Everything that causes the stomach to release food more slowly into the intestines will also result in a slower increase of the blood glucose level (see illustration on page 45). From this, it follows that the composition of the meal will be important, and not only the amount of carbohydrates it contains. Fat and fibre cause the stomach to empty more slowly, while a drink with the meal will make it empty more quickly. A meal containing solid food (such as pasta) is emptied more slowly than liquid food like soup. Swallowing without chewing also causes a slower rise in blood glucose. Extremely cold (4°C, 39°F) or hot (50°C, 122°F) food will also slow down stomach emptying.

The emptying of the stomach is also affected by the blood glucose level. The stomach empties more quickly if the blood glucose is low and more slowly if it is high. Both solid and liquid food are emptied from the stomach twice as fast when the blood glucose drops from a normal level (4–7 mmol/L, 72–126 mg/dl) to a hypoglycaemic level (1.6–2.2 mmol/L, 29–40 mg/dl). This makes sense because if your blood glucose level is low you want your stomach to empty as quickly as possible so that the glucose can be absorbed into the blood.

In this situation, you should take something with a high glucose content, such as glucose tablets, glucose gel, fruit juice or a sports drink.

How is the emptying of the stomach affected?

More quickly	More slowly
Small bites	Large bites
Liquid food	Solid food
Drink with food	Drink after food
	Fatty food
	Food rich in fibre
	Extremely hot or cold food
Hypoglycaemia	High blood glucose
	High levels of insulin
	Smoking
	Gastroenteritis
Light exercise	Heavy exercise

A high blood glucose level causes the stomach to empty more slowly. Even small changes in blood glucose level, well within the normal ranges for individuals without diabetes, seem to affect the rate of stomach emptying. One study of people without diabetes showed a 20% decrease in the emptying rate when the blood glucose level was increased from 4 to 8 mmol/L (72 to 144 mg/dl).

Non-strenuous exercise (like walking) leads to unchanged or more rapid emptying of the stomach, while strenuous exercise or physical exertion stops the stomach from emptying for 20–40 minutes after activity finishes. A possible explanation for this delayed stomach emptying after physical exertion is an increased secretion of adrenaline and morphine-like hormones (endorphins).

Stomach emptying can also be delayed if you have gastroenteritis. This may explain why when some people develop diarrhoea and vomiting, their blood glucose levels remain low for the duration of the illness.

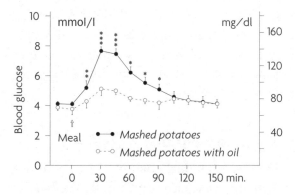

If your meal contains fat, this will delay the emptying of your stomach and cause your blood glucose level to rise more slowly. In this study (Welch, Bruce, Hill & Read), two helpings of mashed potatoes (50 g of carbohydrate) were given with or without corn oil (approximately 30 ml or two tablespoonfuls). The study was done in adults without diabetes, who can increase their amounts of insulin very fast. Notice that the blood glucose level increased very quickly despite this, with a significant change appearing in 30 minutes in the group of people whose mashed potatoes did not contain oil. If you have weight problems, you need to be careful about adding fat to your food.

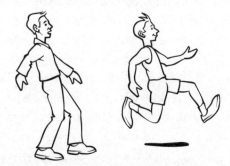

A moderate degree of exercise will not stop the stomach from emptying – and may even speed it up. Strenuous exercise will stop the stomach from emptying while your muscles are working hard.

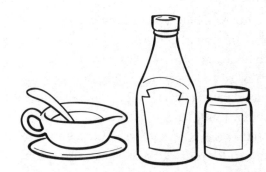

You can have a modest amount of sauce or ketchup with your food without any problems. However, be aware that many commercially produced sauces contain a lot of sugar. You need to keep a count of how much additional sugar you are eating.

Gastroparesis

Gastroparesis is a serious complication of diabetes caused by damage to the nerves that control the automatic muscular activity of the stomach. This disrupts the normal emptying process, and the stomach ends up behaving like a floppy bag. Food is normally squeezed out of the stomach in a matter of hours, but if there is gastroparesis, stomach emptying can be very variable and undigested food may remain in the stomach for days.

Gastroparesis may lead to heartburn, vomiting of food eaten many hours or even days ago and bloating of the abdomen (see also Chapter 31 on Microvascular complications).

Taking fluids with food

You can affect your blood glucose level considerably, depending on what you have to drink with your meals. Sweet drinks like fruit juice can be used to raise your blood glucose if it is in the low range but should otherwise be avoided. Try to drink calorie-free drinks as this will help you to avoid weight gain. If you are going to drink alcohol, don't forget that alcoholic drinks can contain a lot of calories too (see also Chapter 24). If your blood glucose level is high, it is better to have water. You should be wary of too many drinks containing artificial sweeteners, and careful not to let your caffeine intake rise too high either.

Dietary fibre

The fibre content of food is healthy for many reasons. There are two kinds of fibre, soluble (gel-forming) and insoluble. Both help to prevent constipation, but only the soluble fibres (found in fruit, vegetables, legumes and oats) affect glucose control. You will feel full for longer after eating coarse rye or whole-meal bread with a high soluble fibre content than you would after eating the same amount of white bread without fibre. A high soluble fibre content will also decrease the cholesterol level in your blood. Adding fibre (such as oats and barley) to a meal will increase its bulk, causing the contents of the stomach and intestines to empty more slowly. The fibre forms a thin film on the intestinal surface, causing the glucose to be absorbed more slowly.

A European study of 2065 adults with Type 1 diabetes compared a low-fibre diet with a high-fibre diet rich in fruit, legumes and vegetables. Both diets contained exclusively natural foodstuffs. The high-fibre diet resulted in lower blood glucose levels, 0.5% lower HbA_{1c} and a decreased frequency of hypoglycaemia. In a European study on 2065 adults with Type 1 diabetes, the HbA_{1c} in people whose fibre intake was high was found to be approximately 0.3% lower than for the group with a low fibre intake. Although these studies were done in people with Type 1 diabetes, it seems reasonable to suppose that similar effects might be found in Type 2 diabetes.

Sugar content of our food

From a nutritional point of view, we do not actually need pure sugar at all. The liver is quite capable of producing the 250–300 g of glucose that a healthy adult normally needs per day.

Small amounts of glucose along with a meal (for example ketchup or other sauces) do not cause a significant rise in blood glucose. The recommendation to decrease the sugar content in food is based on more general factors:

Sugar gives 'empty calories', i.e. sugar provides energy but contains no other nutrients. If you do not 'burn off' this energy it will cause you to gain weight, while reducing your appetite for more healthy foods. It is therefore important to limit sugary foods where possible.

It used to be common practice to decrease the carbohydrate content in a diabetes meal plan at all costs. Unfortunately, this approach usually causes an increase in fat intake, which in itself is less healthy than a normal diet. Nowadays, the same dietary advice applies to people with and without diabetes, with the recommendation to eat less refined (high GI) carbohydrate and compensate with more low GI carbohydrate. Some people do lose weight by keeping to an ultra-low carbohydrate diet (as in the Atkins diet) but it is important to avoid eating extra fat in compensation. If you decide to give it a try, you should take medical advice first because some medications, such as sulphonylureas or insulin, will cause hypoglycaemia if taken without carbohydrate. A recent study showed that the Atkins diet causes more weight loss than other commercial weight loss programmes at 2 months, but by 6 months the effects of different 'diets' are the same.

Dietary fats

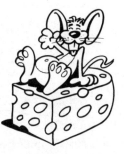

If you have diabetes, a key goal should be to decrease your total fat intake and thus reduce your risk of arteriosclerosis and heart disease (see Chapter 30 on Complications of the cardiovascular system). You need to be particularly careful with saturated fat, which is found in dairy products, red meat and many snack foods such as chocolate, cakes, pastries and crisps. Ordinary margarine and butter are high in saturated fats, so try to use monounsaturated and polyunsaturated fats instead. In general soft or liquid margarines are best, for example margarine containing olive oil and cooking oils such as olive, sunflower and rapeseed.

Many people mistakenly believe that fat directly increases the blood glucose level since people with diabetes are usually advised to cut down on fat in their diet. However, fatty food has no direct effect on the blood glucose level. As fat yields more energy than carbohydrate, the stomach is emptied more slowly when the fat content is high. A meal with a high fat content will therefore cause the blood glucose level to rise more slowly in the initial period. In the long term the higher calorie load in fatty food will lead to increased weight gain which will increase insulin resistance and worsen your blood glucose level.

It is the total amount of fat over time that is important in the long run. As long as you observe a healthy diet for the majority of the time, an occasional celebratory meal out won't cause you too much harm. If you are trying to keep your fat intake low, remember that some 'low fat' foods contain additional carbohydrate, which can raise your blood sugar level. It is worth checking the food label to find out exactly what is in the product.

Food rules of thumb

- Snacks taken between meals are often high-calorie, high-sugar foods which won't leave you satisfied and will increase your weight.
- Eat fresh fruit as a snack rather than drinking fruit juice.
- Cut down on snacks and portion size at every meal if you have weight problems.
- Aim for a high fibre content in your food.

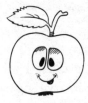

If you want a snack, try a piece of fruit as a healthy option.

Food choices and diabetes
Potatoes

Potatoes, sweet potatoes, taro and yam belong to this type of foodstuff. The carbohydrate content of raw potatoes is absorbed slowly, but boiling causes the cell walls to burst. This allows the carbohydrates to be absorbed more quickly from the intestines. The carbohydrate content of mashed potatoes is absorbed as quickly as pure glucose (see graph on page 45). If you change the surface of a potato (e.g. by frying, deep frying or storing it in the refrigerator), the glucose will be absorbed more slowly than if you eat it freshly boiled. The manufacturing process and the high fat content of potato crisps cause the glucose contained in these to be absorbed very slowly; limit them though because of the increased energy and fat content, which will ultimately promote weight gain.

In one study of adults, chocolate cake was substituted for a baked potato without an increase in blood glucose levels. If the chocolate cake was added to the baked potato, the glucose level increased. However, remember that chocolate cake and baked potato are very different in nutritional and energy value!

Bread

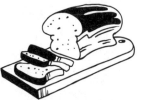

At one time, people with diabetes were strongly advised to eat unsweetened bread. Today, we know that white bread raises the blood glucose level every bit as rapidly as ordinary sugar. However, margarine and something with a high fat content (e.g. cheese) on the bread will slow the rise in blood glucose by delaying the emptying of the stomach. Bread that is high in fibre (e.g. wholegrain) will also slow down any rise in blood glucose levels. Different wholegrain breads have different GI values – choose those with a low GI such as granary or rye.

If you bake your own bread, it is perfectly acceptable to use an ordinary recipe. It should not be necessary to leave out the sugar or

experiment with alternative sweetening agents. It is more important to choose bread that is rich in fibre rather than omitting small amounts of sugar. Gluten-free wheat bread gives a quicker rise in blood glucose compared with the same amount of bread containing gluten.

Cereal

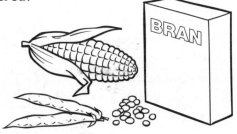

Unsweetened breakfast corn cereal (corn flakes) contains 90% starch, most of which rapidly becomes available as glucose. Sweetened (sugar-frosted) flaked corn cereal, on the other hand, contains around 50% starch and 50% sugar. Initially, both give the same blood glucose rise but sweetened corn flakes give slightly lower blood glucose levels after 3 hours. It comes as a surprise that corn starch raises the blood glucose faster than ordinary sugar. The best cereal to choose is one higher in fibre, such as bran flakes or All Bran. The amount of energy for a given weight of such a cereal is smaller, and the higher fibre content means that the GI is lower.

Rice

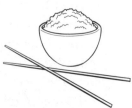

Rice is another staple food that contains carbohydrate. The starch in rice occurs in two main forms: amylose and amylopectin. Amylose is insoluble in water and its linear structure allows it to resist gelatinisation (the greater the gelatinisation, the

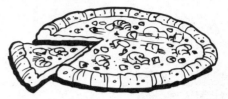

higher the GI). Amylopectin is highly branched and soluble. Different varieties of rice have different ratios of amylose to amylopectin and this ratio affects the overall rate of glucose absorption. For better blood glucose levels, opt for lower GI varieties with a higher amylose content such as Basmati. These high amylose rices stay firm and separate when cooked. 'Sticky' rices such as Jasmine have a high GI. Brown rice often has a surprisingly high GI because the insoluble fibre around the brown rice is micro-thin.

Pasta

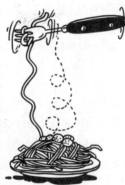

Pasta gives a slow rise in blood glucose since it is prepared from crushed or cracked wheat, and not wheat flour, which causes the starch to be enclosed within a structure of protein (gluten). This makes pasta a suitable food for people with diabetes. Wholewheat pasta is an even better choice. Thinner pasta, such as macaroni, gives a quicker blood glucose response than spaghetti. Cooking time does not affect the rate with which the blood glucose is raised by spaghetti, except in extreme cases of overcooking. Tinned spaghetti increases the blood glucose as quickly as white bread. Because the gluten content of pasta contributes to the slow rise in blood glucose, gluten-free pasta allows blood glucose levels to rise more quickly.

Pizza

Pizza contains bread, cheese, meat or fish and possibly vegetables. However, a pizza usually contains more bread than most meals and often includes lavish helpings of fat – either cheese as a topping or fatty cuts of meat to add flavour. So an occasional pizza as a treat is fine, but don't eat it regularly.

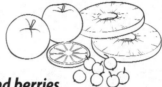

Fruit and berries

Some fruits and berries have a high carbohydrate content, but remember that in general, fruits are good for you. The higher the fibre content, the less effect they will have on the blood glucose level. See the glycaemia index table on page 43 for a guide to the glycaemic effect of different fruits.

Vegetables

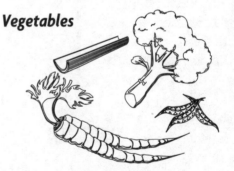

You can eat freely from this food group (except sweetcorn) as the carbohydrate content is very low (see the table opposite). Vegetables are also high in dietary fibre, which helps to smooth blood sugar peaks associated with food intake.

The starch in vegetables is broken down more slowly than other types of starch. Vegetables also contain soluble fibre, which is good for the digestion and prevents constipation.

Vegetables

	Carbs per 100g
Bamboo shoots	4g
Broccoli, cooked	7g
Carrots, raw	5g
Corn, canned	20g
Cucumber	3g
Lettuce	1g
Onions, cooked	11g
Peas, green, cooked	13g
Peppers, green, raw	3g
Radishes	2g
Tomatoes, raw	4g

How quickly is the blood glucose increased?

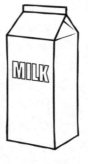

Puffed rice
Corn flakes
Mashed potatoes
Boiled potatoes
White bread
Whole-grain bread
Rice
Pasta
Potato crisps
Beans, lentils, peas

QUICKLY

SLOWLY

Milk

You should switch your milk from whole-fat to skimmed or semi-skimmed milk. The lower fat content in skimmed milk is associated with a reduced calorie burden. Skimmed milk contains a similar content of lactose (milk sugar) and is likely to have the same effect on blood sugar in the short term.

Meat and fish

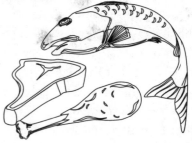

Meat and fish have a high protein content, and in some cases the fat content is also high, so care is needed. However, since they do not contain carbohydrates, they will not cause a direct increase in your blood glucose levels. Dietary protein does not slow the absorption of carbohydrate, and adding protein to a carbohydrate snack does not prevent late-onset or night-time hypoglycaemia.

Eating protein does not increase blood glucose levels. High-protein foods such as lean meat can make you feel full, which may be a real advantage if you have Type 2 diabetes and are watching your weight.

Salt

Salt intake is generally far too high. In Western countries, it is difficult to decrease this as salt is added to many processed foods (only 20% of total intake is added at the table and in cooking). Extra salt in the form of sodium chloride (table salt) will increase blood pressure and can be a risk factor for heart disease, especially as diabetes itself increases the risk of heart and vascular diseases (see Chapter 32). Eating salty food can cause glucose to be absorbed more effectively from the intestine. Salt is also available as potassium chloride, but this is more expensive than common table salt and tastes rather different. It is not suitable for people with renal disease. Sea salt and herb salt usually contain the same amount of sodium as table salt. In many countries, including the UK, iodine is often added to table salt in order to prevent iodine deficiency. If this is available, it is a good choice since iodine is important for the function of your thyroid gland.

Herbs and spices

Herbs will not affect your blood glucose at all. However, it is important to be aware that some herbal 'seasoning' preparations also contain a lot of salt.

Mealtimes

Each family has its own routines for mealtimes, and these are likely to be the ones that particularly suit them. A good dietitian will use the family's own eating habits and routines as a starting point when drawing up dietary advice for a person with diabetes. If you live on your own and aren't interested in cooking, this may be difficult, but the effort of cooking a balanced meal will be rewarded in long-term glucose levels.

'Special' foods

Branded 'diabetic' food?

Diabetic food should be avoided where possible. It quite often contains more calories than 'ordinary' substitutes, and fat may replace missing sugars. It also often contains sorbitol as a sweetener, which may produce side effects such as abdominal pain and diarrhoea. It is much better to learn how to handle ordinary food if you have diabetes.

'Fast food'

Many children, teenagers and adults like 'fast food' and it has become a fixture of modern life. Taking children or grandchildren out to a fast food eating place can be part of a family's social life. However, fast food often contains a lot of fat, so it should only be eaten occasionally.

Vegetarian and vegan diets

A pure vegetarian or vegan diet can sometimes result in a disturbed balance between the amount of protein and carbohydrate in the diet. This is because vegetarian nutrients contain much less protein than animal nutrients. A lactovegetarian diet includes milk products, which result in a higher protein intake but also an increased fat intake, unless you are careful. However, if reasonable attention is paid to achieving a balanced diet, most vegetarians keep very fit and avoid vitamin and mineral deficiencies.

In vegan or lactovegetarian diets, the animal products are mostly replaced by products from leguminous plants. The intake of vitamin B12 will be cut in half when the vitamins in animal products are not replaced. B12 deficiency leads to a number of different medical conditions, including anaemia, and most vegans accept the importance of taking supplements containing B12. You should talk to your dietitian or doctor if you are planning major changes in your diet.

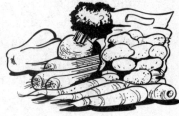

If you are a vegetarian, you will need to talk to your dietitian about your meal plan so that you will get enough of all kinds of essential nutrients.

Party-time

If you eat healthy foods on most days, you can allow yourself some exceptions on special occasions. It is important to teach yourself how to cope with whatever food is served at parties etc. Bringing along your own bag of 'diabetes food' is bound to make you feel uncomfortable. It is better to try and make healthy choices from the food available. If you drink alcohol, this will act as another source of calories, but they are absorbed rapidly and your blood glucose may fall later. If you are taking insulin, then a few extra units should enable you to deal with the party food, but a snack of long-acting carbohydrates such as a bowl of cereal may be advisable when you get home.

Religious fasting days

Many religions have special days when fasting for some or all of the day is required. There is no reason why someone with diabetes should not observe a fast, although anyone taking insulin or a sulphonylurea would be wise to reduce or omit the medication and to monitor the blood glucose while fasting. Consult your diabetes healthcare team if you are at all unsure about how to handle the situation, and keep records in your logbook for the next time!

You can find more information about fasting on the Diabetes UK website (www. diabetes.org.uk).

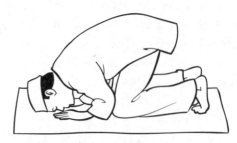

People with diabetes are generally exempt from fasting during Ramadan. If you still want to take part in the fast, it is very important that you seek advice from your doctor before doing so.

Ramadan: the fasting month

During Ramadan, the ninth month of the Islamic year, Muslims fast from dawn until sunset. Sick people, and women who are pregnant, breastfeeding or menstruating are exempt, as are young children. You can find more information about fasting for Ramadan on the Diabetes UK website (www.diabetes. org.uk).

In addition to the problem of fasting during the day, there is risk of overeating high-calorie sweets in the evenings during Ramadan. Although it's difficult to balance your meals during the evening following the fast, you should, where possible, make a healthy choice from the celebration food available.

Sweeteners

Sugar needs to be limited as part of a healthy diet for diabetes. Eating too many sugary foods such as cakes, biscuits, confectionary or sweet drinks regularly, has implications for weight management, heart health and the overall balance of your diet.

Free from sugar?

- Unsweetened
  No compound with a sweet taste has been added to the product. However, it can contain natural sugar (fruit sugar or milk sugar).
- Without added sugar
- No added sugar
- No sugar added
  No sugars have been added. However, it may contain sugar naturally, e.g. pure fruit juice.
- Sugar free
  No more than 0.2 g sugar per 100 g or 100 ml.
- Reduced sugar
  At least 25% reduction on the original product.

There are two main types of sweeteners: intense sweeteners and nutritive sweeteners.

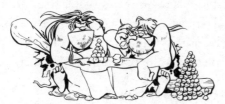

Since prehistoric times, humans have craved sugar. This is believed to be because sweet natural products are seldom poisonous, while many bitter ones can be so.

Intense sweeteners

These were previously known as artificial sweeteners. The five types used most commonly in the UK are aspartame, saccharin, acesulfame K, cyclamates and sucralose. The intense sweetener used in a food will always be listed in the ingredients, either by name or by additive number. Intense sweeteners are both carbohydrate and calorie free. They do not affect blood glucose levels. They are available to buy in tablet, liquid and granulated form and can be used in drinks, on breakfast cereals and to sweeten foods. They are also widely used in manaufactured foods.

Aspartame (E951)

Aspartame is about 200 times sweeter than sugar. It has been studied extensively and its safety in humans has been well established. Despite this, many myths still circulate about its safety.

Brand names include Canderel and Hermasetas Gold.

Saccharin (E954)

Saccharin is 300–500 times sweeter than ordinary sugar. It gives a slightly metallic taste when heated above 70°C (158°F) and should therefore be added only after cooking.

Brand names include Sweetex (tablets) and Original Hermasetas.

Acesulfame K (E950)

This is about 200 times sweeter than ordinary sugar. It withstands heating well and can be used in baking. It is usually used in conjunction with other sweeteners in manufactured products rather than on its own.

Brand names include Hermasetas Gold (with aspartame)

Cyclamate (E952)

This is about 30 times sweeter than ordinary sugar. It is stable at high temperatures and therefore suitable for cooking and baking. It is often used in soft drinks, dairy products and chocolate. The UK Food Standards

Sweeteners without energy

Substance	Trade name	Common in
Acesulfame K	Sunett Hermesetas Gold (aspartame + acesulfame K)	Beverages, jams, sweets baked goods
Aspartame	NutraSweet Equal	Chewing gum Soft drinks Tabletop sweetener
Cyclamate	Sucaryl, Sugar Twin	Tabletop sweetener
Saccharin	Sweet'n Low	Tabletop sweetener
Hermesetas	Original	Tabletop sweetener
Sucralose	Splenda	Tabletop sweetener, drinks, baked goods, frozen and canned fruit

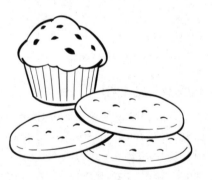

Some artificial sweeteners can be used for baking.

Agency advises that young children (1 ½ – 4 ½ years) should not be given more than three beakers (approximately 180mls each) of diluted soft drinks or squashes containing cyclamate per day and that these drinks should be more diluted than they are for an adult.

Brand names include Sugar Twin.

Sucralose (E955)

Sucralose is 600 times sweeter than ordinary sugar. It tastes like sugar and is heat stable. It can be used both for baking and for cooking.

Splenda is the brand name for sucralose.

Nutritive sweeteners

These include fructose and polyols such as sorbitol, maltitol, mannitol, isomalt, xylitol. They are also known as bulk sweeteners. These all contain calories and carbohydrate so can still cause blood glucose levels to rise. They also have a laxative effect. They are commonly used in diabetic foods and sugar free confectionery. They are not recommended as sweeteners.

Fructose

Fructose is almost twice as sweet as sugar. It does not directly affect your blood glucose level but is converted into glucose in the liver and the calorie content can cause weight gain.

Polyols

Polyols (sugar alcohols) are used by food manufacturers to lower the carbohydrate content of foods such as 'sugar free' sweets and ice cream. They are also found in 'diabetic' products. They provide about half the energy of other carbohydrates. Chemically they are converted into fructose and glucose by the liver. The names of sugar alcohols usually end with '-ol' for example sorbitol, mannitol. The sweetness of sorbitol is about half that of sugar. Sorbitol is a natural component found in some fruit such as plums, cherries and berries. Sorbitol and the other sugar alcohols absorb water from the intestines and provide nourishment for intestinal bacteria. They can cause abdominal pains and diarrhoea when eaten in large quantities.

9

Weight control

Many people with Type 2 diabetes have spent their lives battling against being overweight. They have often put a lot of effort into trying to lose weight by themselves, as well as being told by friends, family members and health professionals that they must lose weight. This chapter looks at the benefits of losing weight and the effects of a number of different diets as measured in randomized controlled studies. We hope that, by the time you have finished reading this chapter, you will be able to come to some practical conclusions about taking control of your weight. If you can find a strategy for losing weight that works for you, you will feel healthier and your diabetes will be easier to manage into the bargain.

What is 'overweight'?

The measure most commonly used to define healthy weight, overweight and obese is the body mass index, or BMI. This is based on a calculation involving your weight and your height. A BMI of between 20 and 25 is healthy, a BMI of 26–30 indicates overweight, whereas a BMI over 30 is a sign of obesity, which is a cause for concern.

Your body shape is also important. People who are naturally 'pear-shaped', who store fat on their bottom and thighs, are at a lower risk of developing Type 2 diabetes than people who are 'apple-shaped' and store fat around their middle. This is called central obesity and

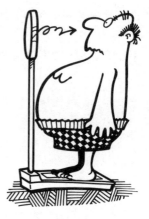

is a risk factor for diabetes and heart disease. This explains why waist measurements can also be taken as a 'risk indicator' for developing Type 2 diabetes.

Younger women are more likely to be 'pear-shaped' than 'apple-shaped'. Unfortunately, hormonal changes around the time of the menopause can change the way fat is distributed so some women may find they change from 'pears' to 'apples' as they get older, thus increasing their risk of developing diabetes.

$$\text{Body mass index} = \frac{\text{weight (kg)}}{\text{height (m)} \times \text{height (m)}}$$

Is weight always a problem?

Although most people who develop Type 2 diabetes are overweight, there are exceptions. If you are of normal weight, or even underweight, when diagnosed, this does not mean

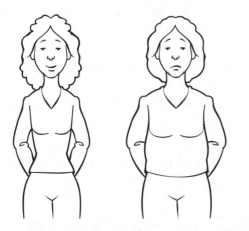

the diagnosis is wrong, though it may come as a surprise. In some cases, weight loss will be recent and is simply one of the symptoms of diabetes. This is caused by the inability to store glucose when diabetes is completely uncontrolled and blood glucose levels are very high. The unused glucose builds up in the bloodstream and overflows into the urine (where it will show up on a dipstick urine test). As much as 500 g (more than a 1 pound bag of sugar) of glucose can be lost in the urine over 24 hours. This is equivalent to 2000 calories per day and, naturally, causes a drain on the body's resources and means that the weight falls off even if you continue to eat the same amount of food (calories).

People who are thin, especially if they have lost weight before diagnosis, are more likely to need tablets at the time of diagnosis and often need insulin within a few months.

Metabolic syndrome

It is common at the time of diagnosis of diabetes for people to have a combination of features which are related to insulin resistance. These are central obesity, raised blood pressure and high levels of cholesterol in their blood. This combination of problems is referred to as the 'metabolic syndrome', and people with it carry a high risk of developing type 2 diabetes. If you have this syndrome, your doctor will encourage you to do everything possible to bring your weight under control. Thus instead of one disease (diabetes), people often discover that they also have high blood pressure and a raised cholesterol level. This can be very depressing especially as it means they are likely to be asked to take a number of new tablets at once.

There are other medical conditions caused by insulin resistance, which cluster with diabetes. These include acanthosis nigricans, fatty change in the liver and polycystic ovary syndrome.

Definition of central obesity

Population group	Waist measurement
Caucasian (white) male	102cm (40 inches)
Caucasian female	88cm (35 inches)
Asian male*	88cm (35 inches)
Asian female*	80cm (32 inches)

*Asian people have a higher risk than Caucasians of developing Type 2 diabetes, so the waist measurement is lower.

Acanthosis nigricans

In this condition, the skin becomes thickened and dark with a velvety appearance. It is seen mainly at the back of the neck and in the skin folds – armpits and groin. It also affects pressure areas such as the elbows and knuckles. It is found in people with central obesity, and is associated with a risk of diabetes. Skin tags are often found in the same patient.

Fatty change in the liver

This is a potentially serious condition, in which excess fat is stored in the liver. This leads to enlargement of the liver and occasionally pain in the right side of the abdomen. Simple liver tests are raised and an ultrasound shows the typical appearance of fatty liver. However, the only way of proving the diagnosis is to do a liver biopsy. The correct name for the condition is non-alcoholic steatohepatitis (NASH) or non-alcoholic fatty liver disease (NAFLD).

The first signs of fatty liver change are mild abnormalities in some of the liver tests but sometimes these slowly deteriorate and liver biopsy may show signs of permanent liver damage, known as cirrhosis. This is a slow process which takes place over many years or decades. There is no proven treatment for NASH although pioglitazone, which reduces insulin resistance, may sometimes be helpful.

Polycystic ovary syndrome (PCOS)

This is a condition affecting women, which causes:

- Irregular periods;
- Reduced fertility;
- High testosterone levels;
- Excess body hair.

Most, but not all, patients with this condition are overweight with central obesity. Treatment with metformin, which is known to improve insulin resistance, often has a dramatic effect and leads to restoration of normal periods and normal fertility. Metformin is not particularly effective at reducing body hair. Women with PCOS carry an increased risk of developing Type 2 diabetes.

Weight loss: the benefits to your health

If you can manage it, a reduction of 5–10% in body weight will make it much easier to control your diabetes and should make your HbA_{1c} fall by 1–2% (10–20 mmol/mol). This will significantly slow down the progression of your diabetes. It will also reduce your total body fat content, particularly central fat, which is a major contributor to insulin resistance. The resulting improvement in insulin sensitivity leads to a reduction in blood pressure and increases the level of good cholesterol (HDL) in the bloodstream as well as being responsible for the improved blood sugars.

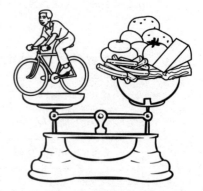

To regulate your weight, you need to balance the number of calories you eat against the calories that you use for daily exercise.

Exercise and weight loss

Unfortunately, there is no magic answer to losing weight or keeping it stable. Put quite simply, weight loss or weight gain depends on balancing the calories you eat against the calories you expend in your day-to-day activity. If you eat more calories than you use up, then you will put on weight. You might not be very keen on joining the gym or starting an exercise programme, but you would be surprised to find that many successful gym attendees started with just that frame of mind. The cost of joining a gym may put you off but some GPs now offer prescribed exercise, and while this might not make your visit entirely free, it should reduce the cost substantially. If the gym just isn't for you, you can try walking. Just getting off the bus one stop earlier, or walking to the paper shop may be enough to create a calorie deficit. Gardening is another efficient way to burn energy. If you have a garden big enough for a vegetable patch, try and rediscover a passion for healthy eating and exercise at the same time.

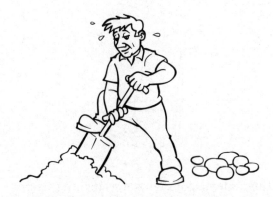

Exercise can take many forms. Gardening, for example, can be very energetic. Growing your own food can have the added benefit of encouraging healthy eating.

Are low carbohydrate diets useful?

This is a well-researched area and the results do appear encouraging for a significant proportion of people. However, although they help people lose a large amount of weight, like most diets, the weight loss is not always maintained and there may be a yoyo effect. If you are on insulin, you will need to reduce the doses dramatically while you restrict your intake of carbohydrate (see Research findings box on page 66).

If you are able to follow a low carbohydrate diet, the results in terms of reduction in insulin resistance, improvement in blood glucose levels, and other problems linked to excess weight such as high blood pressure can be spectacular. However, many people do find it difficult to cut out carbohydrates such as bread, pasta or rice. If this applies to you, it may be that this type of weight loss programme is not your best choice. A conventional low fat diet or meal replacement programme may suit you better. If you feel this type of regime is appropriate for you, there are a number of different websites and books which can help you with carbohydrate reduction.

For a balanced position statement on low carbohydrate diets in diabetes, see the Diabetes UK website, written in March 2011. It points out that low CHO diets lead to an improvement in body weight and HbA_{1c} in the short term (less than one year) but the long-term effects are less effective. There is an increased risk of hypos and you should always take advice from a specialist dietitian.

Are conventional low fat diets useful?

For a number of years, more conventional low fat diet has been recommended for weight reduction in Type 2 diabetes. Many people find it easier than a low fat, low carbohydrate diet as the food bears more relation to a 'normal' diet. Put simply, a reduced intake of saturated fat, with an increased intake of oily fish, complex carbohydrates such as wholemeal pasta or bran and fruit and vegetables is recommended. Meat should be as lean as possible. Studies of conventional low fat diets in Type 2 diabetes suggest that weight loss is around 3–7% at the one-year stage.

There are a number of varied recipes and meal plans that can be downloaded free from the Internet, or found in a suitable low fat diet book.

Partial meal replacement diets

Partial meal replacement implies replacing up to two meals in a structured way with lower calorie alternatives fortified with vitamins and minerals. An example of this type of diet is the Slimfast™ programme. The weight loss achieved appears to be in the region of 7–8% within a year, which is generally slightly more than is seen in conventional reduced calorie diets.

Using the glycaemic index (GI) in dietary planning for weight reduction

Low glycaemic index (GI) diets are now a new dietary trend, following on from Atkins and reduced carbohydrate diets (see Chapter 8 on Nutrition). Low GI foods essentially contain more complex carbohydrate (starches) and more soluble fibre. This means that any glucose peaks after the food is digested occur over a longer period of time and the overall peak reached is also less. A group of researchers tested out the effects of a low GI

diet in Type 2 diabetes. Although the study was very short, they did find that glucose control, lipid profiles and blood thickness were significantly better after only one month of following the diet.

Group therapy

All diets can be hard to keep to, and studies have shown that most people have difficulty in maintaining a diet for more than three months. In response to this problem, a number of organizations, such as Weight Watchers and Slimming World, promote the idea of dieting and lifestyle change through group work. This approach can be very effective in encouraging people to stick to any diet or diet and exercise programme. If you have a friend or another member of the family who is overweight who can attend meetings with you, so much the better. There is no doubt that companionship in dieting makes long-term success much more likely.

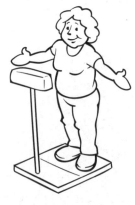

This approach often involves inviting visiting speakers to talk to groups after the regular 'weigh-in' sessions. They may tell motivational stories, give recipe and meal-planning ideas, advise on exercise regimes or reinforce listeners' awareness of the long-term health benefits of weight loss.

Drugs for weight loss

There have been a number of drugs designed to promote weight reduction and hence improvement in control of diabetes. Unfortunately the licences for the two main drugs have been withdrawn by the European Medicines Agency.

Sibutramine (Reductil)

Sibutramine was a fairly effective and widely used appetite suppressant but large surveys showed that people who took this had an increased risk of strokes and heart attacks. In January 2008, the drug was withdrawn since the risks were thought to outweigh the benefits.

Rimonabant (Acomplia)

Rimonabant was launched in 2006 with good evidence in research trials that it was effective in helping people to lose weight. However, it was found to carry a significant risk of depression and in October 2008, the European Agency felt that risks outweighed benefits and the drug was withdrawn. Rimonabant was not licensed for use in the USA but it is for sale over the Internet – a month's supply costs $50.

Orlistat (Xenical)

Orlistat causes weight loss by preventing the absorption of fat from the intestine. If after taking an orlistat tablet, you eat a high fat meal, the fat will appear in your faeces with disastrous consequences. The drug is designed to encourage a patient to stick to a low fat diet in order to avoid the unpleasant side effects. The usual dose is 120 mg three times a day before the main meals.

In 2004, the Zendos trial showed that overweight people taking orlistat had a 37% reduction in the risk of developing diabetes over 4 years. With this strong evidence, orlistat was approved by American and European licensing authorities. NICE supported its use as part of an overall plan to treat obesity but recommended that the drug should be discontinued at 3 months if the patient had not lost at least 5% of their original body weight. The manufacturers provided a telephone helpline which many patients found useful.

Orlistat is no longer widely used as its efficacy has been overshadowed by injectable GLP-1 agonists. However, low dose Orlistat (60 mg) is now available over the counter from high street pharmacists, under the name of Alli. This smaller dose three times a day can in some cases help people lose weight. However, orlistat was most effective when backed up by an exercise programme or telephone helpline so it is unlikely that many people will have the motivation to use the drug to lose weight now these support systems are no longer in place.

Weight loss: summary points

1. The majority of people with Type 2 diabetes are significantly overweight.

2. Many will have tried for many years to modify diet, exercise and general lifestyle to try to encourage a slow loss of weight. A diagnosis of Type 2 diabetes can provide an opportunity to try again, with new impetus.

3. All diets in which the total number of calories taken by mouth is less than the number of calories expended will promote weight loss.

Weight loss: summary points continued

4. No diet is right for everyone. If you've tried one type of diet before and it hasn't worked, try another.

5. Group therapy helps many people, as the support of others can often help them achieve better results than working at weight loss on their own.

6. No matter how hard changing your life seems, it is worth it for the sake of your long-term health. Even modest weight loss can promote great improvements in your glucose control, blood pressure and other risk factors linked to complications of diabetes.

Bariatric surgery

Surgery designed to help a patient lose weight has been performed for over 50 years but in the last 10 years, the numbers of people who have had one of these procedures has increased dramatically and what used to a rare procedure has now become commonplace. In 2006, less than 1000 such operations were carried out in the UK, while in 2011 the total reached 5400. Bariatric surgery includes many different procedures, all of which are designed to reduce the capacity of the stomach. The simplest procedure is to place a silicone band around the stomach. This is inflated to compress the wall and narrow the stomach down to a few centimetres. This procedure is done by keyhole surgery and if necessary can be reversed. In the UK, the most common operation to cause weight loss is a gastric bypass which allows food to be diverted past the stomach and some of the intestine. This is a major operation which cannot be reversed.

All these procedures are designed to cause the patient to eat less food or prevent its absorption. They can all lead to troublesome side effects and it is essential that careful follow-up is provided after surgery.

NICE recommends that anyone with a BMI greater than 40 should have the option of bariatric surgery. If they have an additional risk factor such as diabetes, they should be considered for bariatric surgery if their BMI is between 35 and 40. In practice most funding bodies (health service commissioners) only agree to surgery if the BMI is more than 45, even in people with diabetes.

If you are eligible for gastric surgery and decide to go ahead with it, you should go to a large unit specialising in the procedure. It is important to decide which of the many different procedures available would suit you best and you should only make your choice after detailed discussions with the specialist team. Gastric bypass surgery can have the most dramatic results but like all surgery it is not always successful and may cause unpleasant side effects.

One very positive benefit of gastric bypass surgery is that it may lead to a great improvement in diabetes – or even a cure. Thus a recent research project comparing different procedures showed that after bypass surgery, 21 out of 50 patients had perfect control of their diabetes without the need for tablets or insulin.

10

Exercise

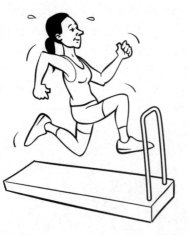

If you have Type 2 diabetes, it is important to take some form of regular exercise. This can help diabetes by increasing the body's sensitivity to insulin. It can also delay the onset of Type 2 diabetes if you have impaired glucose tolerance (see Chapter 11, Monitoring) and are therefore at increased risk of developing it.

Exercise encourages weight loss and leads to improvements in HbA_{1c}, blood pressure, and the profile of fats in the blood. The recommended target is at least 30 minutes of brisk exercise (enough to make your heart race and make you short of breath) on 5 days a week. Exercise can only cause a low blood glucose if you are taking either a sulpho-nylurea or insulin.

What happens during exercise?

Regular exercise stimulates a series of events in the body that result in changes in body composition. It reduces the amount of fat and increases the amount of muscle. Exercise increases your metabolic rate and improves your fitness, which is the amount of exercise that you can do without getting tired or exhausted. Taking exercise not only makes you feel better it also reduces blood pressure and the 'bad' cholesterol (low density LDL) while increasing the 'good' cholesterol (high density HDL). Increasing fitness also increases the body's sensitivity to insulin and lowers blood glucose levels.

If you take insulin to control your diabetes and take up a new exercise programme, you may need to make adjustments to your insulin doses. As you become increasingly fit, your overall daily dose of insulin will fall. The box below gives information about insulin and exercise.

The effects of exercise on the blood level in people treated with insulin

■ Exercise increases absorption of insulin from the injection site that you move during exercise, for example the thigh when running or playing football.

■ It increases the consumption of glucose without increasing the need for insulin. BUT – insulin must be available or the muscle cells will not be able to take up the glucose!

- After prolonged, endurance exercise, there is a risk of hypoglycaemia – for several hours as it takes time for the liver glycogen stores to be replenished.

- People who take the same amount of exercise regularly, are able to estimate what effect this will have on their blood glucose and how much extra glucose to take to prevent hypoglycaemia. However, people who only take exercise on rare occasions must be careful to check their blood glucose to predict hypos.

Planning and maintaining exercise

The first thing about making changes to your lifestyle to increase the amount of exercise in your daily routine is to find a fitness programme that you enjoy. Your aspirations can be very limited, such as taking the dog for a walk. You might set yourself a goal, such as a fun run or a walking holiday, which will require serious training. Exercise does not have to involve sports, and you can usually find something suitable to suit your lifestyle. The staff at your local fitness centre are specially trained to help you with this, and these centres are a good place to start. They will work out an exercise programme with you and show you how to improve your fitness.

Most people with Type 2 diabetes can take part in any exercise they choose, but there are two situations in which exercise needs to be taken up with caution. If you have had significant heart disease in the form of myocardial infarction, it would be sensible to arrange a check of your heart and ask if there are likely to be limits to the exercise you can

do. The other situation is when you have diabetic nerve damage leading to numb feet. A number of new patients always appear in diabetic foot clinics during the holiday season because people have walked much longer distances than usual. As a result, their feet become damaged because they lack the warning signs of pain to make them take a rest. A simple blister can easily turn into an infected ulcer with serious consequences. If you have numb feet, speak to a qualified podiatrist for advice about how far to walk and the most suitable footwear to protect your feet.

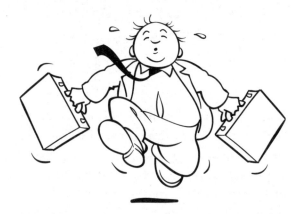

The heavier you are, the more energy you will use when you exercise.

In general, endurance exercise is most effective if you can manage it: 1 hour of walking will burn up 400 calories, jogging 600 and rowing on a machine nearer 700. Of course, the amount you burn up will depend on your weight to start with. The heavier you are, the more energy you use to carry out a particular amount of exercise. It is worth remembering that something which might not seem like a sport, such as digging the garden, may be an efficient way of burning up calories.

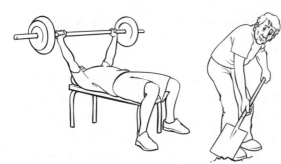

Not everyone likes the same sort of activity. It is important to find a form of exercise you enjoy so you will stick with it.

Exercise and mood

Everyone remembers doing a period of hard exercise, usually something you didn't want to do at school, like a game of rugby or a long run. We all know the feeling of intense exhaustion that you feel during the game and the elation that you experience after the event. You may well not have experienced those feelings for many years, but even modest exercise can bring about a marked improvement in psychological wellbeing.

One study compared the effect on mood of exercise training versus conventional antidepressants in a group of around 150 patients with major depression. After around 16 weeks of exercise training the response in terms of mood and depression scores was the same for the exercise group as it was for the group treated with drugs The amount of exercise undertaken was only three 30 minute sessions per week, but clearly exercise is a very good way to restore positive mood.

Positive mood is also important in the context of Type 2 diabetes. A number of studies have shown that depression and low mood both predispose to getting Type 2 diabetes and are associated with worse blood sugar levels in patients who already have

diabetes. The reason for this is very clear: we have all reached for the comfort foods we enjoy and not wanted to exercise when it seems the world is getting the better of us. See also Chapter 29, Psychological issues.

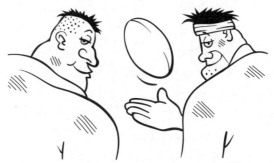

Exercise can have a really positive effect on your sense of wellbeing.

Ways of introducing exercise into your daily life

- Walk whenever you can, and avoid using the car.
- Climb stairs rather than take the lift.
- Walk to and from work.
- Take your dog for more or longer walks.
- Consider buying a bicycle or exercise bike.
- Make a point of taking at least three half-hour walks a week at a fast pace.
- Enrol for a dance class.
- Take up swimming.

Exercise and insulin resistance

Insulin resistance is responsible for causing Type 2 diabetes and a number of other conditions including fatty liver and polycystic ovaries (see also Chapter 9). One of the best ways to reduce insulin resistance is to exercise. Regular endurance exercise, such as walking for a prolonged period, swimming, cycling or jogging for 30 minutes five times per week can have positive effects.

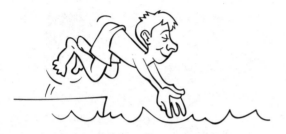

Regular endurance exercise, such as swimming, helps to reduce insulin resistance.

Exercising in this way leads to a reduction in energy fats in the blood, an improved uptake of glucose into muscles and a reduction in blood pressure, particularly the lower (diastolic) figure. In addition it allows the walls of your arteries to relax, so allowing blood flow to get to where it is needed in times of exercise or physical work. This reduces the risk of heart disease.

Benefits of exercise: Research findings

Exercise has been shown to have the following effects:

- Improve blood glucose control.

- Reduce central body fat.

- Increase sensitivity to insulin.

- Reduce blood triglyceride levels.

- Help prevent the development of Type 2 diabetes in those at risk.

Exercise and its effects on blood sugar

A study from Germany confirmed a substantial benefit of exercise on reducing insulin resistance. A group of people with diabetes were asked to exercise for a period of 50 minutes 3 times per week as part of a fitness programme which lasted for 12 weeks. Although the VO2 max (a measure of fitness) didn't change substantially, insulin resistance was reduced by 92% and HbA_{1c} fell by 0.5% at the end of the programme. A highly significant reduction of 5 mmHg in systolic blood pressure and a fall in triglycerides were also seen.

Considering this happened in only 12 weeks, the reduction was very impressive. This demonstrates that, by taking up a modest exercise programme, you may be able to avoid the addition of an extra diabetes medication. Thus, small lifestyle changes can be seen to have a substantial impact on blood sugar levels.

Exercise and muscle strength

Fairly modest exercise in Type 2 diabetes can also have substantial effects on your physical strength. One study looked at 22 patients with Type 2 diabetes who were given a strength training exercise programme of repetition weight lifting on static machines in a gym, for 3 days each week. They had to lift weights for each major muscle group in three sets of 10. Over the course of 4 months the level of weights lifted was slowly increased.

In this short time their muscle strength improved by around 30%. In addition, HbA_{1c} improved by 1.2%, with substantial changes in lipids and blood pressure.

Buy a pedometer

Research studies have shown that providing people with a pedometer is one of the best motivators to help people increase their activity levels. The following information is taken from an activity website promoting pedometers.

Classification of pedometer-determined physical activity in healthy adults

1. Under 5000 steps/day may be used as a 'sedentary lifestyle index'.

2. 5,000–7,499 steps/day is typical of daily activity excluding sports/exercise and might be considered 'low active'.

3. 7,500–9,999 is likely to include some exercise or walking (and/or a job that requires more walking) and might be considered 'somewhat active'.

4. 10,000 steps/day indicates the point that should be used to classify individuals as 'active'.

11

Monitoring

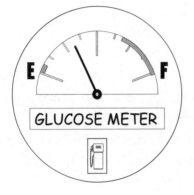

Measuring your blood glucose level is like checking the fuel gauge in your car. The difference is that you don't just need to be careful to avoid running out of petrol (sugar), you also need to make sure that the level doesn't go too high either.

There is a wide range of blood glucose monitors on the market, ranging from very basic to highly sophisticated – a bit like the mobile phone market. If you have recently been diagnosed with Type 2 diabetes, it is likely that you will have thought about getting your own meter – it is even possible that a friend or relative may have bought one for you. It may be surprising to learn that although it is accepted that people with Type 1 diabetes need to monitor their blood glucose regularly so they can adjust their insulin dose, many people with Type 2 diabetes do not need to monitor their blood glucose on a regular basis, if at all. The debate centres around whether people who monitor their blood glucose actually see an improvement in

glycaemic control. This chapter takes a brief look at monitoring, the evidence for doing it, the methods you can use, and the key pitfalls or problems you may encounter.

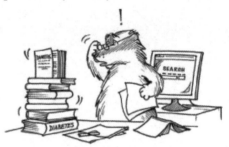

Key questions to ask yourself:

■ Do I need to monitor at all?

■ How many blood tests should I take, and when?

■ What are the most common pitfalls and problems with the equipment?

The blood glucose testing dilemma

Diabetes is a condition in which the main problem is a raised blood glucose. We believe that it is valuable for someone with diabetes to be able to measure their blood glucose and thus discover how they can best keep this under control. Used intelligently, blood glucose testing can help someone find out the effects of different activities such as eating various foods, drinking different types of alcohol and taking exercise. It is also an important way of identifying the problem if the blood glucose is either too high or too low.

On the other hand, most doctors know of individuals who check their blood regularly 3 or 4 times a day but never make any changes if the results are abnormal. It almost seems as if they are testing their blood for the benefit of their doctor or nurse rather than to provide themselves with useful information.

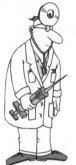

Do you take the tests for your own benefit, or do you take them to have something to show your doctor or nurse when you come to clinic?

Blood glucose monitoring tests can be divided into:

1. **Immediate tests**
   Tests that you can perform at any given moment, in order to measure your blood glucose.

2. **Routine tests**
   Tests that you perform regularly, and which help you to make long-term adjustments in your insulin doses, eating habits and other activities.

3. **Long-range tests**
   Tests that reflect your diabetes control over a long period of time. These include such tests as fructosamine and HbA_{1c}.

Most properly conducted studies designed to investigate the value of blood testing in people whose diabetes is controlled by diet or tablets have not shown that testing leads to improved diabetic control.

Unfortunately, blood glucose test strips are expensive. In an NHS which is under increas-ing financial pressure and in the absence of scientific proof of benefit, it is not surprising that the people who hold the purse strings are keen to restrict the use of blood glucose monitoring strips.

There is disagreement between the scientists and NHS funding bodies on the one hand and people with Type 2 diabetes on the other. Some family doctors believe strongly that blood glucose testing is unnecessary in people with Type 2 diabetes who are taking tablets. Most professionals agree that people with Type 2 diabetes treated with insulin should have the means to measure their own blood glucose levels.

Glucose levels: conversion table mmol/L to mg/dl

mmol/L	mg/dl	mg/dl	mmol/L
1	18	20	1.1
2	36	40	2.2
3	54	60	3.3
4	72	80	4.4
5	90	100	5.6
6	108	120	6.7
7	126	140	7.8
8	144	160	8.9
9	162	180	10.0
10	180	200	11.1
12	216	220	12.2
14	252	250	13.9
16	288	300	16.7
18	324	350	19.4
20	360	400	22.2
22	396	450	25.0

The numbers in this book refer to plasma glucose unless otherwise stated, as this is what most meters now display. Plasma glucose is approximately 11% higher than whole blood glucose.

NICE Guidelines for blood glucose monitoring

National guidelines for blood glucose monitoring in Type 2 diabetes were produced by NICE in 2009. They recognise the value of using blood glucose monitoring to assess the response to lifestyle and treatment changes, but not for routine monitoring except in specified circumstances.

Do you need to monitor at all?

When glucometers were first launched for checking blood glucose at home, doctors believed they would be useful for educating people with Type 2 diabetes. Of course, you may well have a problem with eating too much, eating the wrong types of foods or exercising too little. But the theory went that, by checking your blood glucose after eating a

NICE blood glucose guidelines

NICE Clinical Guideline 87
Pages 12–13

1.4 Self-monitoring of plasma glucose

1.4.1 Offer self-monitoring of plasma glucose to a person newly diagnosed with Type 2 diabetes only as an integral part of his or her self-management education. Discuss its purpose and agree how it should be interpreted and acted upon.

1.4.2 Self-monitoring of plasma glucose should be available:

- to those on insulin treatment
- to those on oral glucose-lowering medications to provide information on hypoglycaemia
- to assess changes in glucose control resulting from medications and lifestyle changes
- to monitor changes during intercurrent illness.

- to ensure safety during activities, including driving.

1.4.3 Assess at least annually and in a structured way:

- self-monitoring skills
- the quality and appropriate frequency of testing
- the use made of results obtained
- the impact on quality of life
- the continued benefit
- the equipment used.

1.4.4 If self-monitoring is appropriate but blood glucose monitoring is unacceptable to the individual, discuss the use of urine glucose monitoring.

Mars Bar or taking a cross-country run, you would learn how this affected the blood glucose and this would help you to maintain a pattern of good behaviour. Unfortunately, the studies reported so far appear to indicate that increased blood glucose monitoring in Type 2 diabetes isn't associated with improved glucose control.

If you are on diet and exercise or tablets, therefore, you may not need to monitor your blood glucose levels at home at all. If you do choose to monitor, you should use it as an educational tool to see what happens to your blood glucose when you eat certain foods or when you exercise or lose weight. There is no value in monitoring regularly if you are not able to make any changes based on the results. If you are taking insulin, then home blood glucose monitoring will be useful in terms of titrating to the right insulin dose and confirming that any symptoms of hypoglycaemia are backed up by a low reading on the meter. You should also do an essential blood glucose test before driving (you can read more about this in Chapter 27). If you are taking a sulphonylurea you may be at risk of hypoglycaemia and, if this is the case, your doctor should let you have blood glucose testing strips.

In the UK, blood glucose monitoring guidelines have been drawn up by Primary Care Trusts in association with GPs. An example is shown overleaf.

Timetable of monitoring

Test	Reflects the blood glucose levels over:
Blood glucose	Minutes
Urine glucose	Hours
Fructosamine	2–3 weeks
HbA$_{1c}$	2–3 months

How many tests should you take?

If you are on diet and exercise, metformin, gliptin, glitazone or GLP-1 treatment

It is probably not necessary to monitor your sugars at home. Your GP will be able to see what is happening from your HbA$_{1c}$, the long-term measure of blood glucose levels. If you do have a monitor, you could use it two or three times a week, at different times and after different activities to get a feel for how particular activities make your blood sugar rise. You can then discover the effect on the blood sugar of foodstuffs that you have been warned against.

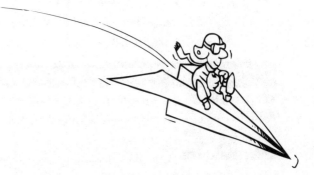

Send your blood glucose charts by mail, email or fax to your diabetes healthcare team and you can discuss them over the telephone.

If you are on sulphonylureas

Sulphonylureas are more likely to cause hypoglycaemia, therefore you may need to test more often than two or three times per week if you are having symptoms of hypoglycaemia. Your doctor will advise on this and will want to see the results. You may need a lower dose of sulphonylurea. If you do experience low blood glucose levels you will need to test before driving (Chapter 27).

Blood Glucose Self-Monitoring Guidelines

These guidelines were developed by Coventry PCT

EDUCATION AND LIFESTYLE

- Advice on diet, exercise and smoking habit key interventions at diagnosis and beyond.

- If necessary, patients should receive education relevant to **appropriate** testing, **understanding when** to test and **what** to do with the result.

ALL PATIENTS WHO ARE SELF-MONITORING SHOULD BE ENCOURAGED TO USE THE MINIMUM NUMBER OF TESTS REQUIRED TO KEEP CONTROL.

NEWLY DIAGNOSED TYPE 2 PATIENT + DIET CONTROL ONLY

RECOMMENDED REGIME: **A**	■ Self-monitoring may be required at diagnosis or as necessary depending on overall diabetes control and management plan. Self-monitoring may **not be necessary** if control is acceptable (e.g. HbA$_{1c}$ to target). ■ Healthcare professional should advise patient when self-monitoring becomes necessary.	Urine testing may be appropriate for some patients in this group provided HbA$_{1c}$ targets are achieved.	*Typical weekly strip usage* **0–6**

TYPE 2 PATIENT, PRESCRIBED ORAL THERAPY

RECOMMENDED REGIME: **A, B, C**	■ Re-assess patient need and educate prior to initiation of single oral therapy or combined treatment. ■ If self-monitoring is necessary, the healthcare professional should tailor monitoring regime to individual patient need, depending on diabetes control. ■ Special focus on testing to prevent hypoglycaemia, especially in sulphonylurea therapy.	If starting self-monitoring at this stage teach patient strip usage before initiating new therapy.	*Typical weekly strip usage* **0–6**

TYPE 2 PATIENT, PRESCRIBED INSULIN

RECOMMENDED REGIME: **B, D, E**	■ Self-monitoring is recommended in all cases with daily testing on initiation of insulin. ■ Once a patient is stable, frequency of profiles can be reduced to 1–2 days a week or daily at varying times (week profile).	Stable patients are those whose blood glucose varies little from day to day and from changes of treatment.	*Typical weekly strip usage* **4–28**

continued on facing page

Blood Glucose Self-Monitoring Guidelines *continued*

TYPE 1 PATIENTS		
RECOMMENDED REGIME: **E, F**	■ Self-monitoring is strongly recommended in all cases. ■ Self-monitoring should be used to adjust insulin dose before meals where this is appropriate (e.g. basal bolus regime, pump therapy). ■ Self-monitoring in Type 1 diabetes may only be required on 1–2 days per week in stable patients and depending on the patient's daily routine.	*Typical weekly strip usage* **8–28**

EXAMPLES OF TYPICAL SELF-MONITORING REGIMES

Regime **A**	One or two tests a week.
Regime **B**	Once daily at various times (week profile).
Regime **C**	Two tests daily.
Regime **D**	Four tests at different times on one day (day profile).
Regime **E**	Day profile twice a week.
Regime **F**	Test before meals and at bedtime each day.

■ Urine testing is appropriate in those:
  – where blood glucose monitoring is not possible
  – or the patient has a preference not to blood test.

■ HbA_{1c} target = below 7.5%.

■ Increase testing frequency during:
  – pregnancy
  – times of illness
  – changes in therapy
  – changes in routine
  – times of poor control
  – when at risk of hypoglycaemia
  – also to rule out hypoglycaemia, especially when driving.

BLOOD GLUCOSE MONITORING TARGETS

Fasting	4–6mmol/L	Bedtime	5–10mmol/L
Pre-prandial	4–6mmol/L	Post-prandial	<10mmol/L

■ Self-monitoring does not replace regular HbA_{1c} testing, which remains the gold standard test, and should only be used in conjunction with appropriate therapy as part of integrated care.

If you are on insulin

It is important to monitor the blood glucose when taking insulin. This helps with insulin dose adjustment and with identification of hypos. Your diabetes specialist nurse will advise, but usually you should aim to check it 2–3 times per day when treatment first starts and adjust your insulin until your sugars are in an acceptable range, (e.g. 5–7 mmol/L in the morning or around 10 mmol/L 2 hours after a meal). Try to estimate what your blood glucose is before checking it so you become familiar with how it feels to be high or low. It is easier to estimate low blood glucose levels than high ones.

Acting on the results

Persistently high or low readings

The important thing about blood glucose monitoring in Type 2 diabetes is to take some action if the results are consistently high or low. This may mean making some diet and lifestyle changes, but it could also mean consulting your doctor or nurse to see if your treatment should be changed. If your blood tests are consistently high, your doctor may add in a tablet that works in a different way to your existing treatment. If you are already on a lot of tablets you may need to change to insulin. If the blood tests are consistently low and you are taking insulin or a sulphonylurea your treatment may need to be reduced.

Isolated high or low readings

When you take a blood test it will reflect your blood glucose level at that moment. However, in some circumstances the blood glucose can go up or down quite quickly. In general, an unexpectedly high blood glucose is not a concern if you are feeling well, but you should check a few hours later to make sure it is falling. All the research projects looking at the risk of complications use the average blood glucose, which is reflected in the HbA_{1c}. Everyone with diabetes has an occasional high blood glucose result, and it is important to realize that an isolated high peak does not do any harm. However, if you are feeling unwell you should consult your doctor. (See Chapter 21, Coping with sickness.)

If your blood glucose is below 4 mmol/L and you are taking insulin or a sulphonylurea you should treat it as a hypo (see Chapter 19).

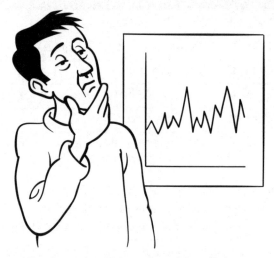

It is easier to estimate low blood glucose values than high ones.

Are some things forbidden?

We are often asked whether you are allowed to do this or that when you have diabetes. The best answer is that nothing is totally forbidden. It is important, however, to experiment in order to find out what you as an individual can and cannot do. It is a good idea to experiment with food, exercise and medication, provided this is done in conjunction with blood glucose monitoring. The only risk you are running is of having a temporarily high or low blood glucose. It may be worth keeping a record of the results of your tests, along with details of the activity you were participating in, for future reference.

Urine tests

Although urine glucose monitoring is no longer recommended as the primary method of glucose monitoring, it does have its advantages. Urine glucose monitoring can be useful in situations where blood glucose monitoring is difficult or impractical. In Type 2 diabetes, it may be used in some elderly patients although, generally speaking, it is not widely used.

How to take blood tests

Wash your hands with soap and water before taking a blood test. This is not just to ensure hygiene (though of course that is important), but to ensure there is no sugar on your fingers giving a false high reading, for example from glucose tablets or fruit. Use warm water if your fingers are cold. Do not use alcohol for cleaning your hands as this will make your skin dry. The risk of an infection from a finger prick is minimal.

There are a variety of different finger-pricking devices for taking blood glucose tests. With some you can adjust the pricking depth. Pricking devices and lancets can vary considerably in size and the way they puncture the skin. Try different types to find out which suits you best. From the point of view of hygiene, you can use the same lancet for a day's blood tests assuming that your fingers are clean. However, the lancet will be very slightly blunted every time you use it, so the

pricks might become more painful with repeated usage.

Lancets for blood glucose tests

Brand	Diameter of needle	Fits to device
BD Micro-Fine+	0.20mm	Standard
BD Micro-Fine+	0.30mm	Standard
Monolet Thin	0.36mm	Standard
Surelite	0.66mm	Standard
ComforTouch	0.45mm	Standard
Unilet G Ultralite	0.36mm	Standard
MediSense lancet	0.36mm	Standard
Softclix II	0.36mm	Softclix
Soft Touch	0.36mm	Standard
Cleanlet Fine	0.36mm	Standard
Microlet	0.50mm	Standard

Standard = Autoclix P, BD Lancer-5, Glucolet, Microlet, Monojector, Penlet II among others.

All lancets can be used for finger-pricking without using them in a device.

All the names mentioned above are ® or ™ of respective company. Other lancets may be available in your region.

If you prick the sides of your fingertips, your sensitivity will be less affected, which may be important if you play the piano or guitar, for example. Don't use your thumbs and right index finger (or left if you are left-handed) for finger pricking. You need the sensation of touch most in these places, and sometimes you will even feel pain the day after a finger prick.

Most blood glucose meters have memories for storing test results and can show the average of your readings over 2–4 weeks. This will give you a good picture of how your blood glucose levels have been during this time. The stored information can be transferred to a computer to view, analyse and print. Some newer meters have built-in blood glucose graphing programmes for summarizing patterns of blood glucose control.

Does continuous finger-pricking cause loss of feeling?

A lot of people are afraid that constantly pricking their fingers to test their blood will cause them to lose all feeling in them. Fortunately, all the evidence suggests that this won't happen. When fingers that had been pricked an average of 1000 times were compared with control fingers not used for pricking, it was only pressure sensitivity that was affected (due to an increased skin thickness). There were no signs of decreased sensitivity to heat or touch.

Why take blood tests?

Advantages

■ It can help you to find out the effect of food and exercise if you are newly diagnosed.

■ It can help to assess the effect of a new treatment if your medication is changed.

■ You can take a test if you think your blood glucose is low. This will help you to learn about hypoglycaemia and its symptoms if you are taking a sulphonylurea or insulin.

■ You can test if you are unwell to see if your diabetes is the reason you feel ill.

■ Lets you know when you need to change insulin doses, e.g. with illness, stress, physical exercise, or going to a party.

Disadvantages

■ Expensive and unnecessary if the blood glucose is stable.

■ Pricking your finger can be painful.

■ Monitoring takes time and extra effort.

Sources of error when measuring blood glucose

False high reading	False low reading
Glucose on fingers	Drop applied too late
	Finger removed too quickly
	Not enough blood on the strip
	Water or saliva on finger

Regular use of the control strip or control solution provided with your meter for calibration is very important to get and maintain reliable values.

Borrowing someone else's finger-pricking device

Borrowing another person's device for pricking your fingers is not a good idea. This is because one small drop of blood left on the device can cause contamination if it is infected. For example, an outbreak of hepatitis B in a hospital ward was caused by using the same pricking device (Autolet) despite switching lancets between each test.

Alternative site testing

- Some new meters are used for testing blood glucose at alternative sites. This may be helpful if you play the piano, for example, and do not want to keep pricking your fingers.

- In the fasting state, the glucose readings from the forearm are similar to the fingertip.

- After an intake of 75 g of glucose, the rise in blood glucose in adults was 2.6–7.6 mmol/L (47– 137 mg/dl) lower on samples taken from the forearm compared with the fingertip.

- When blood glucose fell quickly after an insulin injection, the values from the fingertip were 3.4–6.6 mmol/L (61–119 mg/dl) lower than the values from the forearm.

- Blood glucose changes appeared on average 35 minutes later in forearm tests compared with the fingertip. By rubbing the skin vigorously for 5–10 seconds before pricking, the accuracy from a forearm test was considerably improved, but with large individual differences.

- In another study in which tests were taken after a meal, lower glucose readings were produced from the forearm and thigh compared with the fingertip, in spite of vigorous skin rubbing.

- The differences are caused by a greatly increased blood flow in the fingertip. To be on the safe side, it seems best to rely on fingertip tests when checking for hypoglycaemia, (e.g. when driving a car or after exercise).

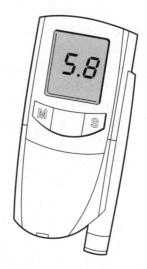

An example of a blood glucose monitoring device.

Does the meter show the correct value?

The margin of error in a correctly used blood glucose meter is approximately 10%. This means that with a blood glucose level of 20 mmol/L (360 mg/dl), the meter can show 2 mmol/L (36 mg/dl) above or below the correct value. However, at a blood glucose of 3 mmol/L (54 mg/dl) the error should not exceed 0.3 mmol/L (5 mg/dl). It is very important to apply enough blood to the strip. Too small a drop will give a false low reading. Don't rub the blood onto the strip. If you have sugar on your fingers when you take the test, this will cause a false high reading.

Which meter?

There is a wide variety of blood glucose meters on the market but unless you are taking insulin you do not need a sophisticated meter. Most meters are available free because the companies producing them make their money from the test strips. For this reason, some PCTs recommend a specific meter so that savings can be made on the cost of the strips, which can be bought in bulk. Your practice nurse will advise you about local policy. Comparing different meters can be confusing as they often show different readings. For example, one may show a blood glucose level of 12 mmol/L (215 mg/dl), while another (used at the same time on the same patient) shows a level of 14 mmol/L (250 mg/dl). However, this difference is well within the error margins stated by the manufacturers of the meters. It is advisable to stick to one meter that works well, as the difference of 1–2 mmol/L is not particularly significant at high readings. Bring the meter with you when you come to clinic, and ask your diabetes nurse to check your meter with glucose control solution at regular intervals. Make sure you calibrate your meter regularly according to the manufacturer's advice. Use the reference test strip and make sure the code numbers correspond.

Self-monitoring around mealtimes

Because of problems with the design of studies, a great deal of debate exists in the medical press about the value of blood glucose monitoring in Type 2 diabetes. The most useful information comes from tests before meals (pre-prandial) or 2 hours after a meal (post-prandial). Both pre-prandial and post-prandial blood sugar levels contribute significantly to your overall blood glucose load, and hence to any risk of long-term diabetes complications. In particular, it seems that in Type 2 diabetes the post-prandial blood sugar level correlates strongly with the risk of cardiovascular disease. We will examine the value of self-monitoring in patients who are and who are not taking insulin.

Self-monitoring around mealtimes if you are not taking insulin

A study which examined the effect of self-monitoring on HbA_{1c} in patients with relatively good control of their diabetes (average HbA_{1c} at the start of the study was around 7.3%) found that the group who monitored their blood sugars had a reduction of just under 0.2% in their HbA_{1c} over a year, versus no change in a control group. This difference is small, and suggests that in people with good control the benefit of blood glucose monitoring is marginal.

We do not have good evidence to demonstrate whether people with less good control benefit from blood glucose monitoring but, undoubtedly, the most important factor would be whether monitoring led to changes in lifestyle or medication to reduce high blood glucose levels.

If you are monitoring your blood glucose and levels are consistently high, you need to speak to your nurse or doctor to discuss what might be done to lower the blood glucose. Proactive working like this can help you and your doctor or diabetes nurse get the most out of your glucose meter.

Self-monitoring around mealtimes if you are taking insulin

If you take insulin for Type 2 diabetes, the rationale for self-monitoring is much clearer and monitoring blood sugar levels can contribute significantly to your HbA_{1c} by enabling you to adjust the insulin dose depending on the blood glucose level.

For patients on twice-a-day insulin injections of mixed (short- and long-acting) insulins, pre-meal and pre-bed blood sugar levels help you decide if you are on the correct dose of insulin. The reading before breakfast and evening meal will tell you whether the dose of long-acting insulin is correct and the readings before lunch and bed reflect the action of the short-acting component of the insulin mix. If all the readings are too high you should increase the insulin. If one is relatively higher than another, you may need a different mix of insulin. You should discuss this with your diabetes nurse or doctor. More information on insulin adjustment is available in Chapter 14. For individuals taking meal-time (bolus) doses of short-acting insulin in combination with one long-acting (basal) injection per day, pre-meal and pre-bed glucose monitoring can be very instructive. You can use monitoring to adjust the amount of insulin you take depending on exercise and activity, as well as meal size, You may also learn how your insulin requirements alter at certain times of the week, for example if you are at work or at home.

Self-monitoring around mealtimes: what it means for you

Too many people have been asked to monitor blood sugars at home without having proper guidance on how to act on the results. With proper education and a management plan, monitoring your blood glucose levels can help improve your overall blood sugar control. It can also help with insulin adjustments related to exercise and healthy eating. If you are able to work out a titration plan for medication, it will allow you to take ownership of your diabetes and make decisions without having to check out everything with your doctor or nurse. However, if you feel that you are not likely to make good use of blood glucose

monitoring, it is better to decline the opportunity. It is not good to let unused blood glucose strips gather dust in a cupboard.

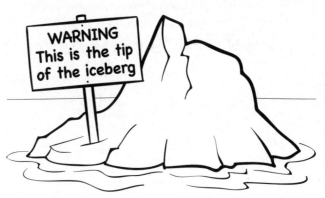

Continuous glucose monitoring

The Medtronic MiniMed CGMS (Continuous Glucose Monitoring System®) is a device that monitors glucose levels (2.2–22 mmol/L, 40–400 mg/dl) every 10 seconds and records an average value every 5 minutes. It measures through a thin plastic tube placed in the subcutaneous tissue, and can be worn for up to 3 days. The latest models allow you to read glucose values in real-time. When the monitor is connected to a computer, the data can be downloaded and viewed on screen. Using this method has made it easier to see patterns of glucose fluctuation, which has in turn led to changes in treatment and improved glucose control in people of all ages. This technique has proved very useful in Type 1 diabetes but at the present time it is not in routine use for Type 2 diabetes

Ketones

Ketones are produced by the body when the cells do not have enough glucose energy. The body then breaks down fat to produce energy and the breakdown products are called ketones. If a person has diabetes, ketones are produced in excess when there is a lack of insulin and high blood glucose levels, indicating a need for more insulin. As even a tiny amount of insulin prevents you from developing ketones and as people with Type 2 diabetes usually have some reserve of insulin production, problems with ketones are very rare, although they can be produced at times of severe illness (see Chapter 21, Coping with sickness). For this reason it is unusual to ask people with Type 2 diabetes to check for ketones.

12

Glycosylated haemoglobin (HbA$_{1c}$)

Glycosylated haemoglobin or HbA$_{1c}$ is the test used to measure average glucose control over several months. Glucose molecules become attached irreversibly to the haemoglobin molecules in the red blood cells, which have a lifespan of 120 days. During the life of the red blood cell, the amount of glucose bound to haemoglobin in the red cell depends on the level of glucose in the blood at any one time. The percentage of haemoglobin that is bound to glucose provides an estimate of the average blood glucose level over the life of the red cell. Since red cells last for 120 days, the average age is 60 days or 2 months.

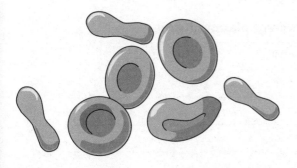

Haemoglobin in the red blood cells takes up oxygen in the lungs and transports it to the cells. The red blood cells also take carbon dioxide from the cells back to the lungs. During the lifetime of red blood cells in the circulation, glucose sticks to the haemoglobin, and the resulting glycosylated haemoglobin (HbA$_{1c}$) can be measured.

HbA$_{1c}$ reflects an average of your blood glucose levels. You can get an acceptable HbA$_{1c}$ reading with a combination of high and low blood glucose values. There is some evidence that HbA$_{1c}$ goes up with age, due to an increase in glucose bound to proteins such as haemoglobin. This may account for the fact that the HbA$_{1c}$ in some elderly patients seems too high when compared with their blood glucose test results.

HbA$_{1c}$

- Glucose is bound to haemoglobin in the red blood cells.

- The level of HbA$_{1c}$ depends on the blood glucose levels during the lifespan of the red blood cells.

- A red blood cell lives for about 120 days.

- HbA$_{1c}$ reflects the average blood glucose during the previous two months.

New way of expressing HbA$_{1c}$

HbA$_{1c}$ was first used to measure average blood glucose in 1979. Many different methods of measuring HbA$_{1c}$ were developed and each laboratory had a different normal range of values; it was therefore impossible to compare results from different laboratories. However, all laboratories reported their results as the percentage of total haemoglobin with glucose attached. Thus, an HbA$_{1c}$ of 8% from one laboratory was not the same as an HbA$_{1c}$ of 8% from a different laboratory. In order to prevent the confusion caused by the use of different methods, a group of international biochemists have worked for several years on a solution to the problem. They have come up with a standardized method of measuring HbA$_{1c}$ and have also changed the units from a percentage to the actual amount of HbA$_{1c}$. The results are now expressed as mmol/mol and cannot be confused with the old percentage units. People who do not have diabetes have an HbA$_{1c}$ of less than 40 mmol/mol. As a guide, an old value of 7% is equivalent to 53 mmol/mol and 10% is 86 mmol/mol. We will only use the new units in this book and have provided a conversion chart for people who are used to using the old units.

What level should HbA$_{1c}$ be?

There is good evidence that people with a lower HbA$_{1c}$ end up with fewer complications of diabetes. Many national bodies have suggested targets for HbA$_{1c}$ in the hope that this will encourage people to keep a low HbA$_{1c}$ and thus avoid complications. American and Canadian Diabetes Associations recommend that the goal of therapy in adults and adolescents should be an HbA$_{1c}$ below 53 mmol/mol and that the treatment regimen should be re-evaluated in patients with repeated HbA$_{1c}$ above goals. The International Diabetes Federation (IDF) now recommends an even lower HbA$_{1c}$ target of 48 mmol/mol. Many studies have shown that with an HbA$_{1c}$ value of less than 64 mmol/mol the risk of long-term blood vessel complications will be considerably lower. If your HbA$_{1c}$ is above 73 mmol/mol

Relationship between HbA$_{1c}$ and blood glucose

HbA$_{1c}$		Average plasma glucose	
%	IFCC mmol/mol	mmol/l	mg/dl
5	31	5.6	103
6	42	7.6	138
7	53	9.6	177
8	64	11.5	208
9	75	13.5	243
10	86	15.5	278
11	97	17.5	314
12	108	19.5	349

This table shows the average glucose value represented by a given HbA$_{1c}$.

you are much more likely to run into problems in the course of time. Studies have also shown that those with a lower HbA_{1c} experience better levels of psychological well-being. This includes less anxiety and depression, improved self-confidence and a better quality of life.

The risk of severe hypoglycaemia makes it difficult and dangerous to achieve very low HbA_{1c} levels. If someone with Type 2 diabetes has an HbA_{1c} within the range for individuals without diabetes, this usually means they are at high risk of severe hypoglycaemia and/or hypoglycaemia un-awareness. In a study of patients with Type 1 diabetes, those with low HbA_{1c} had a threefold risk of severe hypoglycaemia.

Why check your HbA_{1c}?

Is checking your HbA_{1c} worthwhile? For whose benefit is the HbA_{1c} test being done? Many individuals feel as if they are visiting a 'control station' and being examined by health professionals to see how well they have 'behaved themselves'. From the professional point of view, however, the HbA_{1c} test is most valuable to you yourself. When you see the reading, you will know if your way of life over the last three months has allowed you to achieve the average blood glucose level you want for the future.

For how long do blood glucose levels affect HbA_{1c}?

Your recent blood glucose level affects HbA_{1c} much more than that from 2–3 months ago. However, your values during the last week will not show on most methods since this fraction of HbA_{1c} is very unstable. For a given HbA_{1c} value, the contribution of the blood glucose is (counting backwards):

Day	Impact of BG on HbA_{1c}
Day 1–6	very low
Day 7–30	50%
Day 31–60	25%
Day 61–90	15%
Day 91–120	10%

HbA_{1c} goals in Type 2 diabetes

	%	mmol/mol
Person without diabetes	4.1 – 6.1	21 – 43
Adolescents and young adults (normal value)	‹7.5	‹58
Adults	‹7.0	‹53
Needs improving and re-evaluation of treatment	8 – 9	64 – 75
Not acceptable: High risk of complications	›9	›75
May have high risk of severe hypoglycaemia	‹6	‹42

There may be individual differences in the HbA_{1c} value, which is realistically achievable. Discuss with your diabetes team what value may be realistic for you.

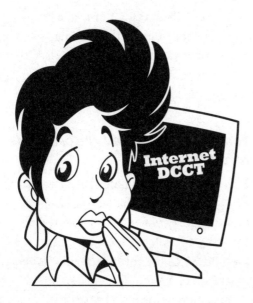

Many countries (US, Australia, UK, Denmark, France, the Netherlands among others) have standardized their HbA$_{1c}$ monitoring methods to show DCCT-equivalent numbers. This means that if you read about studies on the Internet, you can compare like with like between one study and another.

How often should you check your HbA$_{1c}$?

Everyone with Type 2 diabetes should check their HbA$_{1c}$ regularly, every 6 months. A high level (64–75 mmol/mol) is not acceptable, considering the risk of future complications. After a visit to your diabetes healthcare team, you may feel more motivated to 'get your act together' and keep your blood glucose readings low. Use this motivation to address any problems with diet, lifestyle, medication or insulin regimes.

Some clinics send their HbA$_{1c}$ tests to the laboratory, so it may be some days before you get the result while others ask you to send in

a blood sample a week before the clinic. Others use a desktop method that gives a result after a few minutes.

Even if your blood glucose control is improving and your tests are showing lower readings, it will still take some time for this to show in your HbA$_{1c}$. Half the change will show after about a month, and three quarters of the change after 2 months. If you start with a very high HbA$_{1c}$ (108–119 mmol/mol) and normalize your blood glucose levels completely (as often happens at diagnosis), it will go down by approximately11 mmol/mol every tenth day.

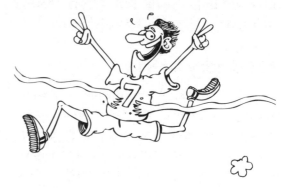

Set your own personal goal for your HbA$_{1c}$ in collaboration with your diabetes team. This goal will be different for different people, and perhaps also different during different times of your life. It may be more difficult to achieve the same HbA$_{1c}$ level at times when, for example, you are having problems at home or at work. By competing with yourself and setting a reasonable goal, you will have a fair chance of winning your race.

Can your HbA$_{1c}$ be 'too good'?

Most doctors who specialize in diabetes care are equally alarmed by a low HbA$_{1c}$ (less than 45 mmol/mol) as by a high result (more than

75 mmol/mol). If you take insulin or a sulphonylurea, you will be asked in detail about hypos. If you are not having daytime hypos but your HbA_{1c} is low, there is a strong possibility that night-time hypos, while you are asleep, are bringing down the HbA_{1c}. You may be asked to set an alarm for 3 AM to do a blood sugar check.

In older people, signs of hypos can be less obvious but equally dangerous and for this reason the target HbA_{1c} should be set higher in people who are beginning to become frail, physically or mentally. In elderly people who are losing their independence, an HbA_{1c} of 68 mmol/mol is perfectly acceptable.

Can the HbA_{1c} measurement give false information?

The HbA_{1c} result relies on the fact that red blood cells last about 120 days. Any medical problem which shortens the life of the red cell will tend to artificially reduce the HbA_{1c} percentage. Such conditions include haemolytic anaemia, kidney failure and pregnancy.

Fructosamine

Measurement of fructosamine is a method of estimating the amount of glucose that is bound to proteins in the blood. The value reflects the blood glucose level during the previous 2–3 weeks. The test is not as reliable as HbA_{1c} and reflects changes in blood glucose over a shorter period of time (2–3 weeks instead of 2–3 months). However, it is valuable when there is an abnormal haemoglobin present, since this invalidates the HbA_{1c} measurement.

People with an abnormal haemoglobin

There are a number of genetic conditions in which the haemoglobin molecule is abnormal. The best known of these is sickle cell anaemia, which is common in people of African origin. About 10,000 people in the UK have this condition. Any abnormal haemoglobin reduces the life span of the red cell and hence interferes with measurement of HbA_{1c} and is usually detected by the HbA_{1c} analyser. In these cases, blood is usually sent for measurement of fructosamine, which is the next best thing to HbA_{1c}.

13

Tablets for lowering blood sugar

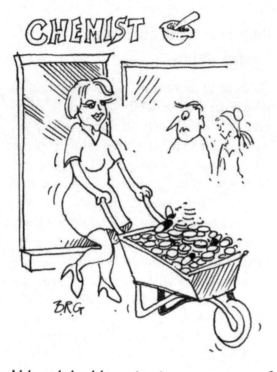

Nine Key Points that you need to know when starting an oral treatment for Type 2 diabetes

- The name of the therapy, or tablet, that the doctor has prescribed for you.
- The dose you need to take.
- The best time of day to take the tablets.
- How the tablets work.
- Why the doctor has started you on this particular medication, and what evidence supports this choice.
- Whether the tablets can cause low blood glucose levels.
- Any other side effects you may experience.
- Possible interactions with other tablets or medications you may be taking (e.g. blood pressure drugs).
- What to do if you have problems (e.g. contact the surgery).

Although healthy eating is a cornerstone of management of Type 2 diabetes, and regular exercise plays an equally important role, it is still very likely that your blood sugar levels will begin to rise over time. Despite the importance of your doctor or nurse exploring every option for lifestyle improvement with you, many health professionals now believe it is a good idea for patients to start taking tablets soon after diagnosis of Type 2 diabetes. Indeed, some authorities recommend that you start to take a tablet called metformin at the time that your Type 2 diabetes is diagnosed.

You may feel perfectly well and this may make it difficult for you to understand why you need tablets. It is very important that your doctor or nurse talks you through the nine key points of your diabetes treatment. If your professionals are not honest with you, and do not communicate clearly, then why should you follow their advice? If you can't understand their explanations, do please tell them.

The following sections mention a number of characteristics and side effects of drug therapies used for lowering your blood sugar. This list can't be exhaustive and is almost out of date as soon as it is written. You can find the latest information on any drug treatment over the Internet from sites such as the electronic medicines compendium (www. medicines.org.uk).

Tablet treatments for diabetes

At the present time, eight groups of drug are used in for treating blood sugar levels in Type 2 diabetes.

1 Biguanides (metformin).

2 Sulphonylureas.

3 Gliptins (DPP-4 inhibitors).

4 Glitazones (also called insulin sensitizers or thiazolidinediones).

5 Postprandial glucose regulators (PPGRs).

6 Alpha-glucosidase inhibitors.

7 SGLT-2 inhibitors.

8 GLP-1 agonists.

Biguanides (metformin)

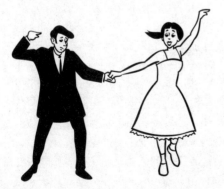

Metformin is a member of the biguanide family of diabetes drugs, and it works by reducing the amount of sugar that is produced by your liver. It is recommended as initial drug treatment for anyone with Type 2 diabetes, unless other medical problems or side effects make its use unwise.

The insulin resistance associated with Type 2 diabetes leads to the release of sugar from glycogen stores in the liver and production of sugar from other energy sources such as lipids (fats). Metformin appears to be most effective in patients who are overweight.

One major advantage of taking metformin is that it does not cause weight gain; indeed, many patients manage a small loss of weight when they take metformin. You should take your metformin with food, as this may reduce the risk of gastrointestinal upset. If you find metformin causes a stomach upset, ask your GP to try the slow-release form.

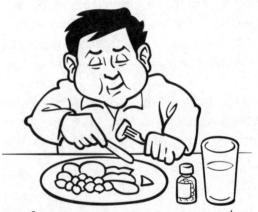

Metformin can cause tummy upsets, but taking your tablets with food will help you avoid this.

When should you not use metformin?

If you have problems with your kidneys, metformin may not be appropriate for you. Your family doctor will probably measure your serum creatinine (a measure of the amount of waste products from the body which are circulating in the blood). When patients have a creatinine level which is more than around 130–150 mmol/L, another drug should be used instead. This is because a very rare side effect of metformin, called lactic acidosis (to do with the acidity of the blood), may be more likely to occur if the kidneys aren't working properly.

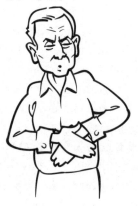

If you have significant problems with your liver, or tend to drink more alcohol than the Department of Health recommended limits (see Chapter 24), metformin may not be suitable for you.

Many patients with diabetes need investigations of their blood vessels at some stage in their lives. These investigations are often done with injection of special dye called contrast medium so that the blood vessels show up on X-ray pictures. When these contrast injections contain iodine, metformin should be stopped at least 24 hours before you have the investigation and not started again until you have recovered from the procedure. If your doctor has booked one of these investigations for you, it is very important to make sure that the X-ray department of the hospital knows you are taking metformin.

Similarly, if you need to have an operation under general anaesthetic, you may need to stop your metformin before the surgery. If you are asked to do this, you should not start metformin again until your doctors are happy that your kidneys are working properly again.

Metformin can be used by pregnant mothers and can also be taken during breast-feeding. Women with Type 2 diabetes who are insulin resistant often take a while to get pregnant in the first place and metformin may improve their chance of ovulation and pregnancy. If you start metformin and don't want to get pregnant, you need to be careful about contraception.

Available metformin preparations

Drug	Brand name	Normal dose
Metformin	Glucophage Glucophage SR (once a day formulation) *Also available in Janumet (sitagliptin and metformin) and Competact (pioglitazone and metformin)*	500mg–3g for the multiple dose form of metformin, 2g for the once-per-day drug.

Who should not take metformin?

- Anyone with kidney problems, particularly if they have a raised creatinine level or a reduced eGFR (estimated glomerular filtration rate), either of which would indicate some degree of kidney damage.

- Anyone undergoing an X-ray involving contrast media or dyes.

- Anyone preparing for a surgical operation – tell the doctors you are on metformin.

Side effects

Gastrointestinal problems (tummy upsets) are the most common problem associated with taking metformin. These may include a combination of nausea, abdominal bloating and diarrhoea. There is every possibility that gastrointestinal problems can be minimised if you and your doctor work to increase the metformin dose gradually over the course of a few weeks. There is some evidence that if you do have problems with nausea or tummy upsets while you are taking metformin, switching to a 'once a day' preparation may reduce these side effects.

You may also find you lose your appetite and this may contribute to some of the weight loss which occurs in metformin users. More unusual problems may include a metallic taste in the mouth, and a lowering of your body's levels of the vitamin B12.

Lactic acidosis can occur very rarely in people taking metformin. Symptoms include lethargy, muscle pains and hyperventilation (overbreathing). Lactic acidosis is associated with increased acidity in the blood and is more likely to occur when metformin is used by people with kidney problems or with heart failure. It is almost unheard of in patients who have healthy kidneys and a well functioning heart.

Side effects may develop soon after you start taking metformin, or may develop after several years. However, many people have taken metformin for decades without experiencing problems.

Evidence for using metformin to manage your diabetes

The main outcome evidence for using metformin comes from the UKPDS (see page 256). In this study, metformin reduced the risk of cardiovascular disease and microvascular complications (kidney, eye and nerve damage). For this reason, it carries the strongest recommendation as initial drug treatment for diabetes. A few other studies have shown that, as well as lowering blood glucose, metformin also has positive effects on blood clotting (reducing the chance of thrombosis) and inflammation.

Other uses for metformin

Metformin is often used in women without diabetes who have polycystic ovarian syndrome (PCOS). In this condition, metformin helps with weight reduction and excessive hairiness and is used to induce fertility.

Sulphonylureas

Sulphonylureas act by making the beta cells of the pancreas release insulin. They do this by binding to a receptor on the surface of the insulin-producing beta cells and this causes insulin to be released. This release of insulin occurs even when blood sugar levels are low, which explains why hypoglycaemia (low blood sugar) may occur with sulphonylureas.

The most commonly prescribed sulpho-nylurea in the UK is gliclazide. Alternatives include glibenclamide, glimepiride, glipizide, and gliquidone. Glibenclamide is less widely used now as the longer duration of action increases the risk of hypoglycaemia.

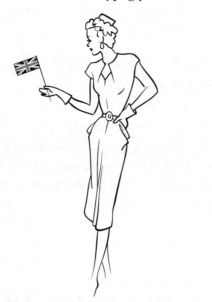

Sulphonylureas were first developed in the 1940s.

Generally, sulphonylureas are no longer recommended as the first choice treatment for Type 2 diabetes. When your doctor is thinking about adding in another tablet to metformin, a sulphonyurea would be pre-ferred if your weight is normal or below average and you have diabetes symptoms. But if you are overweight, a gliptin, a GLP-1 agonist (see page 92) or a glitazone may be a better choice.

The main side effects of sulphonylureas are hypoglycaemia and weight gain. About 20% of patients taking a sulphonylurea have one or more hypoglycaemic episodes in a year. These are usually mild. However, in the course of a year, up to 1% of patients on a

sulphonylurea have a hypoglycaemic attack that is sufficiently severe for them to need assistance from another person. The risk of hypoglycaemia is much greater in the first year and decreases with time.

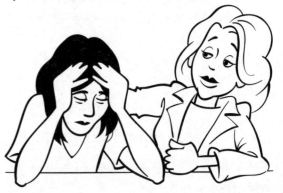

During any year, around 1% of patients taking a sulphonylurea will suffer a hypoglycaemic attack that is severe enough for them to need help from someone else.

Some of the sulphonylureas may be par-ticularly suitable if the kidneys are damaged due to diabetes. For example, gliclazide is broken down by the liver and not the kidneys. When taking a sulphonylurea, you should have the lowest dose possible to control your blood sugar.

When should you take a sulphonylurea, and how much?

Your doctor should generally advise you to take short-acting agents such as glipizide before main meals. Once a day preparations such as gliclazide MR or glimepiride should be taken before breakfast. Small doses of glicazide can be taken once a day, but larger doses need to be taken twice a day. The greatest benefit from a sulphonylurea is seen from a dose at the lower end of the range, and the effect diminishes as the doses are

Commonly used sulphonylureas in the UK

Drug	Marketing names (examples from the UK)	Dose range
Gliclazide (Once or twice a day)	Diamicron	40–160mg daily With breakfast Divide higher doses
Gliclazide MR	Diamicron MR – lower dosing regimen	30 mg MR equivalent to 80 mg of standard preparation
Glimepiride (Once a day)	Amaryl	1–4mg daily With first main meal
Glipizide	Glibenese Minodiab	2.5–20mg daily Before breakfast or lunch up to 15 mg as single dose; higher doses divided

increased. Hence rather than push your sulphonylurea to the highest possible dose, your doctor might consider adding in another medication instead. Generally over time there is a slow drift upwards in HbA_{1c} in patients taking sulphonylureas. For this reason, your doctor will almost certainly need to increase the dose of your medication over time.

When should you not use a sulphonylurea?

Sulphonylureas shouldn't be used if you have severe problems with your liver or kidney function, but your GP will be aware of these contraindications. It isn't generally advisable to take a sulphonylurea for control of diabetes during pregnancy or breastfeeding. One small study has shown that glibenclamide may be an acceptable alternative to insulin for some pregnant women with Type 2 diabetes.

Who should not take sulphonylureas?

- Anyone who has problems with their liver.
- Anyone who has problems with the function of their kidneys.
- Most women who are pregnant or breastfeeding, although it may sometimes be possible for them to take a sulphonylurea drug instead of insulin, provided their doctor monitors them closely.

Side effects

Hypoglycaemia associated with sulphonylurea use tends to be more frequent if you are taking the longer acting sulphonylureas such as glibenclamide, when your eating patterns are erratic (such as if you work shifts) and when your blood glucose levels are close to target. In elderly people, sulphonylureas may lead to severe prolonged hypoglycaemic attacks with confusion or symptoms suggestive of stroke. The diagnosis may be missed if the doctor fails to realize that the patient is taking a sulphonylurea and omits to check the blood glucose level. The annual risk of hypoglycaemia varies from 20% (mild) to 1% (severe).

You are likely to put on weight after you start taking a sulphonylurea. This is usually between 1 and 4 kg, but the increase in weight is at its greatest during the first 6 months of treatment. Hypersensitivity reactions can occur with sulphonylureas, as they can with all drugs, but these are rare. They may manifest as jaundice, skin rashes or problems with the manufacture of blood cells.

Evidence for using a sulphonylurea to manage your diabetes

Evidence from the most robust long-term outcome study for Type 2 diabetes, the UKPDS suggests that reducing blood sugar using a sulphonylurea reduces microvascular complications such as eye disease, nerve and kidney damage. The same study suggests that taking a sulphonylurea does not reduce your risks of cardiovascular disease due to diabetes within the first few years but a follow-up to the initial study, known as the UKPDS 30 year study, found that people who had good control in the early years had a reduced risk of cardiovascular disease many years later. You can read about the UKPDS 30-year study in Chapter 36.

Gliptins

DPP-4 inhibitors (gliptins) act by blocking an enzyme which breaks down glucagon-like peptide-1 (GLP-1). GLP-1 is a hormone produced by the small intestine in reponse to a meal. It has a number of effects (see Chapter 14), which include increasing the secretion of insulin in response to a meal and reducing appetite. This helps to reduce the blood glucose following a meal and can also lead to weight loss. GLP-1 has a shortlived effect as it is rapidly inactivated in the circulation by an enzyme called DPP-4 (dipeptidyl peptidase-4). By inhibiting DPP-4, the effect of GLP-1 can be prolonged. DPP-4 inhibitors appear to lower the HbA_{1c} by about 7 mmol/mol in the short term. This effect persists for at least a year. There is early evidence to suggest that this class of drugs may lower blood pressure and cholesterol.

The DPP-4s will not cause you to put on weight or cause hypoglycaemia. Four preparations are now available – sitagliptin, vildagliptin, saxagliptin and linagliptin. Both saxagliptin and linagliptin are suitable for use in people with kidney disease. More data on their long-term safety will become available over the next few years. The gliptins can be combined with metformin, sulphonylureas, glitazones or insulin.

When should you not use a gliptin

If you have kidney problems the dose may need to be reduced and saxagliptin and linagliptin have been developed particularly for people with impaired kidney function. If you have had an allergic reaction to a gliptin you should avoid other drugs in this class. There have been rare reports of pancreatitis (inflammation of the pancreas) in people treated with a gliptin so if you have a past history of pancreatitis you should avoid these drugs.

Who should not take gliptins?

- Anyone with a past history of pancreatitis.
- Anyone with end-stage kidney failure.
- Women who are pregnant or breastfeeding.

Gliptins

Drug	Brand name	Normal range
Linagliptin	Trajenta	5mg daily
	Also available in combination with metformin as Jentadueto	
Saxagliptin	Onglyza	5mg daily. Reduce to 2.5mg in moderate to severe renal failure
	Also available in combination with metformin as Komboglyze	
Sitagliptin	Januvia	100mg daily. Reduce to 50mg in moderate to severe renal failure
	Also available in combination with metformin as Janumet	
Vildagliptin	Galvus	50mg twice daily. Reduce to once daily in renal impairment
	Also available in combination with metformin as Eucreas	

Side effects

Some people experience diarrhoea and rashes and allergic reactions have been reported but in general, gliptins are very well tolerated.

Evidence for using a gliptin to manage your diabetes

These drugs are very new and there are no studies available yet to show long-term benefit of treatment with a gliptin

Glitazones (insulin sensitizers)

Pioglitazone is the only glitazone currently available in the UK, Europe and the US. Two other drugs in this category – troglitazone and rosiglitazone – have been withdrawn because of safety concerns. The problems which arose with troglitazone and rosiglitazone are not associated with pioglitazone. Glitazones act by helping sugar to get in to muscle and fat, where it can be stored or used for energy. Effectively, this is re-establishing the body's sensitivity to its own insulin. For this reason, glitazones combine well with metformin as they act at complementary sites in the body.

People who are overweight tend to have lower insulin sensitivity, so glitazones may be a good choice for them. Your doctor can use pioglitazone on its own or combined with metformin, a gliptin and/or a sulphonylurea.

When should you not use a glitazone?

Some doctors are cautious about using a glitazone if there is a disturbance of liver function. However, there is evidence that if you have a condition called a fatty liver, with fat accumulating and leading to minor changes in your liver function tests, you might actually benefit from taking pioglitazone. Some of the caution arises because the first glitazone, troglitazone, was withdrawn because of liver problems; but there is no evidence that pioglitazone causes abnormal liver tests.

Pioglitazone

Drug	Brand name	Normal range
Pioglitazone	Actos	15–45mg once daily
	Also available in combination with metformin as Competact	

Because glitazones can increase fluid retention, pioglitazone should be avoided if you have heart failure. Your doctor will be aware of this and if you have heart failure or fluid retention, it is best that you avoid this class of drug. Rosiglitazone was withdrawn because of evidence to suggest it may carry a small increased risk of heart attack. There is no evidence to link pioglitazone with cardio-vascular risk.

Not enough information is available to ensure that pioglitazone is safe to be used in women with Type 2 diabetes who are pregnant or breastfeeding. For this reason they should be avoided in pregnant women or breastfeeding mothers. If you are a young woman with Type 2 diabetes, it is worth bearing in mind that taking glitazones may improve your chances of ovulation, and increase your chances of getting pregnant so you will need to be careful about contraception.

Who should not take glitazones?

- Some people with liver problems. (Anyone who has problems with their liver should have their liver function tested before they start on a glitazone.)
- Anyone who has heart failure or a history of angina or chest pain from the heart.
- Anyone who has problems with fluid retention.

- Most people on insulin treatment, although it may be possible to take a glitazone with insulin in certain circumstances and if your doctor monitors you very carefully.
- Any woman who is pregnant or trying to get pregnant.
- Women who are breastfeeding.

Side effects

One of the main side effects associated with pioglitazone is increase in body weight. This is because the glitazones improve the way that the body stores fats and increases fat stores, particularly around the hips. Most of the weight increase happens in the first 6–12 months of treatment and is around 2–6 kg in total.

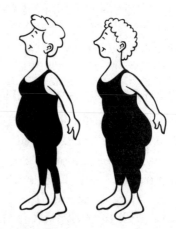

You may find that taking a glitazone tablet moves fat from around your middle (where it is more likely to cause you health problems) to your hips and thighs.

Fluid retention may also be a problem for some people, and is dangerous for those with heart failure. This is why doctors will be unwilling to prescribe pioglitazone to anyone with a history of significant fluid retention. Exact numbers of people with Type 2 diabetes who develop fluid retention are difficult to determine, but in clinical studies it tends to be about 5–10% of participants. Early symptoms of retention of fluid may include a rapid increase in your weight, shortness of breath and swollen ankles.

Another relatively common problem which may occur is anaemia. This is usually mild and occurs mainly because of fluid retention. More recent concerns are an unexplained risk of fractures in people taking pioglitazone and a possible association with bladder cancer – this link is currently being explored.

Evidence for using glitazones to manage your diabetes

Only one outcome study relating to pioglitazone has reported so far. The PROactive Study showed that in addition to lowering blood sugars, pioglitazone gave some protection against cardiovascular disease. This effect was very modest though, and patients did suffer increased fluid retention. One reassuring finding from PROactive was that pioglitazone appears to protect against worsening of blood glucose in some patients. Around half as many patients in the pioglitazone group needed to start insulin to control their blood sugar levels, compared with the group taking the placebo (dummy pill).

Postprandial glucose regulators (PPGRs)

These drugs work in a similar way to sulphonylureas but have a very short duration of action and are usually taken before each meal. They may be useful if you work shifts or eat your meals at odd times of the day. Limitations are similar to those of the sulphonylureas, in that they stimulate release of insulin but do not improve glucose uptake into muscle or fat (improve insulin sensitivity). Two post-prandial glucose regulators, nateglinide and repaglinide, are currently available.

When should you avoid PPGRs?

PPGRs shouldn't be used if you have severe problems with your liver, are pregnant or are breastfeeding. They may be more useful than sulphonylureas where you have a history of kidney problems, because they have a much

Postprandial glucose regulators (PPGRs)

Drug	Brand name	Normal range
Repaglinide Can be used on its own or in combination with metformin	Prandin	500mcg–16 mg Within 30 minutes before main meals Up to 4 mg as a single dose
Nateglinide Can only be used as combination therapy	Starlix	60–180mg three times daily Within 30 minutes before main meals

shorter duration of action and as such are less likely to cause hypoglycaemia.

Side effects of PPGRs

Hypoglycaemia does still occur in patients taking PPGRs, but is less likely than with sulphonylureas because of the shorter duration of action of these drugs. This is more likely when the drugs are used in combination, for instance with metformin.

Weight gain with PPGRs is thought to be less than with sulphonylureas. This may be due to the fact that insulin release is stimulated to a lesser extent because of the shorter duration of action.

Who should not take PPGRs?

- Anyone who has severe problems with their liver.
- Women who are pregnant or breastfeeding.

Evidence for using a PPGR to manage your diabetes

Evidence for the long-term benefit of using a PPGR to manage your blood sugar is limited. There are no outcome studies showing a benefit on cardiovascular disease.

Alpha-glucosidase inhibitors

When you eat complex carbohydrates, such as those you find in pasta, bread or rice, these are broken down by enzymes in the gut called glucosidases. This produces shorter chain sugars which can be more easily absorbed by the body and used for energy. If the action of the glucosidases is inhibited, the complex carbohydrate cannot be broken down and therefore cannot be absorbed. This prevents a rise in the blood glucose. Acarbose is an alpha-glucosidase inhibitor, currently used in the UK.

Who should avoid taking acarbose?

Acarbose is not recommended in patients with significant bowel troubles. If you have had abdominal surgery or inflammatory bowel disease such as Crohn's or ulcerative colitis, then acarbose may not be a good idea for you. If you have problems with the function of your kidneys or liver, you are unlikely to be prescribed this drug. Acarbose shouldn't be used by women who are pregnant or breastfeeding.

Side effects of acarbose

The main problems associated with acarbose tend to be gastrointestinal side effects. The sugars which are prevented from being digested by acarbose pass into the large bowel. There, they provide a very readily available food source for the naturally occurring bacteria that live in your large bowel. The bacteria that use them as a food source then produce large amounts of gas.

Alpha-glucosidase inhibitors

Drug	Brand name	Normal range
Acarbose *May be used alone or in combination with other drugs*	Glucobay	50–600mg The dose should be increased slowly to improve tolerability and reduce problems due to gastric upsets

This gas leads to abdominal wind and bloating, pain because of distension of the colon, flatulence and 'blowy' diarrhoea.

Care needs to be taken if acarbose is used in combination with drugs which may cause hypoglycaemia. Many of the products used to treat hypoglycaemia contain sucrose, the absorption of which is blocked or slowed by acarbose. If you are taking acarbose in combination with other drugs then you may need to carry glucose, rather than sucrose, as a treatment for hypoglycaemia.

Who should not take acarbose?

- Anyone who has bowel problems such as inflammatory bowel disease.
- Anyone who has a hernia or who has had abdominal surgery.
- Anyone who has severe problems with the function of their liver or kidneys.
- Women who are pregnant or breastfeeding.

What is the evidence for using acarbose to treat Type 2 diabetes?

There is evidence that acarbose is effective in reducing blood glucose, particularly in early Type 2 diabetes. But it has not been a popular choice, due to the side effects described above. Studies in pre-diabetes show that acarbose can both prevent progression to Type 2 diabetes and reduce cardiovascular events in this important group of patients.

Sodium-glucose transporter-2 (SGLT-2) inhibitors

This is a new class of drugs, just becoming available in the UK. They act by blocking transport systems within the kidneys so that the kidneys leak glucose into the urine. This can lead to a loss of about 50 g of glucose per day, which effectively lowers the blood glucose and can also lead to weight loss. Side effects are those which might be predicted – infections such as candida can affect both men and women and there is an increased incidence of urine infections.

GLP-1 agonists

Exenatide (Byetta) and liraglutide (Victoza) are the first type of medication in a class of drugs called 'incretin mimetics' or GLP-1 agonist. The term GLP-1 agonists sounds rather frightening but they are an exciting treatment for Type 2 diabetes that has made a great difference to the lives of many people, The initials GLP-1 stand for Glucagon Like Peptide 1, which is a hormone produced naturally by the cells of the small intestine. A GLP-1 agonist is the name for a group of drugs which mimic the action of natural GLP-1.

Each GLP-1 agonist is produced synthetically and works in four different ways:

1. It helps your body produce more insulin when it is needed.

SGLG-2 Inhibitor

Drug	Brand name	Normal range
Dapagliflozin	Forxiga	10mg once daily

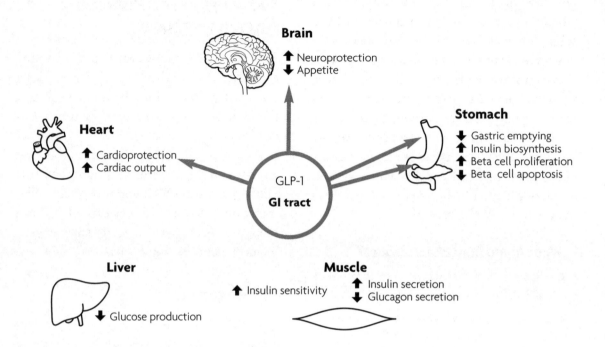

Brain
↑ Neuroprotection
↓ Appetite

Heart
↑ Cardioprotection
↑ Cardiac output

Stomach
↓ Gastric emptying
↑ Insulin biosynthesis
↑ Beta cell proliferation
↓ Beta cell apoptosis

GLP-1
GI tract

Liver
↓ Glucose production

↑ Insulin sensitivity

Muscle
↑ Insulin secretion
↓ Glucagon secretion

How GLP-1 affects the beta cells.

2. It reduces the amount of glucose being produced by your liver when it is not needed.
3. It reduces the rate at which your stomach digests foods and empties. This means that the rate at which glucose from your food is released into your blood is lowered.
4. Reduces appetite and the amount of food you eat.

GLP-1 agonists are different from diabetes tablets and insulin injections. Although taken by injection, they are not insulins. They are also likely to cause nausea as a side effect which usually wears off with time.

GLP-1 agonists on their own cannot cause hypoglycaemia as they only stimulate insulin production in response to food. However, if they are taken in conjunction with insulin or a sulphonyurea, there is a risk of hypoglycaemia. People taking one of these combinations should be aware of this and should test their blood glucose at times when hypoglycaemia is a possibility.

Exenatide

Exenatide has been available in the UK since 2006 and because of its costs (£68.24 per month in 2012) it has not been freely available. However, NICE has recommended its use in patients when metformin and a sulphonylurea have failed to keep the HbA$_{1c}$ below 58 mmol/mol and when the patient's BMI is greater than 35 (see Chapter 9, Weight control). NICE has agreed that if a patient works in a job which makes insulin use a problem, such as driving an HGV, then exenatide may be used if the BMI is less than

35. NICE also recommends that exenatide can only be continued if, after 6 months, the weight has fallen by 3% and the HbA_{1c} has fallen by 1% (11 mmol/mol in the new units).

The starting dose of exenatide is 5 mcg by injection twice a day. After 4 weeks, the dose is increased to 10 mcg, which is the final and most effective dose. Ideally exenatide should be given at any time within 60 minutes of eating a meal – but not immediately after eating.

At first NICE did not license the use of exenatide with insulin, even though a large number of patients would clearly benefit from this combination. In March 2012, however, NICE approved the combination of exenatide and basal insulin so people who also take mealtime insulin are still not covered by the NICE regulations. In practice, many patients who take multiple insulin injections and exenatide often achieve very good clinical results in the form of weight loss, improved diabetes control and a reduction in the dose of insulin.

The main side effect of exenatide is nausea and, occasionally, vomiting. This is frequently a problem at the start of treatment but usually becomes less severe over the first few weeks and may recur when the dose is increased. The vast majority of patients who continue with exenatide only have rare attacks of nausea. A common effect of the drug is to make people feel full after eating a small amount of their meal. Thus exenatide has the effect of forcing people to do what every dietitian advises, namely to reduce portion size. In a research study less than one patient in ten who was taking exenatide had to stop because of persistent nausea.

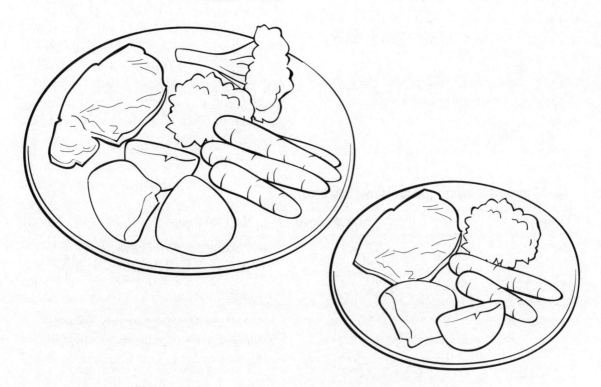

Patients taking exenatide often find they want to reduce the size of their food portions.

Liraglutide

Liraglutide became available in the UK in 2009 under the name Victoza. It has the advantage of requiring only a single daily injection. It costs slightly more than exenatide at £76.75 per month for the normal daily dose of 1.2 mg daily. It is standard practice to start liraglutide with a daily dose of 0.6 mg and increase the dose to 1.2 mg which is continued indefinitely.

Just like exenatide, liraglutide causes nausea but head to head studies have shown that nausea wears off more quickly with liraglutide than exenatide. In practice, however, there seem to be some patients who can only tolerate one of these drugs, so that if either drug causes troublesome side effects, it is always worth trying the other.

Liraglutide can only be prescribed under the same restrictions as exenatide:

■ Patients with poor control (HbA$_{1c}$ > 58 mmol/mol) on metformin and a sulphonylurea.

■ Body mass index of 35 or more – unless their employment precludes the use of insulin, in which case it may be used at a lower body weight.

■ Only continue use after 6 months if body weight has fallen by 3% or more, and if HbA$_{1c}$ is 1% or 11 mmol/mol lower.

Once weekly exenatide

This became available in 2012 under the name of Bydureon. It overcomes the main drawback of the earlier version of exenatide (Byetta) which requires twice daily injections. Bydureon costs £73.36 for a month of treatment. It is a new drug so clinical experience is limited. Early reports suggest that some patients are very enthusiastic about Bydureon, while others are not so. Some described swelling and itching at the injection site.

Oral treatment pathways for blood glucose: what is the best form of treatment?

The International Diabetes Federation (IDF) has published guidelines recommending the gold standard way to manage blood glucose with tablets in Type 2 diabetes. Previous targets for HbA$_{1c}$ have been relaxed following results from trials which have suggested that very low HbA$_{1c}$ targets may be associated

GLP-1 agonists alpha-glucosidase inhibitors

Drug	Brand name	Normal range
Exenatide	Byetta	Starting dose 5mcg twice daily Increasing to 10mcg after 4 weeks
	Bydureon	2mg once weekly
Liraglutide	Victoza	Starting dose 0.6mg once daily Increasing to 1.2mg after 1 week
Lixisenatide	Lyxumia	Starting dose 10mcg once daily Increasing to 20mcg after 1 week

with increased mortality (see Chapter 12). The IDF-recommended threshold for introducing further treatment is now an HbA_{1c} of more than 53 mmol/mol, although in England NICE recommends a target of 48 mmol/mol for patients on diet alone or metformin, rising to 58 mmol/mol if more than one medication is in use. Both IDF and NICE guidelines support the use of metformin as initial drug therapy if diet and lifestyle measures do not achieve the target HbA_{1c}. They then recommend that either a sulphonylurea, a glitazone (referred to as thiazolidinedione), a gliptin or an alpha glucosidase inhibitor be added next.

If your HbA_{1c} remains above target when you are taking two blood glucose lowering drugs, the guidelines suggest that you start insulin, consider triple oral therapy or a GLP-1 agonist. They stress the importance of

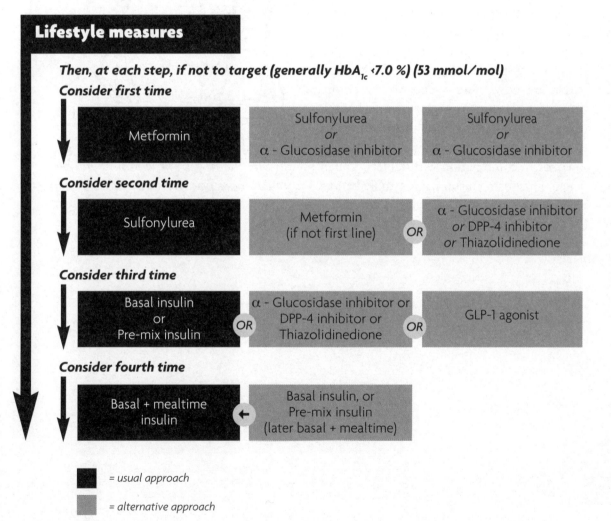

The IDF treatment algorithm summarizes the recommendations for treatment of Type 2 diabetes.

considering insulin therapy at an early stage if your symptoms are increasing or your blood glucose levels are becoming harder to control.

Most diabetes experts recommend tailoring treatment according to the weight of the patient concerned. There is evidence that, if you are overweight and taking metformin, you may benefit more from addition of a gliptin, or possibly a glitazone rather than a sulphonylurea. If your BMI is greater than 35 you may benefit from a GLP-1 agonist, which can promote weight loss.

Unfortunately, no tablet treatment currently available to treat Type 2 diabetes can stave off insulin therapy forever, although there are now more agents to try before turning to insulin. Your doctor may broach the subject of starting insulin treatment with you at some stage. Insulin may be used on its own, or in combination with tablets. When you are first using insulin, it may only be one

injection a day to supplement the tablets. If this does not appear to be working sufficiently, then two or more injections of insulin per day may be used.

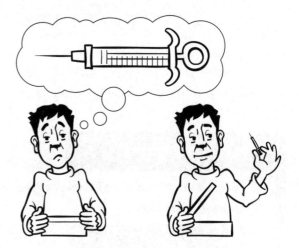

It is natural to feel afraid of starting insulin therapy, but the reality will be much more positive than you may expect.

14

Insulin treatment

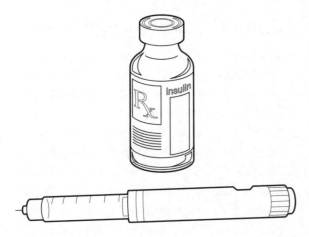

Animal, human and analogue insulin

In the past, bovine (beef) and porcine (pork) insulin were the only forms of insulin available. Nowadays, human insulin is the most commonly used, but more recently insulin analogues ('designer insulins') have been introduced to provide insulins with more rapid onset or longer duration of action to suit individual needs. Human insulin has a chemical structure identical to the insulin produced by the human pancreas. This can now be produced on a large scale so it is no longer necessary to produce insulin from cows and pigs and manufacturers are withdrawing production of animal insulins. Human insulin is produced using gene technology, which involves the insertion of human insulin-producing genes into a yeast cell or bacterium. In this way the yeast cells or bacteria are tricked into producing insulin instead of their own proteins.

The pancreas of a person without diabetes secretes a small amount of insulin into the bloodstream constantly throughout the day and night (called basal secretion). After a meal, a larger amount of insulin is secreted to deal with the glucose coming from the food (called the bolus secretion; see graphs on page 106). If you have Type 2 diabetes, your pancreas will eventually become unable to produce enough insulin to overcome the resistance to its action and will not respond to the rise in blood glucose after a meal. Although there are now a variety of non-insulin treatments available, these become ineffective with time and the majority of people with Type 2 diabetes will need insulin eventually. The goal of all insulin replacement treatment is to mimic normal pancreatic function and provide insulin to the bloodstream in the most appropriate way.

Production of human insulin: biosynthetic DNA-technology method

Production from baker's yeast	Novo Nordisk insulins
Production from coli-bacteria	Eli Lilly insulins Sanofi-Aventis insulins

Insulin comes in the form of short or rapid-acting insulin, for use with meals, and longer acting insulin, which provides the background (or basal) requirement throughout the 24 hours. Short- and rapid-acting insulins are pure insulin without any additives. They are in the form of a clear liquid and do not require stirring or mixing before use. Different additives such as protamine or zinc are used to make the insulin longer-acting, and in most cases these make it cloudy. The cloudy component collects as sediment at the bottom of the bottle or cartridge. This sediment should be mixed again with the rest of the contents by turning over or rolling (but not shaking) the cartridge 20 times before use. The newer (analogue) basal insulins are clear because they are solutions. Analogue insulins have a prolonged effect because changes to their molecular structure slow down absorption.

Methods of slowing the action of insulin

NPH insulin (isophane) Insulatard, Humulin I	Binds to a protein from salmon (protamine).
Lantus	Clear solution but precipitates (becomes cloudy) after injection due to a higher pH in the subcutaneous tissue.
Levemir	Binds to a protein (albumin) in the bloodstream.

Intravenous insulin is often used during surgery or if a person is suffering from diarrhoea and vomiting. It also gives us a practical way of working out how much insulin the person needs over a 24-hour period, for example when changing from intravenous treatment during illness to subcutaneous insulin injections on recovery.

Since the half-life of insulin in the circulation is very short, only about 4 minutes, the blood glucose will increase sharply if intravenous insulin is stopped. When intravenous insulin is used, the blood glucose must be checked every hour (even during the night) to monitor the correct dosage.

Units and insulin concentrations

Insulin is measured in units, abbreviated to U (international units, previously abbreviated IU). One unit of insulin was originally defined as the amount of insulin that will lower the blood glucose of a healthy 2 kg (4.4 lb) rabbit that has fasted for 24 hours to 2.5 mmol/L (45 mg/dl) within 2.5 hours. Quite a complicated definition, don't you think? Today, the most common insulin concentration around the world is 100 units/ml (U-100). In some countries other concentrations are used, mostly 40 units/ml (U-40). Insulin units are counted in the same way, regardless of the concentration. A weaker insulin will be absorbed more quickly. Insulin of 40 units/ml gives approximately 20% higher insulin levels 30–40 minutes after injection compared with the same number of units of 100 units/ml. People taking insulin need to be aware that it will take effect more quickly if they switch from 100 units/ml to 40 units/ml. If you are abroad and need to obtain insulin, you need to check that the concentration of insulin (normally U100) is the one you normally take.

Short- and rapid-acting insulin

Short-acting insulin (e.g. Humulin S®, Actrapid®) is taken to deal with the rapid rise in blood glucose after a meal. However, regular short-acting human insulin is a bit slow in onset of action and lasts longer than it ideally should. As a result, the insulin level in your blood is not high enough during the meal but can be higher than necessary a couple of hours later, This can lead to a low blood sugar 2–3 hours after a meal and may mean that you need to snack between meals, which can be a problem if you are trying to lose weight.

Rapid-acting insulins (e.g. Humalog®, NovoRapid®, Apidra®) are insulin analogues which have been designed to work more quickly and last for a shorter time than regular 'short-acting' human insulin. The rapid onset of action coincides more closely with the rate of glucose absorption from meals and, because of the shorter action span, it is possible to achieve lower (more normal) insulin levels between meals, lessening the need for snacks.

Basal insulin

People without diabetes always have a low level of insulin in their body between meals and even during the night (see graphs overleaf). The steady release of insulin from the pancreas takes care of the glucose that is released between meals from the store in the liver. This constant low level of insulin is known as basal insulin or background insulin. People with diabetes do not have this steady production of insulin and in order to produce a steady supply of basal insulin they need to take intermediate or long-acting insulin to replace it. The intermediate-acting insulin (sometimes known as NPH or isophane) has been modified by the addition of a protein (protamine) so that its action is prolonged and it only needs to be taken once or twice daily.

New basal insulins

Once a day injections of existing inter-mediate-acting insulin preparations do not provide a 24-hour basal insulin level (between meals and during the night) in most people with diabetes. The long-acting analogue Lantus (glargine) was introduced in 2000. By altering the insulin molecule, the blood glucose-lowering effect has been spread more evenly over up to 24 hours, re-sembling the background insulin secretion in a person without diabetes. The subcutaneous uptake of insulin is more stable from day to day with Lantus compared with human intermediate-acting insulin (Humulin I or Insulatard.)

Levemir (detemir), another basal insulin, was introduced in 2004. A 6-month study of adults using NovoRapid as pre-meal insulin showed that, with Levemir, the HbA_{1c} level was the same as with intermediate insulin (7.6%) but with a lower risk of hypoglycae-mia, especially during the night. Overnight glucose profiles were more even with Levemir, and body weight was significantly lower after 6 months in the Levemir group. In another study the variability of insulin effect from day to day was smaller with Levemir compared with intermediate insulin and Lantus. More recent studies have shown that Levemir appears to be associated with less weight gain than other long-acting insulins. One possible explanation is that Levemir may have a greater effect on the liver and less effect on places where fat is laid down.

A review of several studies comparing Levemir and Lantus in adults found the duration of action to be very much the same (21.5–23 hours for Levemir and 22–24 hours

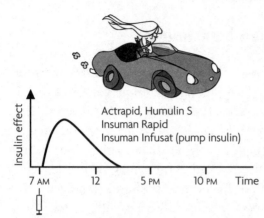

Actrapid, Humulin S
Insuman Rapid
Insuman Infusat (pump insulin)

Regular short-acting insulin

Regular short-acting insulin (also called soluble insulin) is given as a bolus injection before meals. The listed brand names are examples of insulins.

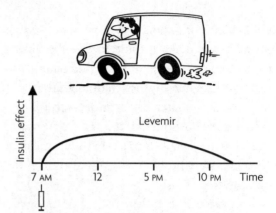

Levemir

Basal insulin analogues

Basal insulin analogues have effect for up to 24 hours. Older forms have been superseded by new long-acting insulins Levemir and Lantus which give a more stable Insulin effect and are injected once or twice daily.

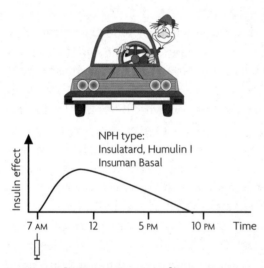

NPH type:
Insulatard, Humulin I
Insuman Basal

Intermediate-acting insulin

Intermediate-acting insulin is used as basal (background) insulin when injecting twice daily and once or twice daily in a multiple daily Injection regimen.

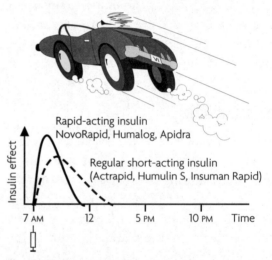

Rapid-acting insulin
NovoRapid, Humalog, Apidra

Regular short-acting insulin
(Actrapid, Humulin S, Insuman Rapid)

Rapid-acting Insulin

The newer rapid-acting insulin analogues (NovoRapid, Humalog, Apidra) have a much more rapid action than regular short-acting insulin. You can inject them just before a meal and still get a good insulin effect at the time when the glucose from the food reaches the bloodstream. However, the insulin will have less effect after 2–3 hours, and the blood glucose may therefore rise before the next meal. Because of this, a basal insulin that takes effect during the day is usually given.

for Lantus) but Levemir gave a more stable insulin effect from day to day in the individual person. A 6-month study in adults comparing Levemir (given twice daily) and Lantus (given once daily) as basal insulin found no difference in HbA_{1c} or weight gain, but the Levemir group had a lower fasting glucose level and less severe night-time hypoglycaemia.

Research findings: Levemir

- A study of adults using Levemir (detemir) found the time of action to be between 6 and 23 hours when doses between 0.1 U/kg and 0.8 U/kg were given.

- The use of Levemir is associated with less weight gain than NPH insulin.

- One possible explanation for this is that Levemir's chemical structure causes it to have a greater effect in the liver than conventional insulins. This may increase the glycogen store and affect hunger signals.

Research findings: Lantus

- Lantus has been shown to give similar levels of basal insulin over 24 hours to an insulin pump.

- In one study, adults with Type 1 diabetes compared Lantus (given once at bedtime) with NPH (given once or twice daily). Fasting glucose was 2.2 mmol/L (40 mg/dl) lower when using Lantus.

- In the group using NPH once a day, the doses of Lantus were similar. But Lantus doses for the group using NPH twice daily were 6–7 units lower than the sum of the NPH doses.

- A recently published study of treating to target with Lantus in Type 2 diabetes has shown neutral or only slight weight gain, with acceptable levels of nocturnal hypoglycaemia.

Pre-mixed insulin

Pre-mixed insulin available for insulin pens contains different proportions of rapids or short-acting insulin mixed with intermediate-acting insulin of NPH type. It is normally taken twice a day. With pre-mixed insulins, the proportions of the two insulins cannot be adjusted, so if you increase or decrease the dose you will get more or less of both types of insulin. If you are taking a pre-mixed insulin you will need to take care to eat at fairly regular times during the day – if you delay a meal, your blood sugar may become low because the insulin has already been taken and will continue to work even if you have not eaten.

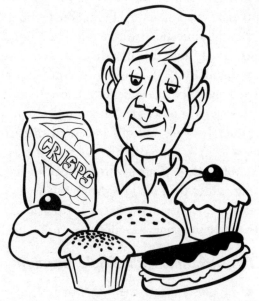

Snacking to deal with hypoglycaemia will lead to weight gain.

Twice-daily treatment

Twice-daily injections of pre-mixed insulin are still widely used in Type 2 diabetes. It is often difficult to adjust mentally to taking insulin during the early stages of insulin therapy, and injections twice daily help a high percentage of people with Type 2 diabetes to reach their targets. However, a twice-daily injection regimen usually means that there is less flexibility for planning mealtimes. When targets aren't achieved, increasing twice-daily insulin may risk hypoglycaemia during the late afternoon or night. Snacking to deal with hypoglycaemia will cause weight gain.

Multiple injection treatment

Multiple injection treatment implies taking rapid-acting (NovoRapid, Humalog, Apidra) or short-acting (Actrapid, Humulin S, Insuman Rapid) insulin before each main meal, and one or two doses of intermediate-acting (Insulatard, Humulin I, Insuman Basal) or long-acting (Lantus, Levemir) insulin to cover the need for insulin between meals and during the night.

Multiple injection treatment has been used since 1984, and the first insulin pen was introduced in 1985. Studies in adults with Type 1 and Type 2 diabetes have shown that it is possible to improve glucose control with this regimen. If using multiple injections doesn't give you an improved HbA_{1c}, it may at least give you more flexibility with your day-to-day living, rather than planning your day around your insulin. This arrangement is particularly easy to use in people who do shift work.

Research findings: multiple injections

- Studies indicate that more than 90% of participants have found multiple injections acceptable.

- Results from the DCCT study in Type 1 diabetes show that using an intensive treatment regimen can have positive effects, particularly on microvascular complications.

Injections before meals (bolus insulin)

Bolus insulin is the rapid- or short-acting insulin taken before a meal. Rapid-acting insulin begins to act after 10 minutes and is at its most effective after just one hour. If you are using rapid-acting insulin, you will not need to be as strict about mealtimes if you also have a dose of basal insulin in the morning (see page 105). Short-acting regular insulin (Actrapid, Humulin S, Insuman Rapid) begins to act 20–30 minutes after a subcutaneous injection and has its maximal effect after 1.5–2 hours. The blood glucose lowering effect lasts for about 5 or more hours. One difference between rapid- and short-acting insulins for multiple injections is that with rapid-acting insulin you may notice a rise in your evening blood sugars if you eat a large afternoon snack, unless you are playing sport, digging the garden or doing some other activity. With short-acting insulin, the opposite is the case and activity may mean that you need a sandwich in the middle of the afternoon to avoid hypoglycaemia. Check your blood glucose level to help you decide what dose you need.

Results from the Lantus 'treating to target' algorithm study suggest that intensive treatment with a long-acting insulin analogue regime results in improved control and only a small rise in the incidence of hypoglycaemia, accompanied by little significant weight gain.

When should you take your pre-meal dose?

The regular short-acting insulins (Actrapid, Humulin S, Insuman Rapid) have the same time action and start to have an effect 15–30 minutes after injection. Ideally, these short-acting insulins should be administered 20–30 minutes before meals since they do not affect the blood glucose immediately.

Rapid-acting insulins (Apidra, Novo-Rapid, Humalog) start working within a few minutes of injection. The abdomen is the most common injection site for pre-meal injections. If you take regular pre-meal insulin in the thigh (or buttocks) you may need to add another 15 minutes to these time limits since insulin is absorbed more rapidly from the abdomen than the thigh. The time limits given in this chapter refer to abdominal injections of regular short-acting insulin if not otherwise stated. If you use rapid acting insulin you must adjust the time intervals as indicated above.

Can regular short-acting insulin injections be taken just before a meal?

To find out, take the injection just before your meal and measure your blood glucose before and 2 hours after the meal. The blood glucose should have risen 4.0 mmol/L (70 mg/dl) at the most. If it has risen more, the effect of your regular insulin is too slow.

Try the same thing when you take your insulin 15 and 30 minutes before eating, to find out which suits you the best. If the blood glucose is too high, even when you have taken the insulin 30 minutes before the meal, you will probably need a higher dose.

> ## Timing your injections
>
> *The rapid-acting insulins (Apidra NovoRapid, Humalog) are very quick to take effect and can be given immediately before the meal. However, since it takes 20–30 minutes for regular short-acting insulin (Actrapid, Humulin S, Insuman Rapid) to begin its action, you must give the insulin a head start or the race will be very uneven. The carbohydrates from your meal will enter the bloodstream first and raise your blood glucose level. The insulin will enter your bloodstream later, but will remain in the system after the food has been absorbed. This will lead to a high blood glucose initially but put you at risk of a low blood glucose before your next meal. Taking your injection 30 minutes before the meal is particularly important at breakfast time, but if you recognize these problems, you should take your injection 20–30 minutes before all meals.*

What do I do if my premeal blood glucose is high or low?

If your premeal blood glucose is higher than your target (usually less than 7mmol/l), you may wish to take some extra short- or rapid-acting insulin to correct for the high level. As a rule of thumb, we normally recommend a starting correction dose of 1 unit of insulin to reduce the blood glucose by 3 mmol/L. In practice, many people with Type 2 diabetes are insulin-resistant and need significantly more insulin to achieve this effect – you need to find out what works for you. We suggest that you experiment to discover how many units of insulin you need to reduce your blood glucose by 3 mmol/L. You will then be able to use this information to work out how much extra insulin you need to take when your blood glucose is high.

If your premeal blood glucose is low (less than 4 mmol/L), you have two choices. If you are feeling well, your blood glucose is above 3 mmol/L and you are about to eat a meal containing rapidly-absorbed carbohydrate, you may wish to go ahead with the planned meal but to reduce the insulin dose by 2–3 units to take account of the low blood glucose. As with a high blood glucose, you will need to find out what works for you. If your blood glucose is below 3 mmol/L, or if you are feeling low, it is sensible to take some rapid-acting carbohydrate in the form of a glucose drink to treat the hypo before you eat. If you do this you should be careful not to delay your meal and ensure that it contains adequate carbohydrate – take your normal insulin dose immediately before you eat.

If you inject regular short-acting insulin just before your meal, it is important that the food is not absorbed from the intestine immediately. If it is, your blood glucose will rise before the insulin reaches your bloodstream. Any fat content of the meal will slow down the gastric emptying rate. For example, ice cream made with milk products has a higher fat content and will therefore give a slower rise in blood glucose than water ice. See also Chapter 8 on Nutrition.

The blood glucose reading before a meal will indicate when it is appropriate to take the injection. If your blood glucose is high, you can wait 45–60 minutes before eating if this is convenient. If you have a low blood glucose, you should leave the injection until it is time to eat or wait 15 minutes at the most (see table below). If you use rapid-acting insulin (Novo Rapid, Apidra or Humalog) it should normally be injected just before the meal.

If your background insulin lasts 24 hours (which should be the case), the timing of the bedtime dose won't matter.

Can I skip a meal?

Your body needs to have some insulin in the blood, even between meals, to take care of the glucose produced by the liver. Your background insulin should ensure that the blood glucose does not rise if you miss a meal. If your blood glucose does rise, you may need a small corrective dose of rapid-acting insulin. As decribed above, you could try taking 1 unit of insulin to bring your blood glucose down by about 3 mmol/L, but you will need to find what works for you.

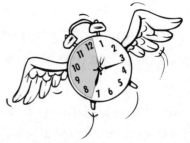

You can usually adjust your timetable for meals and injections provided you are taking the correct dose of a 24-hour background insulin (Lantus, Levemir or twice-daily Isophane). If you are taking a one-daily isophane in combination with a short-acting insulin at mealtimes, you should try to avoid going for more than 5 hours between meals as you may run out of background insulin.

If the blood glucose falls you will need to take some glucose. Missing a meal, or taking a carbohydrate free meal, is a good way of checking whether the dose of background insulin is right. If it is, your blood glucose will stay steady, even if you do not eat.

Bedtime insulin

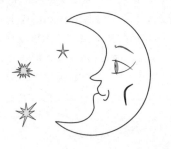

The bedtime insulin injection is the most difficult dose to adjust. Although we do not eat during the night, our bodies need a continuous low level of insulin to prevent the liver releasing glucose freely into the blood-stream. The most common bedtime insulin with multiple injection treatment used to be intermediate-acting insulin of NPH (iso-phane) type. Insulin with longer effect (Lantus or Levemir) is now used widely instead. Modern long-acting insulin ana-logues such as Lantus or Levemir are designed to have a 24-hour profile, but in practice this is not always the case and small doses of Lantus or Levemir may not last the full 24 hours. Working out the correct dose of background insulin can have a great impact on HbA_{1c} and on your quality of life.

When should the long-acting injection be taken?

The long-acting insulin analogue Lantus can be taken at the evening snack, at bedtime or even in the morning. Because it has a long half-life, your levels of Lantus are likely to reach a steady state after the first few injections. Most people find one evening dose of Lantus is sufficient, but some may need to split the dose and give part of it in the morning. Levemir (detemir) has a similar long duration of action, requiring one or two injections per day. Both these newer analogue insulins are associated with much less hypoglycaemia at night than traditional inter-mediate-acting insulins.

Since long-acting insulins act for up to 24 hours, sometimes even longer, it is important not to change the dose more often than 2 (or 3) times a week.

Mixing insulins

Insulin of NPH type (Insulatard, Humulin I, Insuman Basal) can be mixed with both rapid-acting NovoRapid and Humalog and regular short-acting insulin. You should not mix the new long-acting insulin analogues Lantus and Levemir with rapid-acting insu-lin in the syringe.

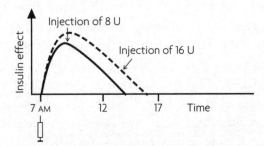

A larger insulin dose (dashed line) gives both a stronger, and a longer-lasting effect.

Depot effect

If only intermediate- or long-acting insulin is used, a depot (store) of insulin is formed in the subcutaneous fat tissue, corresponding to about

24 hours of insulin requirements. If the dose of bedtime insulin is changed, the size of the insulin depot makes it necessary to allow 2–3 days for your body to adjust until you see the full effect of the change.

The disadvantage of a large insulin depot in Type 2 diabetes is that, if your levels of long-acting insulin have built up to too high a level over a long period, there may be problems with hypoglycaemia lasting for more than 24 hours. Differences in the rate of absorption can vary when you change injection position, for example from the top of the legs to the abdomen, where people with Type 2 diabetes may have rather more subcutaneous fat.

How accurate is your insulin dose?

If used correctly, an insulin pen will give a very accurate insulin dose with an error of only a few per cent. However, the effect of a given insulin dose also depends on a number of other factors. The effect of an identical dose of insulin, given to an individual at the same site, can vary by as much as 25%. It can vary by nearly 50% when the same dose is given to two different individuals. This explains the frustrating fact that you can eat the same food, do exactly the same things and give identical doses of insulin for two days in a row, but get quite different blood glucose results. There is less variation in the action profile of the newer insulin analogues.

Insulin absorption

The absorption of insulin from the injection site can be influenced by a number of factors. Heat will increase the absorption. If the room temperature increases from 20° to 35° C (68–95° F), the speed of absorption of short-

acting insulin will increase by 50–60%. Taking a bath or a sauna at a temperature of 85° C (185° F) may increase the absorption by as much as 110%! In other words, you could be at risk of hypoglycaemia if you inject short-acting insulin shortly before taking a hot bath. A temperature of just 42° C (108° F) in a shower, spa bath or jacuzzi may double the insulin level in your blood, while a cold bath (22° C, 72° F) will decrease the absorption of insulin. Massage of the injection site for 30 minutes has been found to give higher insulin levels and lower blood glucose, with both short-acting and long-acting insulins.

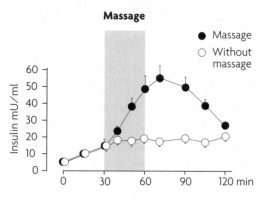

Massaging the injection site will considerably increase the absorption of insulin. Short-acting insulin (10 units) was given at 0 minutes. You can utilize this if you want your short-acting insulin to take particularly rapid effect, for example if you have a high blood glucose.

The skin temperature is also important. In one study, the same insulin injection gave twice the concentration in blood after 45 minutes when a skin temperature of 37°C was compared with that of 30° C (same room temperature). In the same study, individuals with a thicker subcutaneous fat layer (10 mm) had lower insulin levels than those with a thin subcutaneous fat layer (2 mm). The above mentioned factors have less of an effect on the absorption of new insulin analogues.

Factors influencing the insulin effect

1. **Insulin resistance**
   Insulin resistance probably has the most effect on insulin efficacy and the dose required for control in Type 2 diabetes. Resistance to the effects of insulin underpins the development of the disease in overweight patients.

2. **Subcutaneous blood flow**
   (increased blood flow will give a faster insulin absorption).
   Increased by
   Heat, e.g. sauna, jacuzzi, hot shower, hot bath or fever.
   Decreased by
   Cold, e.g. a cold bath. Smoking (constriction of the blood vessels). Dehydration.

3. **Injection depth**
   Faster absorption occurs after an intramuscular injection.

4. **Injection site**
   An abdominal injection of short-acting insulin will be absorbed faster than a thigh injection. The absorption from the buttocks is slower than from the abdomen but slightly faster than from the thigh.

5. **Insulin antibodies**
   Insulin antibodies can bind the insulin, resulting in a slower and less predictable effect. These are of much more clinical relevance in Type 1 diabetes.

6. **Exercise**
   Exercose increases the absorption of short-acting insulin even after you have finished exercising.

7. **Massage of the injection site**
   Massaging the injection site promotes increased absorption of short-acting insulin, probably due to a faster breakdown of the insulin.

8. **Subcutaneous fat thickness**
   A thicker layer of subcutaneous fat gives a slower absorption of insulin.

9. **Injection in fatty lumps**
   (lipohypertrophy) Slower and more erratic absorption of insulin.

10. **Concentration of the insulin**
    40 units/ml is absorbed faster than 100 units/ml.

What if you forget to take your insulin?

You can try the following suggestions if you have had diabetes for some time and are confident about how the insulin you inject works.

If you are even slightly unsure, you should seek expert advice.

Forgotten pre-meal injection (multiple injection treatment)

It is unlikely in Type 2 diabetes that missing one mealtime injection of insulin will cause you much of a problem, but of course if this happens over a number of occasions, your average control will be poorer and your HbA_{1c} will begin to rise. The best thing to do is to check your blood glucose at your next mealtime and take a corrective dose of insulin if it is high. Start by taking one extra unit of short-acting insulin for every 3 mmol/L above 10, but if you are insulin resistant you may need significantly more insulin, and you should experiment to find out what works for you.

Forgotten bedtime injection (multiple injection treatment)

If you normally take NPH (isophane) and you wake before 2 am, you can still take your bedtime insulin, but you should decrease the dose by 25% or 2 units for every hour that has passed since the normal time of injection. Unlike in Type 1 diabetes, it isn't likely that missing one night-time injection will cause you too much harm. Naturally, your blood sugar level may be significantly higher the following day.

If you have forgotten your evening or bedtime Lantus or Levemir dose, you can take it when you remember it, if only a few hours have passed. If you remember in the morning, take approximately half of the dose you should have taken in the evening. However, if you take Levemir or Lantus twice daily, just take your usual morning dose. In addition, if your blood glucose level is high, you should take extra mealtime insulin to correct this.

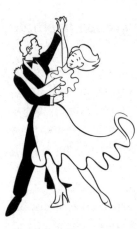

If you are out clubbing or at a party, remember that dancing is exercise too. Don't forget to eat something during the evening. You may well need to reduce your bedtime injection of insulin or eat a bedtime snack, such as a bowl of cereal.

What if you take the wrong type of insulin?

At bedtime

Taking your pre-meal insulin instead of the bedtime insulin by mistake when going to bed is not uncommon. This may happen if your day and night pen injectors are very similar. Long-acting Levemir and Lantus insulins are clear solutions so it can be easy to mistake short-acting or rapid-acting insulin for the long-acting variety if both are drawn from vials and given with syringes.

This can be very frightening, but it is not a catastrophe! You will need to check your blood glucose regularly during the night and it would be sensible to eat some long-acting carbohydrate (bowl of cereal and milk). If possible make a partner or other family member aware of the problem.

It would be a good idea to have food available to eat extra meals during the night, preferably food that is rich in carbohydrates but contains as little fat as possible. If you need to take glucose to counter hypo-glycaemia, the effect will be much slower if you have a fat-rich meal in your stomach. Taking the wrong type of insulin will only be dangerous if you take short- or rapid-acting insulin at bedtime without noticing it. If you are used to low blood glucose levels, your body might not give any warning symptoms until the blood glucose is dangerously low (see 'Hypoglycaemia unawareness' on page 143). Remember that the effect of rapid-acting insulin usually diminishes after 4–5 hours (a little later if you have taken a dose larger than 10 units). Short-acting insulin will last a little longer. Because the shorter-acting insulin wouldn't last through the night, your morning blood sugar level is likely to be high. This isn't anything too much to worry about and will settle when you take your usual long-acting insulin the following evening.

During the day

If you happen to take a dose of intermediate-acting instead of rapid- or short-acting insulin during the day, it will not give you much of a blood glucose-lowering effect for that meal. The effect will come some hours later. It would be best, therefore, to factor in a mid-morning or afternoon snack to avoid hypoglycaemia.

Having a lie-in at weekends

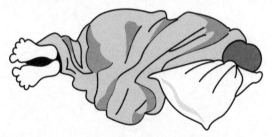

You may want to sleep in a little longer at weekends. This is rarely a problem but you will notice that your morning blood glucose is a little higher. This is unlikely to cause problems in practical terms in Type 2 diabetes.

Staying awake all night

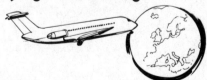

Being up all night is not common practice, but it is sometimes unavoidable for shift workers or people who are travelling. During intercontinental flights, people often have to stay awake for long periods (see 'Passing through time zones when on insulin' on page 206).

If you stay awake all night, you should take your normal dose of Lantus or Levemir. However, you should probably not take your bedtime insulin if it is isophane. Instead, you should inject pre-meal insulin when you eat every 4 or 5 hours. Adjust the dose according to how much you eat (compare the carbohydrate content of your meal with your usual lunch, dinner/tea or evening snack). You should not use the amount of insulin taken at breakfast for comparison because more insulin is commonly needed for breakfast. If you use rapid-acting insulin (NovoRapid or Humalog), and twice daily intermediate acting basal insulin (Insulatard, Humulin I, Insuman Basal), you may need to take half the night-time dose to cover your basal need of insulin during a long-distance flight. If you use long-acting insulin (Lantus or Levemir), this will probably give sufficient basal effect throughout the flight.

Shift work

It may be difficult to combine diabetes with shift work. After returning home from a night shift, you need insulin to cover both the meal you are about to eat as well as background insulin for the time you sleep during the day. Rapid-acting insulin (Apidra, NovoRapid or Humalog) is a better mealtime insulin in this situation as its effect will be wearing off as the basal insulin takes effect. With regular short-acting insulin, there will be a risk of overlapping effects, which could cause hypoglycaemia after 3–4 hours. If you switch to a work pattern with lots of shifts, consider asking your diabetes nurse for advice first.

Safe use of insulin and insulin passports

You will realize from reading this chapter that there are a number of different insulins available and in some cases the names are very similar (for example Humalog, which is a rapid-acting insulin and Humalog Mix 25, which is a mixture of rapid- and intermediate-acting insulin in a 25:75% ratio). There is potential for confusion over these names and this can lead to errors in prescribing and dispensing. If the wrong insulin is prescribed, this can have very serious consequences. There is a great deal of concern about insulin errors and, as a result of the number of errors reported to the National Patient Safety Agency (NPSA), this organization has ordered that all people taking insulin should be provided with a leaflet about the safe use of insulin, along with identification documenting which insulin(s) they are taking – known as the insulin passport. At the request of the NPSA, the insulin manufacturers have produced cards which clearly identify the name and appearance of each insulin. If you are taking insulin you should be given an insulin identification card (or some similar form of documentation) which clearly states which insulin(s) you are taking. Your pharmacist may ask to see the documentation before handing over the prescribed insulin, so that they can check that you have been given the correct insulin.

15

Administering insulin

Insulin acts by binding to the receptors on the cell surface and it reaches these receptors via the bloodstream. The only practical methods of administration are by injection under the skin or infusion into a vein. A great deal of money and energy has gone into developing alternative ways of giving insulin. Inhaled insulin (Exubera from Pfizer) became available in the UK in 2006 and a number of patients found it a useful way of avoiding injections. However, the vast majority of patients taking insulin decided to continue with injections and in 2008, Pfizer stopped production because of poor sales figures. There were also some safety concerns about inhaled insulin.

Injection technique

Fear of injections is normal and most people would put off insulin injections if they could. However, once it is obvious that insulin is important to maintain good health and other options have failed, most people accept the need to inject themselves. When we review patients a month or so after starting insulin, at least 90% accept injections philosophically and tell us that they are not really a problem. For the small percentage of people who continue to find injections a burden, there are ways of helping. It is obviously sensible to reduce the frequency of injections to as few as possible and perhaps a partner can be pulled

in to give injections. In the very few patients who continue to suffer with needle-phobia that is making their lives miserable, psychological help in the form of cognitive behavioural therapy (CBT) can be tried.

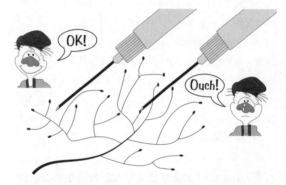

Nerve fibres look like thin branches of a tree. If you hit a nerve, you will feel more pain than if you inject between the nerve fibres.

Taking the pain out of injections

Pain is generated by the pain receptors just under the skin and the sensation is carried along fine nerves to the spinal cord and up to the brain. The nerves spread like the branches of a tree. If you hit a pain receptor directly, this will be painful. It is a matter of chance whether your needle hits a pain receptor and there is nothing much you can do about it – either continue with the injection and get it over and done with or try another site. The experience of most patients is that about one injection in ten in painful in this way. Certain areas on your abdomen and thighs will probably hurt less than others. However, the disadvantage of always using the same places for injections is that you will soon start to develop fatty lumps (lipohypertrophy; see page 138). In time, these fatty lumps can become as large as a clenched fist and they cause serious disturbance in the way insulin is absorbed from under the skin. The advantage of the fatty lumps is that injecting into them is always painless but the drawback is that insulin is absorbed very slowly and erratically from these lumps. They are a common cause of poor control of diabetes and seem to weaken the effect of insulin.

For many years, people with diabetes have been using the same needle time and again but current advice is that for each injection, you should use a new needle. Needles are finer, shorter and lubricated to make inject-ions as painless as possible.

Research findings: injection technique

- Even with an 8 mm needle, there is a considerable risk of injecting into the muscle when using a perpendicular injection technique (despite lifting a skin fold with a correct two-finger technique).
- The safest way to inject with the 5–6 mm needles is to lift a skin fold with two fingers and inject at a 90° angle.

Is it best to inject into fat or into muscle?

Insulin is designed to be injected into the fatty layer under the skin. In the past, needles up to an inch in length were used and it was common for such needles to penetrate through the fatty layer into the muscles below. Injecting into muscle is usually painful and because it has a high blood flow, insulin is absorbed much more rapidly than it is from the fatty layer. Insulin needles are now only 4 or 5 mm long and are designed to be pushed through the skin at right angles. In general they are too short to reach the muscle layer, unless there is very little fat under the skin.

Longer 8 mm needles are still available and with these, there is a possibility of injecting into muscle. It is hard to see the advantage of a longer needle and it seems sensible to use only 4 mm needles.

Recommended injection sites

Rapid-acting insulin	Abdomen (tummy)
Short-acting insulin	Abdomen (tummy)
Intermediate-acting insulin	Thighs or buttocks
Long-acting Lantus or Levemir	Abdomen, thighs or buttocks

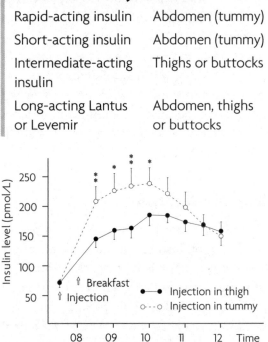

In an American study, adults took the same dose of short-acting insulin before breakfast in the tummy one day and in the thigh one day. The injection in the tummy gave both a faster onset of insulin action and a higher peak level of insulin in the blood.

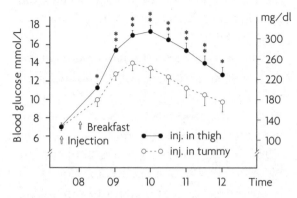

Blood glucose levels from the same study as above. Because insulin enters the blood more quickly after an injection in the tummy, this will cause the glucose content of the breakfast to enter the cells more effectively, resulting in a lower blood glucose level.

In the tummy or the thigh?

These are the sites most people use for injecting insulin and for ease of access, the abdomen is the usual choice. As a general rule the fatty layer in the abdomen has a better blood supply that the thigh and so insulin is more rapidly absorbed from an abdominal injection. When speed of insulin action is important, the abdomen is therefore the choice site for rapid-acting mealtime insulin. However, these differences in rate of absorption do not make much difference in practice and other factors can influence how rapidly insulin is absorbed from under the skin. The following activities increase blood supply to the limb and speed up insulin absorption from the thigh:

- Exercise such as running, cycling, swimming
- Sunbathing
- A hot bath or shower

In practice, people using multiple daily injections often use the abdomen for their mealtime insulin and their thigh or buttocks for the long-acting insulin taken at bedtime or first thing in the morning.

Subcutaneous injection technique
4–5 mm needle

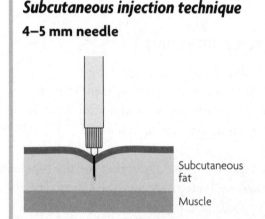

1. Eject a tiny amount of insulin (½–1 unit with a pen) in the air to ensure that the tip of the needle is filled with insulin.
2. The 4–5 mm needle should be used for perpendicular injections. If the subcutaneous layer is very thin, you may need to pinch up a fold of skin.
3. Penetrate the skin at an angle of 90°.
4. Inject the insulin.
5. Count to 10 slowly before removing the needle.

Is it necessary to disinfect the skin?

There is no need to disinfect your skin with alcohol before injecting with an insulin pen or syringe. The risk of skin infection is negligible, and alcohol disinfection often causes a stinging pain when the needle is inserted. Good hygiene and careful hand-washing are more important. If you use an insulin pump or indwelling (Insuflon®)

catheter, you should wash the skin with an antiseptic solution or use chlorhexidine in alcohol or a similar disinfectant if you have problems with skin infections. Some skin disinfectants contain skin moisturisers which may cause the adhesive to loosen more easily.

Storage of insulin

Insulin withstands room temperature well. Most manufacturers recommend that insulin in use should be discarded after 4 weeks at room temperature (not above 25–30° C, 77–86° F).

Check the package leaflet for the type of insulin you are using and the expiry date on the bottle or cartridge. At room temperature, insulin will lose less than 1% of its potency every month. According to one study, regular Lente and NPH insulin used for up to 110 days kept their insulin concentration at 100 units/ml. Even after a year or more of being stored at room temperature, as long as it is kept in darkness, the insulin will lose only 10% of its effect. Check the expiry date on the bottle or cartridge.

A practical routine is to have your spare insulin supplies stored in the refrigerator (4–8° C, 39–46° F), and the bottle or cartridge that is currently in use, stored at room temperature. Don't put your insulin too close to the freezer compartment in the fridge as it cannot withstand temperatures below 2° C (36° F). Don't expose insulin to strong light or heat, such as the sunlight in a car or the heat of a sauna. Insulin loses its effect when it is stored at temperatures above 25–30°C (77–86° F). Above 35° C (95° F) it will be inactivated four times as fast as it is at room temperature. It is easy to get hold of insulated boxes or wallets, specially designed to carry your

diabetes supplies and to prevent insulin from over-heating. The Diabetes UK website has a wide selection.

You need not store human insulin in the dark as it keeps just as well in daylight (but not bright sunlight). Human insulin carried in a shirt pocket for 6 months did not deteriorate significantly more quickly than when it was stored at room temperature. Never use insulin that has become cloudy if it is meant to be clear (applies to rapid- and short-acting, Lantus and Levemir). Inter-mediate- or long-acting insulin that contains clumps or that has a frosty coating on the inside of the vial should not be used either.

Syringes

Disposable syringes have been used since the 1960s and are still the standard injection device in many countries. They are graded in units for U-100 insulin, containing 30, 50 or 100 units. Syringes are used when mixing two types of insulin into the same injection or for types of insulin that are not available in pen cartridges. You will need to be careful when travelling, especially if you are visiting countries that use a different concentration of insulin. It is particularly important not to use U-40 insulin in a U-100 syringe or vice versa. In countries where pen injectors are less common, syringes are used for multiple injection therapy. In many countries with lower economic standards, non-disposable glass syringes with needles that require manual sharpening are still used.

Injections with syringes

Cloudy insulin (intermediate- and long-acting) needs to be mixed before use. This is done by gently turning or rolling the bottle between the hands 10–20 times. Do not shake the bottle as this will lead to problems with air bubbles in the syringe. Start the injection by drawing air into the syringe corresponding to the dose of insulin you will inject. Then inject the air into the insulin bottle, turn it upside down and then draw up the correct dose of insulin. Hold the syringe with the needle upwards, and then tap on it a couple of times to get rid of the air bubbles.

Pen injectors

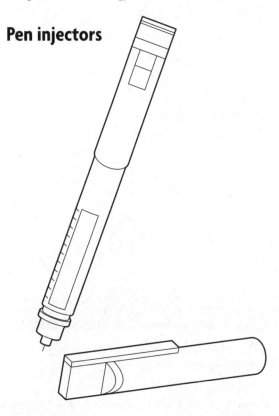

An insulin pen.

A pen injector (insulin pen) is a practical tool that is loaded with a cartridge of insulin for repeated injections. The standard cart-ridges contain 300 units (3 ml). Pen injectors will give a more accurate dosage compared with syringes, especially in the low doses. Some pens can be adjusted to half units.

Insulin pens are the standard way of giving insulin in the UK. They are slightly more expensive than a syringe and vial but are much more convenient and make insulin administration less "medical". It is much simpler when eating out to discretely give insulin using a pen compared with drawing up insulin into a syringe.

Disposable pens are also available for most insulins. They are a practical alternative for carrying spare insulin, for example when you are travelling. People who take multiple daily injections usually keep spare insulin pens at their place of work. Traditional intermediate- and long-acting insulins are cloudy and the bottle must be turned or rolled (not shaken!) at least 20 times before the insulin is injected to mix it up well. The pen cartridge contains a small glass or steel marble that will help stir the insulin when the pen is turned.

Replacing pen needles

Sterile, disposable pen needles and syringes are designed for single use only, but many patients re-use them for several injections. The risk of infected injection sites when re-using disposable needles seems to be negligible. However, the injections may hurt more since the needle becomes blunted due to tip damage after repeated use, and the silicon lubricant wears off. There is also some evidence that re-using needles with damaged tips causes repeated small injuries to the tissue when injecting. This can cause a release of certain growth factors that may lead to the development of fatty lumps (lipohyper-trophy) which may affect the amount of insulin required and its absorption.

Isophane insulin may solidify in the needle, so either change the needle every time or at least eject 2 or 3 units into the air before each injection to make sure the needle is clear.

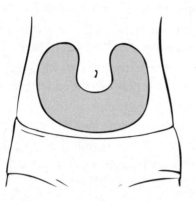

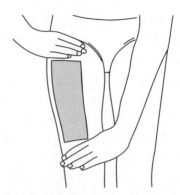

The abdomen is usually used for injections of short-acting and rapid-acting insulin (Apidra, NovoRapid or Humalog). It will be absorbed slightly faster above the tummy button compared with other areas of the abdomen. Always use the same area for a given type of insulin, e.g. the tummy for short-acting insulin, and the thigh for bedtime insulin. It is important to rotate the injection sites within each area to avoid the development of fatty lumps (lipohypertrophy, see page 138).

Put one hand above the knee and the other below your groin. The area between your hands is suitable for injections into the thigh. Remember that insulin will be absorbed more slowly from the thigh than from the tummy.

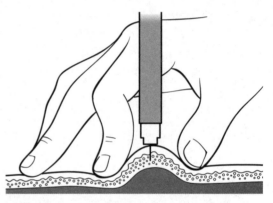

If you lift the skin with a whole-hand grip, there is less risk of a superficial injection with a 4–6 mm needle. This technique, however, should not be used with the longer 8 and 13 mm needles since the muscle will be lifted as well as resulting in a risk of intramuscular injection.

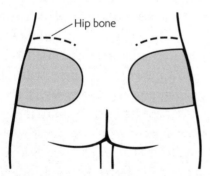

Hip bone

You can also use your buttocks for injections. Inject a few centimetres below the edge of the hip bone. The absorption of insulin is slightly slower from the buttocks than from the tummy. The illustrations are from the reference by Henriksen and colleagues.

Different pens for daytime and night-time insulin

It is easy to take the wrong pen injector by mistake if the pens for daytime and night-time insulin are similar. To avoid taking the wrong type of insulin, we recommend that you always use two completely different pens for daytime and bedtime insulin, so that you can feel the difference even if it is completely dark. If you have experienced taking the wrong type of insulin even once, having two completely different pens can be a simple preventative solution.

Air in the cartridge or syringe

When the cartridge warms up with the needle attached (e.g. when you carry it in an inner pocket), the liquid in the cartridge will expand and a few drops will leak out through the needle. When the temperature falls again, air will be sucked in. In one study, the surrounding temperature was lowered from 27° to 15° C (81° to 59°F). This caused air corresponding to 4 units of insulin to be sucked into the cartridge.

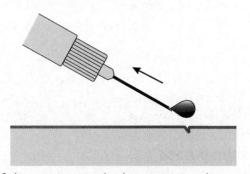

If there is air inside the pen cartridge, you may see a drop of liquid coming out from the needle tip after you have redrawn the needle from your skin.

A particular problem will occur with intermediate-acting insulin when the temperature is lowered. As the insulin is in the cloudy substance that sinks to the bottom of the cartridge, only the inactive solution will leak out through the needle. The result will be that the remaining insulin will become more potent, up to a concentration of 120 or 140 units/ml. If the pen is stored upside down, the problem will be reversed. The insulin crystals will then be closest to the needle and leak out when the temperature increases and the liquid expands. The remaining insulin will then be diluted. In one study, the insulin concentration in used vials and cartridges of NPH insulin that had not been mixed thoroughly varied between 5 and 200 units/ml.

How to get rid of the air in the insulin cartridge

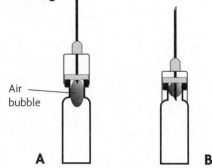

Air bubble

A   B

When you replace the needle you can get rid of the air by the following method:

Push the needle slowly through the membrane to allow the air to leak out (A). When the needle is pushed in too quickly, a small pocket of air forms within the neck of the cartridge (B).

The problem of altered concentration will not occur with clear insulins as the insulin is completely dissolved in the liquid. However, the air can still cause problems with accuracy. You can get round this problem by removing the needle after each injection since the cartridge has an air-tight rubber seal. It is possible, on occasion, to accidentally inject a bubble of air from the syringe or cartridge along with the insulin. Subcutaneous air is quite harmless to the body and will soon be absorbed by the tissue. The real problem is that you will have missed out on a certain amount of insulin (as much as was misplaced by the air). You may need to take a unit or two extra to compensate for this. The same also applies if you are using an insulin pump (see below). Air injected through the tubing is completely harmless, but you will have missed a certain amount of insulin at the same time which may cause problems.

Insulin is sensitive to heat and sunlight, so be careful not to leave it in direct sun or allow it to become overheated.

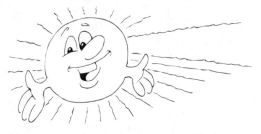

Insulin is sensitive to heat and sunlight, so don't leave it in the sun or a hot car.

Insulin on the pen needle

Sometimes a drop of insulin will leak from the tip of the needle after it has been withdrawn from the skin. The drop contains up to 1 unit of insulin and is caused by air in the cartridge which is compressed when you press the pen mechanism. You can avoid this problem by waiting about 15 seconds for the air to expand before withdrawing the pen needle. You can also remove the needle after each injection, which will prevent air from being sucked into the cartridge. This problem will not occur when you are using a syringe because you inject all the insulin it contains. Remove the air in the pen cartridge according to the illustration on the previous page. Even if all the air is removed, it is a good idea to

hold the needle in for 10 seconds to prevent insulin dripping from the tip of the needle.

Used needles and syringes

Discard used syringes, pen needles and finger-pricking lancets in a special sharps box so that no one will be pricked by mistake. Sharps boxes and their disposal should be the responsibility of the local council. If you have trouble with this service, ask your diabetes specialist nurse for advice. You can get a special cutter (B-D Safe- Clip, see below) to remove needle points.

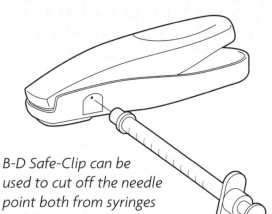

B-D Safe-Clip can be used to cut off the needle point both from syringes and from pen needles.

Insulin pumps

The rationale for using insulin pumps has been extensively studied for patients with Type 1 diabetes. There is good evidence that patients using them have better blood glucose control, and fewer hypos, and a number of studies have shown an associated improvement in quality of life. Not surprisingly, as by far the greatest proportion of patients have Type 2 diabetes, clinicians have begun looking at the value of using insulin pumps in this group. Here we'll look at the rationale and evidence for using pumps, particularly in an older patient group with Type 2 diabetes.

What is an insulin pump, and should you use one in Type 2 diabetes?

An insulin pump is a small battery-operated infusion pump which delivers insulin continuously via a small catheter device under the skin. The pump is set up to deliver a background lower rate of insulin delivery to cope with requirements outside mealtimes, and there is a facility on the pump to deliver an extra burst of insulin to cope with a meal. The amount of insulin needed at mealtimes is estimated by the pump user according to the carbohydrate content of the meal. Every snack can also be covered by a small dose of insulin, which can be given via the pump in a matter of seconds.

What do the studies say about using pumps in Type 2 diabetes?

The best study to look at is one where older patients with Type 2 diabetes (above 60 years of age, with poor glucose control or on one or more insulin injections a day), were randomized to go onto either the Minimed insulin pump or onto multiple injections of insulin when they were failing on at least one injection of insulin per day to get their glucose to a target HbA_{1c} of 53 mmol/mol. Very overweight people with a body mass index (BMI) of more than 45 were excluded from entering this study.

What the study showed was that both an intensive regime of lots of insulin injections and pump therapy achieved a significant improvement in HbA_{1c} of around 16 mmol/ mol over a year. There wasn't a great deal of difference between patient groups in how they scored quality of life, the amount of weight they put on or the number of times they suffered from low blood sugars. Several other case studies have been presented and suggest that pump therapy may be a good option for more obese people as there is less tendency to over-use

insulin and end up having to eat to avoid a hypo, which causes more weight gain. Unfortunately, a good study like this one but in the very overweight doesn't actually exist.

What's the conclusion?

In the UK, this is an academic question as NICE does not recommend insulin pumps for Type 2 diabetes and the cost is high. If you decide to use a pump, you will have to pay for it yourself. Most insulin pumps cost about £2000 and they last about 4 years. There are additional costs for the consumable attachments, e.g. infusion sets, batteries and pump reservoirs, which you may also have to pay for yourself. This amounts to about £100 a month. However, some people with Type 2 diabetes might want to make the investment to simplify their insulin delivery and give themselves the opportunity of achieving perfect diabetes control. The evidence published so far suggests that in people who can cope with multiple injections, the data for blood glucose control are just as good. There are no long-term data on blood glucose or the prevention of complications of diabetes. There is also no evidence for early introduction of the insulin pump in Type 2 diabetes as the majority of studies have been conducted with people already on at least one insulin injection per day.

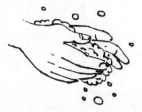

Hygiene is particularly important if you use an insulin pump. Always wash your hands before replacing the catheter. We recommend using chlorhexidine in alcohol for disinfecting the insertion site.

Also, pump users have to be motivated, interested and be prepared to have a machine attached to them day and night. They must also be careful about hygiene and hand-washing.

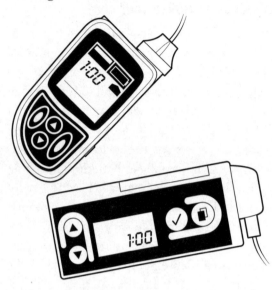

Modern insulin pumps are small and easy to manage.

Until the price of the technology reduces and the evidence base grows, pump therapy is likely to remain out of reach, certainly for most patients. In the longer term, as the technology for continuous glucose sensing improves, there may come a time when an integrated sensor for glucose can be built into the insulin pump, with an algorithm for the computer to automatically regulate the insulin delivered. This would finally bring about the prospect of greater improvements in quality of life for a significant number of patients.

New methods of insulin delivery

Inhaled insulin

The Exubera story was told at the start of this chapter. When Pfizer decided to withdraw their production of inhaled insulin, other manufacturers who were developing similar devices followed suit and gave up on this method of insulin delivery.

Nasal insulin

In 1991 a company developed a system for giving insulin in the form of a nasal spray. After an initial burst of optimism, it turned out that the absorption of insulin from the lining of the nose was too variable and it was impossible to achieve a consistent dose. The nasal spray was abandoned.

16

Changing insulin requirements

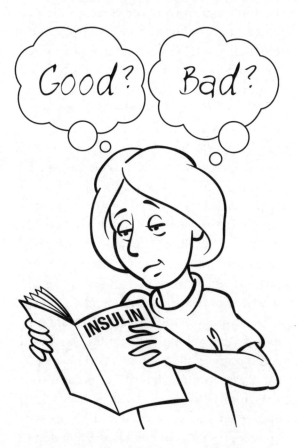

Good? Bad?

Type 2 diabetes is a progressive condition. At the time of diagnosis, most people can achieve very good control of their blood sugars by increasing their activity and making changes in the food they eat. Metformin may or may not be given at the very beginning.

As time goes by, it is normal for people with Type 2 diabetes to need more and more tablets to enable them to keep their blood glucose results within the normal range. This is because the cells in the pancreas that

produce insulin slowly degenerate. The average time from diagnosis for people to need insulin used to be 6 years but with the appearance of new therapies for controlling blood glucose, including GLP-1 agonists, this time is often much longer.

Even when insulin is first needed, the pancreas is usually able to produce a certain amount of insulin in response to food so good control can be achieved with a single injection of long-acting insulin.

Moving on to insulin

If you are taking a number of treatments for diabetes and your HbA_{1c} is creeping above the target range (usually 58 mmol/mol), the question of insulin will be raised by your doctor or nurse. At this stage you might ask for a few months' grace while you make a special effort with diet and lifestyle to improve the result. This is an ideal time to take some careful measurements of your blood glucose values. This may give you the answer to the rise in HbA_{1c}. For example, certain types of food may send your sugars sky high or you may discover that taking more exercise may lead to normal results.

You should also take regular blood glucose measurements at the standard times (before meals and before bed) and it may be possible to see a pattern in the blood glucose values, as shown in the graphs below.

These different patterns will influence the type of insulin you need to achieve good control. The easiest way of starting insulin is to give some long-acting insulin at bedtime and this is likely to be effective if you have pattern 1 with a high fasting glucose. If on the other hand your morning glucose is near normal, there is a possibility that bedtime insulin will actually lead to hypoglycaemia in the night. If you have pattern 2, you are likely to need mealtime insulin to control the sugars. This can either be in the form of short-acting insulin with each meal (the prandial regime) or you can try taking a mixture of insulins twice daily.

Combination therapy – basal insulin combined with other treatments

Insulin can be introduced as a single injection of long-acting (basal) insulin such as Insulatard, Humulin I, Lantus or Levemir, combined with any tablet regime. The basal insulin lowers the fasting blood glucose so that you start the day with a lower reading and the tablets are therefore able to work more effectively. If your blood test show a high fasting glucose (pattern 1 above) this will probably be the best choice for you.

Insulin and metformin

Metformin is used in combination with insulin to reduce your total insulin requirements and minimize any weight gain associated with insulin treatment. One study of Type 2 diabetes involved starting people on insulin alone, or starting insulin and continuing metformin treatment. Those people who continued metformin gained less weight

and required a smaller total daily dose of insulin. Unfortunately not everyone can tolerate metformin and at least one in five of those who take it experience troublesome side effects.

Insulin and other tablets

Insulin can be used in combination with any other tablets or injections used to control blood glucose. It is routine practice to continue metformin with insulin as it may reduce insulin requirements and provide some cardiac protection. If only background insulin is being taken, either as a single injection at night or in the morning or both, it is normal to continue all other tablets with the expectation that the extra insulin will lead to improved blood sugar levels. If on the other hand mealtime (prandial) insulin is taken, the need for tablets should be reviewed. Sulphonylureas (e.g. gliclazide and glimepiride), which work by stimulating insulin release with food, become redundant if mealtime insulin is taken. Pioglitazone may reduce the amount of insulin needed to achieve good control and in some cases it should be continued. DPP-4 inhibitors (e.g. sitagliptin) have only been available since 2007 and there is not much evidence for their use with insulin. Gliptins should probably be stopped when prandial insulin is started.

Insulin and GLP-1 agonists

When exenatide and liraglutide were first introduced for use in the UK, they were only licensed to be used with metformin, sulphonylureas or both. At that time, there was no research evidence to show that they worked well in combination with insulin. Once the value of GLP-1 agonists was established, people who were overweight and had poor control of their diabetes could be offered exenatide or liraglutide rather than insulin. Many patients who had been started on insulin before GLP-1 agonists became available, had put on a lot of weight after starting insulin. It seemed harsh not to give them the chance of losing some of the weight by adding a GLP-1 agonist to the insulin. In practice many doctors have prescribed this combination and have found that patients were able to lose weight and significantly reduce or even stop the insulin. In 2011, exenatide and liraglutide were licensed for use with insulin.

Treatment with insulin alone

With time, your own insulin reserves will dwindle and you will need a full insulin regime. If the pattern of your blood tests shows that you are high after meals (pattern 2 above), you will need to take an insulin which can respond rapidly to food. If your lifestyle is fairly routine from day to day with fixed meal times, you may want to start with twice daily injections of pre-mixed insulin (see below). If on the other hand you want to be flexible with mealtimes, the only practical option is to take short-acting insulin before each meal and background insulin at bed-time.

Pre-mixed insulin

The most common pre-mixed insulin consists of 30% short-acting insulin and 70% long-acting, taken twice a day. This system of giving insulin suits people who lead fairly regular lives without much variation in meal-times. If you give a pre-mixed insulin before breakfast, say at 8am, the short-acting

component will provide insulin to cover the carbohydrate that you eat during this meal. The long-acting component will come into play about 4 hours later, causing your blood glucose to dip at this time. This means that with pre-mixed insulin, lunch cannot be delayed without risking a hypo. An alternative way of keeping your blood sugar in a safe range before lunch is to have a mid-morning snack. However, that means taking in more calories which is not good if you are trying to lose weight. The second injection of pre-mixed insulin is taken before your evening meal; the short-acting component will cover the meal and the long-acting insulin will provide overnight background insulin.

Splitting the evening dose of mixed insulin

People taking twice daily mixed insulin sometimes find that the amount of short-acting insulin in the mix may not be enough to cover a high carbohydrate meal resulting in a high blood glucose before bed. If the morning blood glucose is normal, increasing the evening dose of mixed insulin leads to a risk of night hypo. The only way to deal with this problem is to "split the evening dose" into its components of short- and long-acting insulin. This means giving a dose of quick-acting insulin before the evening meal, aiming to keep your bedtime blood glucose in the normal range, This is followed by some long-acting insulin at bedtime. Taking three different insulins a day can be confusing and you need to devise a system of identifying each pen so you give a mixture before breakfast, short-acting insulin before dinner and long-acting insulin at bedtime.

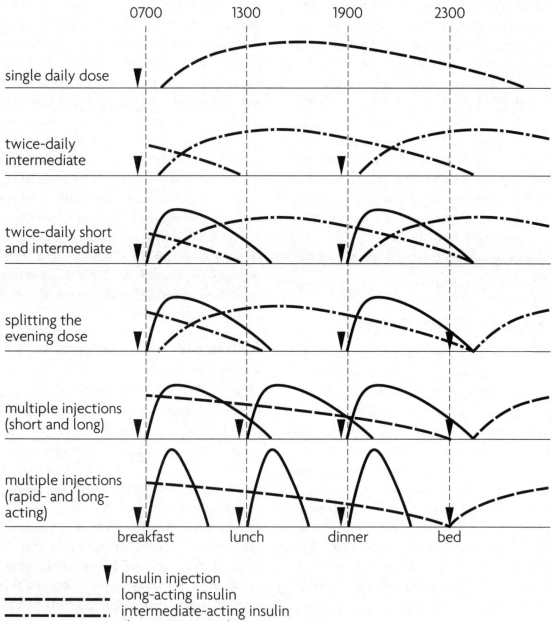

	0700	1300	1900	2300

single daily dose

twice-daily intermediate

twice-daily short and intermediate

splitting the evening dose

multiple injections (short and long)

multiple injections (rapid- and long-acting)

breakfast   lunch   dinner   bed

▼ Insulin injection
- - - - - - - long-acting insulin
- · - · - · - intermediate-acting insulin
——————— short-acting insulin

Why do blood glucose results vary from day to day?

Most people who take insulin describe their frustration at the variability of the insulin effect. Someone can do everything in their power to make two days identical in terms of physical activity, mealtimes and food eaten only to discover that their blood glucose results vary significantly on the two "identical" days. The more effort that goes into keeping everything the same, the more frustrated the person with diabetes becomes. We know some of the factors responsible for this variability but, even if every scientific precaution is taken to remove variables, there may still be a variation in blood glucose values.

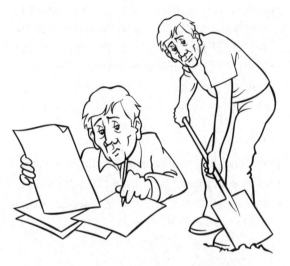

Your lifestyle can change dramatically when you retire: so can the nature and amount of activity you do.

These are some of the known variables:

- Food intake and its glycaemic index (see page 39);
- Skin temperature;
- Physical activity;
- Site and depth of insulin injection;
- Illness;
- Stress.

Food intake

It is hard to maintain an identical food intake and the rate at which food is absorbed has a major impact on blood glucose. As described in the section on glycaemic index, we have some detailed knowledge about the rate at which different foods are absorbed and thus

their effect on blood glucose. However, there are many unknown factors which affect the speed that food moves down the intestine and how rapidly it enters the bloodstream. These can affect the blood glucose levels in unpredictable ways.

Skin temperature

The rate of absorption of insulin following an injection depends mainly on the blood supply to that particular area of fatty tissue. When the skin becomes hot, for example when sunbathing, the blood supply increases to help the body lose heat from the skin. Conversely, when the skin is cold the blood vessels constrict to conserve heat. If insulin is injected close to a high flow blood vessel, it will be absorbed more rapidly than into a small, sluggish blood vessel. Anything that increases the local blood flow will speed up insulin absorption. Lying in the sun or in a hot bath leads to a higher blood flow and more rapid insulin uptake.

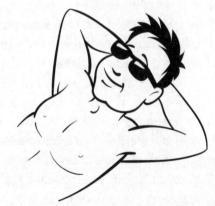

Absorption of insulin will be affected by the skin temperature. For example, when the skin becomes warm, the blood supply increases to help the body lose heat from the skin. The resulting higher blood flow will cause the insulin to be absorbed more rapidly.

Exercise

We have all had the experience of setting out on a cold winter's day and doing something energetic. Within a short time, we feel hot and sweaty and want to discard some of our warm clothes. This is due to a reflex action which increases the blood supply and sweating, which are both designed to prevent the body from over-heating. This effect will be even greater if for instance we inject insulin into our thigh and then go for a run or a bicycle ride. The muscles involved need extra blood to fuel the activity and the blood supply to the leg is further increased. This partly explains why insulin is absorbed so rapidly during exercise.

Depth of insulin injection

When insulin is injected into a resting limb, there are still differences in the blood supply depending on the depth the needle reaches. If the injection is very shallow (a matter of one or two millimetres), it is possible to inject into the outer layer of skin. This is called an intradermal injection and will result in very slow absorption of insulin. These are always rather painful and raise a bleb on the surface of the skin. With modern very short needles, an intradermal injection is a real risk, which is why people are taught to insert the needle at 90^0 to the skin. The correct level for an injection is into the fatty layer of skin. Below this is the muscle layer which has a much higher blood supply and also tends to be more painful than injection into fat. It is important to avoid injecting into muscle since the high blood supply will lead to very rapid insulin absorption.

Site of injection

Strictly speaking, you can inject into any area of fat lying under the skin. However, in practice the most common sites are thighs and abdomen, mainly because they are more accessible. In the past the arm was commonly used for insulin injections but since the fatty layer is usually very thin, it meant that many injections went into muscle and were then absorbed too rapidly. Of the two commonly used sites, insulin is absorbed more rapidly from the abdomen than from the thigh but any form of exercise may increase the blood supply to the thigh and increase the absorption rate.

Illness

Illness is likely to increase insulin resistance, resulting in higher blood sugars. This effect is seen as a result of any illness such as 'flu, a chest or urinary infection, a heart attack or a surgical operation. There is no hard and fast rule about the increase in insulin requirement from any particular disease or ailment but, as a general indication, the background insulin rate will be doubled. Because of this, people taking insulin are at risk of losing control of their diabetes during an illness and sometimes need to be rescued in hospital. It is thus important to keep a close check on your blood glucose when ill and to be prepared to give extra doses of short-acting insulin to prevent your glucose spiralling out of control (see Chapter 21, Coping with sickness).

Stress

Everyone with diabetes discovers that if their lives become stressful due to major problems at work or at home, their diabetes is more difficult to control and they usually need more insulin to maintain control of their sugars. Most attempts to prove this in a research setting are unsuccessful and there is no clear explanation for the effect of stress on diabetes.

It may be that the levels of catecholamines are raised and these oppose the action of insulin. Alternatively when daily living is disrupted by a stressful situation, this will knock diabetes off the top of your priority list and the necessary routines of testing, giving insulin in the correct dose and carbohydrate counting are pushed to one side.

Blood glucose goals

The American Diabetes Association recommends that blood glucose goals should be individualized and that lower goals may be reasonable on benefit–risk assessment. If you find your blood glucose level is low (less than 4 mmol/L) at a time when you have no symptoms of a hypo, you may have lost warning signs of hypoglycaemia. This is a serious situation and affects your ability to drive. You need to discuss this with your doctor as there are strategies available to help you regain your warning signs. If you find you are low at 2 am, this has particular significance and may mean that this is happening regularly without you being aware of this. This low blood glucose at night is thought to be a cause of high morning blood sugars as the result of a rebound effect. If you discover that this is happening to you, it is important to seek advice. You will need to alter the dose of background insulin and possibly need a change of insulin type.

Managing your insulin doses

When you are on insulin and there is need for a change in treatment due to high blood glucose levels or increased hypoglycaemia, you need to monitor more often. Before altering doses, it is best to check your blood glucose pattern across the day – before meals, two hours after food and at bedtime.

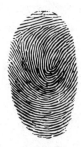

Just as all fingerprints are different, insulin doses vary, and unfortunately they often seem to work differently every day. This is perfectly logical if you think about it – we are all very different as individuals, and insulin must be adjusted to fit the individual lifestyle.

Keeping good records

Register all blood glucose readings in your notebook, otherwise you can never make an adequate judgement. If you have difficulties remembering to write them down, an electronic notebook can be a good alternative. Most blood glucose meters have memories and can be connected to a computer to be read. In an American study, patients who recorded their blood glucose readings properly had lower HbA_{1c} values (54 mmol/mol compared with 63 mmol/mol) than those who did not record their tests.

There are useful i-Phone apps for recording blood glucose levels and generally keeping a log of events relating to diabetes. These are either free or cost less than £1.

What to do if your blood glucose level is high

You should not worry if you have a single high blood glucose reading. It is important to look for patterns of blood glucose in the course of a day. Having done so, you should make a decision about changing insulin to correct the results that are outside target. If you constantly chase high and low blood glucose results with changes in your insulin dose, you may find you never know which insulin is causing the problem. You can end up chasing your tail. You also have to accept the irritating fact that sometimes, when you are trying very hard and doing everything according to the book, you will have an unexplained high or low glucose level.

Whatever your problem with glucose control, it can usually be solved by working with your doctor or diabetes nurse.

17

Side effects and problems with insulin

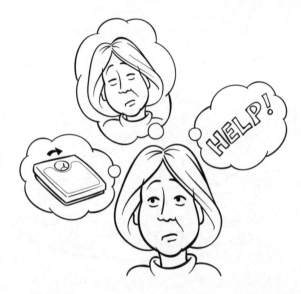

This chapter discusses some of the potential side effects and problems with insulin. The main problems for people with Type 2 diabetes are weight gain and hypoglycaemia. The chapter also discusses why people with Type 2 diabetes may need more insulin than those with Type 1 diabetes, along with problems which may affect your injection sites.

Many people are concerned about the idea of having to inject themselves, in fact it would be abnormal not to be worried about this in advance of taking insulin or a GLP-1 agonist. However the vast majority of people come to terms with this and after experiencing it, anxiety levels nearly always subside. You can find more information about administering insulin, including injection techniques and other methods and equipment that are available in Chapters 14 and 15 of this book.

Key concerns people have about insulin treatment

- How will I cope with the injections?
- Will I gain weight on insulin treatment, why does this happen, and how can I limit it if possible?
- What about hypoglycaemia and insulin treatment?
- Why do people with Type 2 diabetes need more insulin than those with Type 1 diabetes?
- How do I avoid problems with injection sites?

Insulin and weight gain

You will now be aware that Type 2 diabetes is closely associated with being overweight, particularly around the abdomen (central obesity). As described in earlier chapters, this results in insulin resistance, which in turn leads to failure of the beta cells in the pancreas. As a result, your glucose begins to rise and you find yourself with symptoms of diabetes.

After a variable number of years, insulin production from the pancreas dwindles despite increasing numbers of tablets. At this point the blood glucose will rise and you will be advised to take insulin in some shape or form. When the blood glucose is high, the excess glucose in the blood passes out of the body in the urine and this urine loaded with glucose is a major source of energy loss. In Chapter 9, we explain that the daily glucose loss may be 500 g or more, and this amounts to about 2000 calories. This explains why people with uncontrolled diabetes lose weight. Once the insulin has restored the blood glucose to more normal levels, glucose will no longer be lost in the urine so the calories will stay in your body to be stored as fat. To prevent weight increase after starting insulin, you would need to reduce your food intake to compensate for the calories previously lost in the urine. This is a big ask and most people do put on weight after starting insulin.

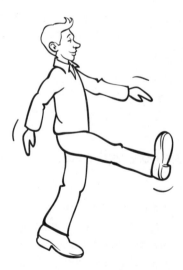

You will need to be careful about keeping your weight under control when you start on insulin. Making sure that you get enough exercise will help.

Does insulin increase appetite?

There is evidence that insulin itself increases the desire to eat and makes people feel hungry. There is also a suggestion that high insulin levels have an effect on the brain and reduce that "full up" feeling which is called satiety and which makes people stop eating. GLP-1 agonists (see page 97) on the other hand have the opposite effect on the brain and by increasing the satiety effect, encourage people to reduce their portion size.

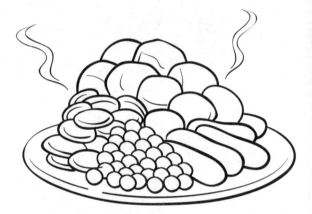

Think carefully about portion size at mealtimes.

If you are about to start insulin, it is important to be realistic about the effect it will have on your weight and your appetite. People are usually asked to start with small doses of insulin, which are increased until the blood glucose level is normal. Once the blood tests are nearing the normal range, the dose of insulin should not be increased further as it is likely that the extra insulin, which is surplus to requirements, leads to the increase in body weight and appetite.

There is some evidence that the new long-acting insulin analogues, Lantus (glargine) and Levemir (detemir) may be associated with less weight gain. Various theories have been put forward to explain this observation. Levemir, in particular, binds to human albumin, a protein found in the blood. This may mean it is less likely to get through to the brain and cause hunger. Levemir may also have a different effect on the liver compared with other insulins.

Sometimes pioglitazone is used in combination with insulin treatment. Studies have shown that the combination improves control of blood glucose and reduces the amount of insulin needed to achieve control of the blood glucose. Unfortunately, the risk of fluid retention and further weight gain must be taken into account when deciding on this combination.

In contrast, combining metformin with insulin leads to less weight gain and better control than using insulin alone. If metformin upsets your stomach, you may find the slow-release preparation suits you better.

Hypoglycaemia

People who take tablets for diabetes are only at risk of hypos if they take sulphonyureas or repaglinide, both of which work by stimulating insulin production by the pancreas. The risk of hypos from these tablets is highest when they are first being used, or in older people who may not eat properly after taking these tablets. In such cases, hypos can be prolonged and dangerous. However, none of the other tablets used to control diabetes can cause troublesome hypos. People with Type 2 diabetes treated with insulin are at risk of hypos, though the problem is usually less challenging than in Type 1 diabetes.

In one population-based study, patients with Type 2 diabetes taking insulin suffered around 16 hypoglycaemia events per year. This would translate into one event about every 23 days. Severe events which required the patient to have help from another person were much more rare, with a rate of 0.35 per year. In other words, a patient could expect one event about every 3 years.

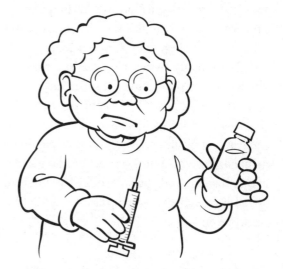

Don't put up with frequent hypos. Consult your diabetes team for advice on how to avoid hypos while keeping your blood glucose under good control.

While this may seem a relatively minor problem, if you are working as a commercial driver, it may put your livelihood at risk (see the section on driving and diabetes, page 201). If you live alone or are elderly, the prospect of having a hypoglycaemic attack becomes very scary indeed. As a consequence, some people do not to take as much insulin as they need in order to avoid hypoglycaemia. Thus, sugars begin to rise and overall control is not as good as it should be. With the right support from your diabetes team, you should be able to work through these problems and reduce the likelihood of hypoglycaemia while preserving good glucose control.

Long-acting insulin analogues, Lantus and Levemir, may cause less hypoglycaemia as well as reduced weight gain. A number of studies have shown that Lantus and Levemir have gentler peaks of action. This reduces the chance of having too much long-acting insulin, which reduces the risk of a hypo. If you take a twice-a-day mixed insulin preparation and you have troublesome hypoglycaemia without reaching your target HbA_{1c}, you should probably switch to three injections of short- or rapid-acting insulin and one injection of long-acting insulin per day. Depending on the policy in your local area the long-acting insulin may be a human insulin or an analogue type. If it is one of the older long-acting insulins and you still suffer from hypos, switching to an analogue insulin would be the next option.

Why do patients with Type 2 diabetes have to take such large amounts of insulin?

As we discussed earlier in this book, one of the primary defects associated with Type 2 diabetes is insulin resistance. Put simply, this means that you need more insulin to reduce your blood glucose to a given level than someone who is insulin sensitive.

Insulin resistance lies at the heart of the pathway to developing Type 2 diabetes. In Type 2 diabetes, there is a genetic predisposition to developing diabetes, with the additional risk of becoming insulin resistant coming from a sedentary lifestyle and over-eating. This leads to an over-accumulation of fats in the body, particularly in the liver and muscles. It also interferes with the ability of the pancreas to produce insulin.

Insulin resistance syndrome

People with Type 2 diabetes develop the insulin resistance syndrome, which is characterized by obesity, particularly an accumulation of fat around the abdomen, raised blood sugar levels, raised levels of fats or triglycerides, and raised blood pressure.

In the presence of insulin resistance, it is usually possible to control the blood glucose by giving large doses of insulin.

Reducing the insulin dose

You can do something to reduce your insulin dose. There is some evidence that drugs which increase insulin sensitivity, namely metformin and pioglitazone, can reduce your insulin requirements. Adding metformin may lead to a small reduction in the dose of insulin but will not cause further weight increase. Pioglitazone may spectacularly reduce the amount of insulin you need to control your blood sugar, but this will always be at the expense of increasing weight. Combining insulin with pioglitazone may increase the risk of fluid retention and should be avoided in the presence of heart failure.

Problems at the injection sites
Lipohypertrophy

If insulin is injected repeatedly into the same area, fat is laid down at this site (known as lipohypertrophy). This can interfere with insulin absorption, leading to unpredictability in the speed of insulin action and variable blood glucose levels. As a general rule, injecting insulin into a fatty lump causes very slow entry into the bloodstream and glucose levels usually rise.

A group of patients with lipohypertrophy

who had poor glycaemic control were followed in one study after a period of education about rotating injection sites and avoiding injecting into fatty lumps. In this study, within three months, HbA_{1c} fell from 7.9% to 7% and total insulin requirements were significantly reduced.

If you are unsure about which sites to use for injecting insulin, or about how you rotate them, ask your healthcare professional for help.

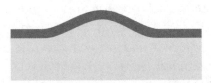

Insulin causes the subcutaneous tissue to grow if you inject frequently into the same spot. You will get a 'fatty lump' (lipohypertrophy) in the skin that feels and looks like a soft bump.

Redness at injection sites

Redness, sometimes with itching, occurring immediately or within hours of an insulin injection can be due to an allergy towards the insulin or a preservative. Tell your doctor if you have this problem. A special skin test is available to find out whether you are allergic to the insulin or the preservative. If this redness continues, the simplest solution is to change the type of insulin. Fortunately, it is extremely rare for someone to be allergic to more than one type of insulin.

It is important to make sure your insulin has not passed its use-by date and that it is stored correctly (see page 120). Inappropriate storage conditions can result in the insulin breaking down and give rise to harmful substances that can cause local allergic reactions.

Allergy to the nickel in pen and syringe needles can cause redness after injections. The needles are covered with a layer of silicone lubricant. If you are allergic to nickel you should not use the needles more than once as the silicone layer wears off and the nickel will come in closer contact with the skin. Needles on syringes have a thicker silicone layer since they need to penetrate the membrane of the bottle when drawing up insulin. For this reason, they will be more appropriate if you are allergic to nickel. You can have a skin test to see whether this is the case. If you are allergic to nickel, you will usually react to it in other items as well, for example earrings, belt buckles or wrist watches.

Stinging after insulin injections

Lantus (glargine) is a long-acting analogue insulin. The long-acting characteristic is achieved by slowing down absorption after injection. Lantus in solution has an acidic pH (4.0). When it is injected into the subcutaneous fat, which has a pH of 7.4, Lantus comes out of solution and forms crystals. This slows down the rate at which it enters the blood stream. The acidity of Lantus sometimes causes a stinging sensation after it is injected.

Bruising after insulin injections

The fatty layer that is used for injections contains a number of very fine blood vessels (arterioles) which are far too small to be visible, and it is impossible to know if your needle has entered an arteriole. If this happens, there is bound to be a small leakage of blood from the damaged blood vessel and once the needle has been removed, blood will continue to ooze out into the fat until the normal process for stopping bleeding has

Normal cell

Insulin   Glucose

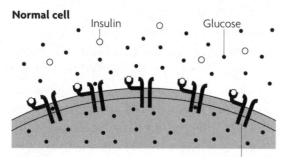

Insulin receptor

This diagram shows the surface of a normal cell, which contains around 20,000 receptor sites. The receptors attract the molecules of insulin and glucose, containing them.

Insulin-resistant cell

Insulin   Glucose

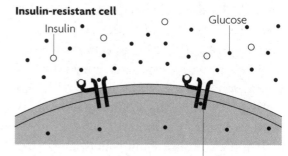

Insulin receptor

This diagram shows an insulin-resistant cell. This contains only about a quarter of the number of receptor sites to that in a normal cell. As a result, only around 25% of the glucose and insulin molecules can be contained, leading to a lot of (unstable) glucose and insulin.

come into effect. After a few hours, this will appear as a bruise under the skin. It is easy to prevent this from happening but you have to assume that each injection damages an arteriole and after removing the needle, you must quickly apply downward pressure onto the skin with a finger.

The leakage from the blood vessel is only under low pressure and enough finger pressure to indent the skin by about 1 centimetre will stop any new bleeding. Any minor bleeding which has already occurred will clot in about one minute and you should keep on pressing for this period of time.

Insulin antibodies

Your body will produce antibodies to 'defend' itself against foreign substances. Insulin antibodies were common with pork and beef insulin. With the use of human insulin, it is not common to have sufficiently high levels of antibodies to cause problems. In Type 2 diabetes, insulin antibodies do not interfere with the action of insulin.

18

Hypoglycaemia

Hypoglycaemia means 'low blood glucose'. A number of different symptoms can be experienced when the blood glucose is low, and some of these may occur with other conditions or as a response to other problems in the body. Most people, particularly those in the first few years of diabetes, get 'sensations' warning of hypoglycaemia (hypos) before their blood glucose falls to dangerously low levels.

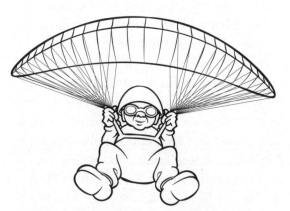

Avoid situations where hypoglycaemia could have catastrophic consequences. This does not mean that it is impossible for people with Type 2 diabetes who are taking sulphonylurea combination therapies or insulin to engage in risky sports such as mountain climbing, paragliding or scuba diving. What it does mean, however, is that they should prepare carefully, thinking about the sorts of adverse situations that could arise, tailoring their food intake and medication towards the expected activity.

In addition, hypoglycaemia is extremely rare in Type 2 diabetes unless people are treated with suphonylurea tablets or insulin. Patients may not experience a severe attack of hypoglycacmia for many, many years. With the use of modern insulin regimes and shorter-acting sulphonylureas, significant hypoglycaemia is becoming rarer still. It is very unusual for patients on metformin, gliptins, GLP-I agonists or glitazones to experience hypoglycaemic attacks unless they are taking these treatments in combination with a sulphonylurea or insulin, when the risk of a hypo is higher. For this reason, a number of problems and solutions described in this chapter may never apply to you.

Not everyone will have the same symptoms when they develop hypoglycaemia. However, the symptoms usually follow the same pattern for each person. In the early stages of drug treatment for Type 2 diabetes it is very unlikely you will suffer hypoglycaemia at all. At this stage, regular home monitoring of glucose levels is not necessary unless you are trying to find out what effect a lifestyle change or a new treatment has had on your blood glucose level. Patients with Type 2 diabetes who are most at risk of attacks of hypoglycaemia are those patients taking sulphonylureas or on insulin treatment. When you start either of these two treatments, your doctor or nurse will explain about the symptoms of hypoglycaemia and should encourage you to test your glucose at home. This will help you learn how to recognize the way your body reacts to hypoglycaemia. If you start insulin treatment, it is worth explaining to partners or other close family members what they need to do to treat hypoglycaemia in a safe and effective manner.

Usually, symptoms of hypoglycaemia are divided into two categories:

- symptoms caused by the body attempting to raise the blood glucose level, by producing adrenaline for example (known as 'autonomic' or 'adrenergic' symptoms);
- symptoms originating in the brain as a result of a deficiency of glucose in the central nervous system ('neuroglycopenic' symptoms).

See the boxes on page 144 for details of symptoms of low blood sugar.

When a person with diabetes starts to become hypoglycaemic, the first symptoms they are likely to notice are those caused by production of adrenaline from the adrenal glands (shakiness, heart pounding or sweating). However, observers may notice symptoms such as irritability, and behavioural changes, which indicate the brain is being affected. The brain's reaction to hypoglycaemia is usually triggered at a slightly lower blood glucose level than the symptoms caused by adrenaline.

The brain is very sensitive to hypoglycaemia so the body automatically reacts to try and avoid this. Adults generally experience neuroglycopenic symptoms (i.e. symptoms from the brain; see above) at blood glucose concentrations of 2.8–3.2 mmol/L, 50–58 mg/dl).

Hypoglycaemia is usually an unpleasant experience, involving loss of control over your body. This is indeed what happens as the brain does not function well without glucose.

Some people become unusually irritable, while others may look pale, sick or sleepy. Occasionally, people do something uncharacteristically dangerous or stupid that may damage themselves or someone else. Traffic accidents on a bicycle or in a car can sometimes be caused by hypoglycaemia (see page 201). Sometimes people do really strange things, so it is very important for your family and friends to understand that you are not quite in control of yourself when you are having a hypo, and you cannot help what you are doing. Even if individuals with diabetes are aware of having symptoms of hypoglycaemia, they may find it difficult to eat or drink. This can still be a problem if food is right in front of them. Observers find this difficult to understand, but patients describe the feeling as: 'You know you should drink the juice, but your body just does not obey the orders from the brain'.

If the blood glucose is lowered quickly, even if it stays within the normal range, some people will feel hypoglycaemic. This type of reaction is more common in people with a high HbA_{1c} and can occur people with Type 2 diabetes starting insulin. In one study, in a group of adults with diabetes with an HbA_{1c} of 11%, the blood glucose was lowered from 20 to 10 mmol/L (360–180 mg/dl) using intravenous insulin. These subjects showed the same type of increased blood flow to the brain that both people in good control and people without diabetes had at a blood glucose of 2.2 mmol/L (40 mg/dl).

Stages of hypoglycaemia

1. **Mild hypoglycaemia**
   Minor symptoms. Self-treatment is possible, and blood glucose levels are easily restored.

2. **Moderate hypoglycaemia**
   Your body reacts with warning symptoms of hypoglycaemia (autonomic symptoms) and you can take appropriate action. Self-treatment is possible.

3. **Hypoglycaemia unawareness**
   You experience symptoms from the brain (neuroglycopenic symptoms) without having had any bodily (autonomic) warning symptoms beforehand. However, it is obvious to people observing you that something is wrong.

4. **Severe hypoglycaemia**
   Severe symptoms of hypoglycaemia disable you temporarily, requiring the assistance of another person to give you something to eat or a glucagon injection. Severe hypoglycaemia can cause you to lose consciousness and have seizures.

Blood glucose levels and symptoms of hypoglycaemia

Symptoms of hypoglycaemia may not be recognized by a person with diabetes, particularly when the focus of their attention is elsewhere. For example, some people report that they are less likely to recognize symptoms of hypoglycaemia at work than when relaxing at home.

Your brain contains a kind of blood glucose meter that triggers defence reactions in your body and raises a low blood glucose level. It works in a similar way to a thermostat ('glucostat') and is triggered at a certain blood glucose level. This reaction depends very much on where your blood glucose level has been during the last few days. If your blood sugar has been high for some time, symptoms of hypoglycaemia and the release of counter-regulating hormones (hormones which are produced to raise a low blood sugar, such as adrenaline, glucagon, cortisol and growth hormone) will appear at a higher blood glucose level than usual. If your HbA_{1c} is high, you may start having symptoms of hypoglycaemia when your blood glucose level is 4–5 mmol/L (70–90 mg/dl) or even a little higher. On the other hand, if you regularly have a blood sugar below 4 mmol/L (70 mg/dl) your body may not produce counter-regulating hormones until the blood glucose is much lower. This can lead to loss of the adrenaline warning signs of a hypo – a condition known as hypo unawareness.

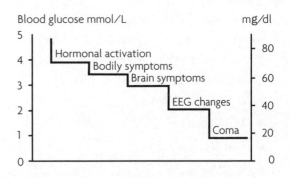

When your blood glucose is lowered, the reactions in your body and brain take place at different levels. These levels are in turn dependent on your recent blood glucose levels, i.e. if you recently have had higher blood glucose readings. The symptoms will occur at a slightly higher blood glucose level and if you recently have had lower blood glucose readings and hypoglycaemia, the symptoms will occur at a slightly lower blood glucose level. The graph is taken from work by Amiel (1998).

Symptoms of hypoglycaemia related to adrenaline production

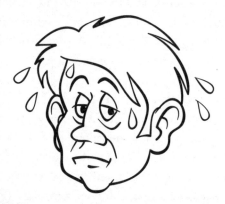

Bodily symptoms (autonomic and adrenergic symptoms) are the result of both adrenaline secretion and the autonomic nervous system. They usually start when the blood glucose concentration dips below 3.5–4 mmol/L (65–70 mg/dl). The threshold for triggering these symptoms will change depending on the person's recent blood glucose concentrations (the 'blood glucose thermostat').

- Irritability.
- Hunger, feeling sick.
- Trembling.
- Anxiety.
- Heart palpitations.
- Throbbing pulse in the chest and abdomen.
- Numbness in the lips, fingers and tongue.
- Looking pale.
- Cold sweats.

Symptoms of hypoglycaemia from the brain

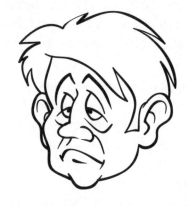

The blood glucose concentration at which your brain begins to show symptoms of impaired function (neuroglycopenic symptoms) is lower than that for adrenaline symptoms, and unlike adrenaline production, it does not vary depending on recent blood glucose levels. The last two bullet points occur in extreme cases only.

- Weakness, dizziness.
- Difficulty concentrating.
- Double or blurred vision.
- Disturbed colour vision (especially red–green colours).
- Difficulties with hearing.
- Feeling warm or hot.
- Headache.
- Drowsiness.
- Odd behaviour, poor judgement.
- Confusion.
- Poor short-term memory.
- Slurred speech.
- Unsteady walking, lack of coordination.

For some unknown reason, caffeine can increase your awareness of the symptoms of hypoglycaemia.

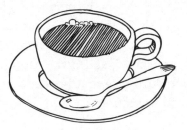

Caffeine in coffee and cola can increase your awareness of hypoglycaemic symptoms.

Research findings: effects of low blood glucose

- In one study, tests involving associative learning, attention and mental flexibility were the ones most affected at a blood glucose level of 2.2 mmol/L (40 mg/dl).

- Women were less affected than men in this study. This may be explained by women having lower levels of adrenaline and less pronounced symptoms of hypoglycaemia than men.

- Changes in EEG (brain wave) activity will occur when the blood glucose falls below 2.2 mmol/L (40 mg/dl) in adults.

- Unconsciousness occurs when the blood glucose level drops to approximately 1 mmol/L (20 mg/dl).

- Symptoms of hypoglycaemia can change over time, depending on your average blood glucose levels (see text).

Severe hypoglycaemia

Severe hypoglycaemia is defined as a hypoglycaemic reaction with documented low blood glucose (3.5 mmol/L, 62 mg/dl) or reversal of symptoms after intake of glucose, with symptoms sufficiently severe for the person to need help from another person or even admission to hospital. In some cases, the person with diabetes will lose consciousness (either fully or partially) and may have seizures. Insulin coma results from severe hypoglycaemia with loss of consciousness. Approximately 10–25% of individuals with Type 1 diabetes experience a severe hypoglycaemic episode during a period of one year but severe hypoglycaemia is very uncommon in Type 2 diabetes. Sulphonylureas may sometimes cause low blood sugar, particularly when used in combination with insulin. Other factors that will increase your risk of severe hypoglycaemia include taking the wrong dose of insulin, missing a meal, and drinking alcohol after an unusual amount of activity such as energetic dancing at a party. Even planned activity, such as digging over the vegetable patch, can cause hypoglycaemia when you are taking insulin, unless you take steps to avoid it by eating extra food or taking less insulin before and after exercise.

What caused your hypoglycaemia?

- Too little to eat or delayed meal?
- Skipped a meal?
- Physical exercise?
  - the risk of hypoglycaemia is increased for several hours after heavy physical exercise.
- Too large a dose of insulin?
- Too large an increase in your dose of sulphonylurea?

- New site for your insulin injections? e.g. from thigh to abdomen or to a site free of fatty lumps (lipohypertrophy).

- Recent hypoglycaemia?

- Glucose stores in the liver may be depleted. This can lead to more hypoglycaemia and fewer warning symptoms of hypoglycaemia (hypoglycaemia unawareness).

- Very low HbA$_{1c}$?

- Increased risk of hypoglycaemia unawareness (as low blood glucose can lead to reduced warning signs).

- Drinking alcohol?

- Small quantities of alcohol do not lead to hypos but larger amounts can impair the liver's ability to release glucose in reponse to a fall in the blood sugar.

- Variable insulin absorption (see 'How accurate is your insulin dose?' on page 112). Rates of insulin absorption can vary if you have recently moved to a new injecting area which may have more or less subcutaneous fat.

- Gastroenteritits or tummy upset?

Seizures

Seizures may occur if the blood sugar is very low and can be very alarming for those who witness them. The person having the seizure should be turned onto his or her side (the recovery position), after making sure that the airway is free. This is the safest position for someone who might be sick. Call an ambulance immediately if you can. You should not leave the person alone so delegate this task to someone else if at all possible, especially if you do not have a mobile phone with you.

If you have access to a glucagon injection, this should be given as soon as possible. However, people with Type 2 diabetes do not usually carry glucagon so you may not be in a position to help in this way. After recovery, the insulin or sulphonylurea dose should always be reviewed, and if the cause of the low blood glucose cannot be identified, the dose should be reduced.

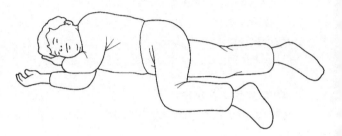

The recovery position, with the patient lying on his or her side, is the safest position for someone who is unconscious.

Hypoglycaemia unawareness

Hypoglycaemia unawareness is defined as a hypoglycaemic episode that comes on without the usual warning symptoms associated with a low blood glucose. If you have frequent hypoglycaemic episodes, the threshold at which you recognize symptoms will occur at a lower blood glucose level. If the threshold for secreting counter-regulatory hormones falls below the blood glucose level that provokes a reaction in the brain, you will not have any physical warning symptoms. Because of this, you will not react in time (by taking glucose) so your hypoglycaemia can rapidly become severe. Sometimes you will not even remember afterwards that you had hypoglycaemia.

Hypoglycaemia unawareness will increase the risk of severe hypoglycaemia and is more common among those prone to severe hypoglycaemia. It should be part of your routine to check your blood glucose as soon as you start getting symptoms that might indicate hypoglycaemia and, more importantly, to treat a low blood glucose promptly. If your readings are below 3.5 mmol/L (65 mg/dl), this is a warning sign that your risk of becoming severely hypoglycaemic may increase considerably. If you delay treatment, this increases the risk of developing hypoglycaemia unawareness, because your body gets used to the sensation of a low blood glucose and stops providing warning signs.

If you have hypoglycaemia unawareness, you should aim for a higher average blood glucose. Above all, you should avoid a blood glucose level that is lower than 5.0 mmol/L (90 mg/dl). If you can manage this for at least a fortnight, you should begin to recognize symptoms of hypoglycaemia again. By training yourself to recognize subtle symptoms as your blood glucose is decreasing, you will increase your chances of treating your hypoglycaemia in time. Many people with long-standing diabetes will have a reduced adrenaline response to low blood glucose, which reduces the warning symptoms they receive from their autonomic nervous system. Thus, these people have less effective counter-regulation when their blood glucose is falling. A number of people report a loss of their hypo warnings when changing from pork or beef insulin to human insulin. Several studies have looked at this issue, and there is no scientific proof of a relationship between human insulin and hypoglycaemia unawareness.

Driving and insulin

Driving is the most widely-practised activity that can be seriously affected by hypoglycaemia. Each year a number of people with diabetes, treated with insulin, are involved in road accidents. It is often clear that these took place while the driver's blood glucose was below normal. In some cases, the driver or an innocent third party may be seriously injured. The Driving and Vehicle Licensing Authority (DVLA) is aware of this and people using insulin have to renew their driving licence every 1–3 years and declare that they are not subject to hypos without warning. More information about the regulations related to diabetes and driving is provided in Chapter 27.

Tips for safe driving

- Have glucose, sweets or Lucozade to hand.
- Test your blood glucose before driving and every two hours on long journeys.
- If you feel you could be hypoglycaemic, pull off the road, get out of the car or move from the driver's seat. This is to demonstrate that you are not driving the car to the police.
- Take concentrated sugar to correct the hypo immediately and wait 15 minutes before testing to prove that your sugar is above 4 mmol/L.
- Consider running your blood glucose levels a little high while driving.
- Following a hypo your judgement may be impaired for up to an hour afterwards, even though you feel normal and your blood glucose levels are above 4 mmol/L.

Rebound phenomenon

Your body will try to reverse hypoglycaemia by using counter-regulatory responses (see Chapter 6, Regulation of blood glucose). Sometimes this counter-regulation will be too effective and the blood glucose will rise to high levels during the hours following hypoglycaemia. This is called the 'rebound phenomenon'. People who live alone may be unaware of nocturnal hypoglycaemia and may misinterpret a high morning glucose, believing it to be due to insufficient insulin, when it is actually a result of a rebound from a night-time hypo. When the HbA_{1c} is near to target and the morning blood glucose levels are very high, rebound phenomenon should be considered.

Too little food or too much insulin?

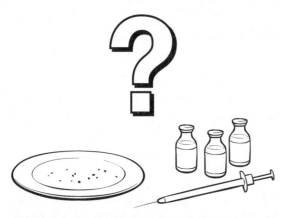

Both can result in a low blood glucose level, but the way the body handles the situation is different. The effect of glucagon in breaking down the stored glucose (glycogen) is counteracted by insulin. Insulin acts in the opposite direction, by transporting glucose into the liver cells to be stored as glycogen. From this, it follows that the more insulin you have injected (resulting in a higher insulin level in the blood), the more difficult it will be to release glucose from the liver. This means that a low blood glucose caused by a large insulin dose (e.g. if you have taken extra insulin) will be more difficult to reverse than a low blood glucose due to inadequate food intake.

Night-time hypoglycaemia

Night-time hypoglycaemia may occur if background insulin doses are increased to help achieve target blood sugar levels. Adrenaline responses are reduced during deep sleep, which may contribute to the failure to wake up. Night-time hypoglycaemia can be caused by too large a dose of bedtime insulin. Another cause can be too high a dose of short-acting insulin to correct a high bedtime blood glucose which will result in hypoglycaemia early in the night. There are several studies with Novo-Rapid and Humalog insulins which suggest that reducing the action time of the short-acting insulin (by the use of rapid-acting insulin) helps to decrease night-time hypo-glycaemia. Evidence is also accumulating that use of long-acting insulin analogues (Lantus/ glargine and Levemir/ detemir) may also be associated with a reduced incidence of night-time hypoglycaemia in Type 2 diabetes. Attacks of night-time hypoglycaemia can also be caused by vigorous afternoon or evening exercise.

Night-time hypoglycaemia may be caused by:

- The dose of short-acting insulin before the evening snack being too high (hypoglycaemia early in the night).
- The dose of bedtime insulin being too high (hypoglycaemia around 2 am or later with NPH insulin).

- Not enough to eat in the evening, or an evening snack containing mostly 'short-acting' foods being absorbed too quickly.

- Exercise in the afternoon or evening without decreasing the dose of bedtime insulin.

- Alcohol consumption in the evening.

Symptoms indicating night-time hypoglycaemia

- Nightmares.

- Sweating (damp sheets).

- Headache in the morning.

- Tiredness on waking.

- Bed-wetting (can also be caused by high blood glucose during the night).

A good basic rule for avoiding night-time hypoglycaemia is always to have something extra to eat if your blood glucose is below approximately 7 mmol/L (120–130 mg/dl) before going to bed. See also 'Bedtime insulin' on page 111. Taking extra food before going to bed reduces the risk of night hypoglycaemia but does not abolish it completely. If in doubt, it is worth doing one or two 2 am blood checks, which will answer the question. If you are taking twice-a-day mixed insulins for your Type 2 diabetes and can't reach your target without being at risk of night-time hypoglycaemia, it might be sensible to consider splitting the evening dose to take short-acting insulin with your evening meal and long-acting at bedtime. This allows you to adjust the doses to fit with the mealtime and overnight requirement. Remember, taking extra calories because of the inflexibility of a twice-a-day insulin regime and needing to snack may contribute to further weight gain.

Taking the wrong type of insulin

- Be careful not to mix up different bottles or types of insulin when using syringes.

- Make sure that the pens you use for daytime and night-time insulin are so different that you cannot accidentally use the wrong pen, even if it is completely dark.

- Often only the colour coding will differ between pens from the same company. You may want to consider using disposable pens for one type of insulin and a regular pen for the other or use pens from two different manufacturers.

Can you die from hypoglycaemia?

Major hypoglycaemia associated with Type 2 diabetes is very rare. Death as a result of hypoglycaemia has not been reported in Type 2 diabetes as even severe hypos are normally reversible. Modern insulin therapy regimes are associated with episodes of severe hypoglycaemia with an incidence of 1% or less per year. Long-acting sulphonylureas such as glibenclamide, known to cause problem low blood sugars, are now rarely used in routine clinical practice. People with Type 2 diabetes do not fall victim to the 'dead in bed' syndrome, which has been reported in Type 1 diabetes. Some potentially dangerous activities put people in danger if they are hypoglycaemic at the time. The most important of these is driving, as discussed above on page 147. See also Driving and diabetes, page 201.

19

Treating hypoglycaemia

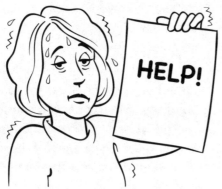

Although giving pure glucose may be the preferred treatment for hypoglycaemia, any form of carbohydrate that contains glucose will raise blood glucose levels. Ten grams of glucose will raise the blood glucose of an adult by about 2 mmol/L (35 mg/dl) after 15 minutes. The blood glucose will rise over 45–60 minutes and then start to fall. It is important not to take too much glucose 'just to be on the safe side' since the blood glucose will then rise too steeply. If you have hypos regularly and eat too much when your blood sugar is low, you will put on weight.

Which dose of insulin contributed to your hypoglycaemia?

Practical instructions

1. Test your blood glucose. The sensations of a hypoglycaemic reaction do not necessarily imply that your blood glucose is actually low. If your symptoms are so intense that it is difficult to measure the blood glucose, you should of course eat something containing glucose or sugar as soon as possible. If your blood glucose happens to be high, a little extra glucose will not make much difference.

2. If your blood glucose is low (less than 4.0 mmol/L, 70 mg/dl), have some glucose tablets or something sweet to drink. Start with a lower dose according to the table on next page and wait 10–15 minutes for the glucose to take effect. If you don't feel better after 15–20 minutes and your blood glucose has not risen, you can take a repeat dose of the same amount of glucose.

3. Glucose will lead to a more rapid rise in blood glucose than other types of carbohydrate. Avoid food and drink containing fat (e.g. chocolate, biscuits, milk or chocolate milk) if you want a rapid response. Fat causes the stomach to empty more slowly, so that the glucose reaches the bloodstream later (see page 152). If your blood glucose is only slightly low (3.5–4.5 mmol/L, 65–80 mg/dl), you may need to make a decision about eating some carbohydrate, postponing exercise or changing your insulin dose.

4. Don't take any physical exercise until all symptoms of hypoglycaemia have vanished. Wait at least 15 minutes before you do anything that demands your full attention or quick understanding, such as driving, operating a machine or taking a meeting at work.

5. If eating something containing glucose or sugar doesn't bring the blood glucose level back to normal, it may be because the stomach isn't emptying its contents into the intestine (where the glucose is absorbed). If your blood glucose doesn't increase sufficiently within 15 minutes, try drinking some carbonated lemonade to encourage the relaxation of the muscle (pyloric sphincter) that controls the exit of food from the stomach to the intestines.

6. If there is no apparent explanation for why the hypoglycaemia occurred and you are taking insulin, you should decrease the 'responsible' dose of insulin the next day. For more information, see Chapter 16, Changing insulin doses.

7. If the person is conscious but has difficulty in chewing, give glucose gel (e.g. HypoStop) or honey.

8. If the person is unconscious or has seizures, give a glucagon injection. Never give an unconscious person food or drink because it might be accidentally inhaled and cause suffocation or subsequent pneumonia.

Treatment of hypoglycaemia (as recommended by the DAFNE study)

ALWAYS TREAT HYPOS IMMEDIATELY!
When you feel the symptoms of a hypo coming on, take some quick-acting carbohydrate as soon as you can. This will stop the symptoms and prevent your needing help from anyone else. Even if you do not have symptoms, if your blood glucose level is below 4 you must treat it with quick-acting carbohydrate.

■ The best treatment is fruit juice or a sugary drink, equivalent to 20 g of carbohydrate, for example:

■ Lucozade (100–130 ml/half a teacup).

■ Fruit juice (150–200 ml/one small carton).

■ Lemonade or cola (150–200 ml; approximately one teacup full).

■ Glucose tablets can be useful too, but some people find chewing and swallowing them difficult when they are hypo.

How many glucose tablets are needed to treat hypoglycaemia?

'RULE OF THUMB'
20 g (six tablets of glucose) will raise your blood glucose approximately 4–6 mmol/L (70–110 mg/dl) i.e. your blood glucose will be approximately 4 mmol/L (70 mg) higher after 15–30 minutes than it would be without extra glucose. Usually, an increase of 2 mmol/L (35 mg/dl) will be enough, but if you have recently taken insulin and your blood glucose level is falling, you may need more glucose. Check the type of glucose tablets you use as they are likely to contain 3–4 g of glucose.

Timing and hypoglycaemia

The time interval between the bout of hypoglycaemia and your next meal will determine how you should treat the hypo.

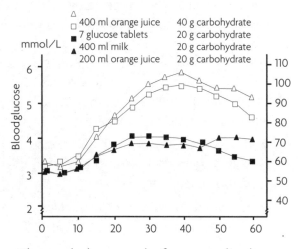

The graph shows results from a study where 13 adults with diabetes were given different types of sugar to reverse hypoglycaemia. Four hundred ml (2/3 pint) of water was given with the glucose tablets. Milk contains fat and gives a slower rise in blood glucose as fat leads to a slower emptying of the stomach.

Hypoglycaemia just before you eat

Take glucose in liquid form (Lucozade or fruit juice) since this passes through the stomach and will be absorbed more rapidly than tablets. Remember that glucose from the food must reach the intestines before it can be absorbed into the blood.

Hypoglycaemia 45–60 minutes before your next meal

The same advice applies as in the example above for a rapid reversal of your hypoglycaemia. Afterwards, you will need something to eat (a piece of fruit, for example) to keep your blood glucose level up until the next meal.

Hypoglycaemia 1–2 hours before your next meal

Take glucose and wait 10–15 minutes before you eat anything else in order to reverse your hypoglycaemia quickly. Since it will be a while until your next meal, it is important to eat something that contains more 'long-acting' carbohydrates. If hypoglycaemia develops slowly, you can skip the glucose and have a glass of milk and/or a sandwich instead. An alternative approach is to take fast-acting sugar only, and repeat if necessary. This has the advantage of helping to avoid unwanted weight gain. Try to find out what works best for you and discuss this with your diabetes team.

Helping someone with diabetes who is not feeling well

If you find yourself in the situation of helping someone else with hypoglycaemia, it is very unlikely you will know what the person's blood glucose level is, and you may lose precious time trying to measure it. The best course of action is to give something containing sugar as quickly as possible and then call for help. Make sure that people who may need to help know this simple advice.

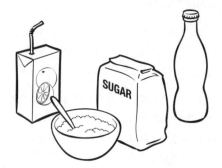

If someone you are with develops hypoglycaemia, the best thing you can do is give them something containing sugar – and fast!

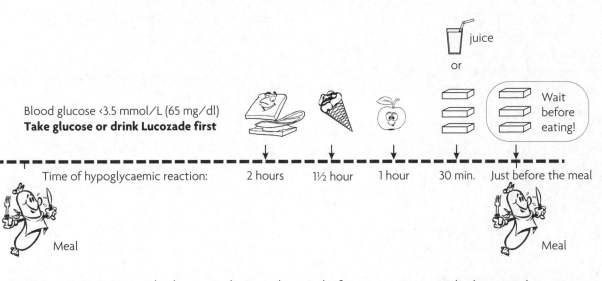

It is important to consider how much time there is before your next meal when you have hypoglycaemia. Don't eat more than you will need to get you through to your next meal. It is all too easy to have too much to eat since it takes a while before the blood glucose rises and makes you feel better. If your blood glucose is below 3.5 mmol/L (65 mg/dl) or the symptoms of hypoglycaemia are troublesome, it is best to take only glucose and then wait 10–15 minutes before eating anything else to cure the hypoglycaemia as soon as possible. If you become hypoglycaemic while sitting with a meal in front of you, it may be quite a while before you feel better again if you eat immediately. It is better to eat something with a higher sugar/glucose content (e.g. glucose tablets), wait 10–15 minutes or until you feel better, and then enjoy your meal.

Remember that the little packets of sugar available in cafes and fast food restaurants will be very effective in this situation, as will fruit juice or fizzy drinks such as lemonade or cola (as long as they are not the 'diet' variety).

If a high blood glucose is making someone feel ill, taking extra glucose will not make them feel any worse. But they DO need to take insulin.

Glucose

Pure glucose has the quickest effect when correcting hypoglycaemia. Emergency glucose is available in tablets and gel form (for example, Glucogel). It is important to think of glucose as a medicine for hypoglycaemia and not as a 'sweet'. Everyone with Type 2 diabetes who is taking insulin should always have glucose handy and must know when they need to take it. Friends must also know in which pocket the glucose tablets are kept. If you are taking acarbose, particularly in combination with other drugs, hypoglycaemia may rarely occur. If it does, acarbose blocks the metabolism of complex sugars, so you will need to take glucose tablets, not ordinary sugar, to reverse hypoglycaemia.

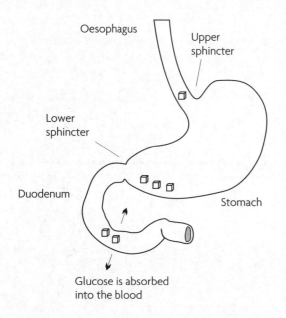

Oesophagus

Upper sphincter

Lower sphincter

Duodenum

Stomach

Glucose is absorbed into the blood

Sugar must reach the intestine to be able to be absorbed into the bloodstream so that it can raise the blood glucose level. Glucose cannot be absorbed through the lining of the mouth (oral mucosa), or from the stomach. The lower sphincter (pylorus) regulates the emptying of the stomach. Different factors influence how quickly the stomach empties, and this will have a direct effect on the speed with which glucose can be absorbed into the blood to correct hypoglycaemia.

Sports drinks contain different mixtures of sugars and give a quick increase in blood glucose. Pure fruit juice contains mostly fructose, which gives a slower increase in blood glucose. A glass of juice containing 20 g (2/3 ounce) of carbohydrate gives a slower increase in blood glucose than glucose tablets containing the same amount of carbohydrate. Ordinary sugar is sucrose (also called saccharose) which is composed of both glucose and fructose. It will therefore not give the same increase in blood glucose as an equal amount of pure glucose, but it is useful if glucose is not available.

Should you always eat when you feel hypoglycaemic?

1. Measure your blood glucose.
2. If it is 3.5 mmol/L (65 mg/dl), eat something sweet, preferably glucose.
3. If it is greater than 3.5–4 mmol/L (65–70 mg/dl), eat something if your next meal is more than ½–1 hour off or if you know that your blood glucose is decreasing, e.g. after physical exercise.

But beware!

■ This advice must be taken in context.
■ Blood glucose meters are not always accurate, especially at low levels, so a measured 4.5 may well already be below 4.
■ Blood glucose levels can fall particularly fast if you are doing something active like running or swimming.
■ You CANNOT afford a low blood glucose if you are driving, for example.

Fructose

Fructose has a sweeter taste than ordinary sugar. It is absorbed more slowly from the intestine and is not as effective as glucose in raising the blood glucose level. This is because it does not affect the blood glucose directly. It is mainly taken up by the liver cells (without the help of insulin) where it is converted into glucose or triglycerides. A high intake of fructose will increase the body fat. Fructose can also raise the blood glucose by stimulating glucose production in the liver. Honey contains 35–40% glucose and the same amount of fructose. Sorbitol, found in many sweets, is converted in the liver to fructose.

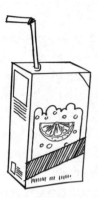

A carton of juice can come in handy if your blood glucose drops. It is easy and discreet to carry with you. If you don't feel like eating, or are in a public place, it is often easier to sip from a carton than to take glucose tablets or gel.

Sweets containing chocolate and chocolate bars raise the blood glucose very slowly and should not be used to treat hypoglycaemia. This is particularly important when blood glucose levels are below 3.5 mmol/L (65 mg/dl) as you need to raise your level rapidly.

After hypoglycaemia

You will usually feel better within 10–15 minutes after you have eaten something containing glucose. However, it will often take 1–2 hours after the blood glucose has normalized before you find yourself returning to a level of maximum performance again.

Headaches are common after recovering from hypoglycaemia, particularly if your blood glucose level was very low. If the hypo is very severe, you may also experience symptoms in the nervous system, though this is less common. These may include temporary weakness or difficulties in speaking and are caused by swelling in part of the brain following hypoglycaemia. If you find yourself experiencing any symptoms like these, you should contact your doctor.

Sometimes people feel sick or vomit after hypoglycaemia, especially if the blood glucose has been low for some time. This may be associated with raised levels of ketones in the blood and urine. Both ketones and nausea are caused by the hormone glucagon, which is secreted from the pancreas during hypoglycaemia. This is the same type of side effect that can be experienced after a glucagon injection. If the vomiting continues, you should seek medical advice.

Research findings: recovery from hypoglycaemia

- In a study of adults without diabetes, insulin was used to induce hypoglycaemia (blood glucose 2.7 mmol/L, 50 mg/dl, for 70 minutes). The reaction time was decreased for 1½ hours and only returned to normal 4 hours after the blood glucose had normalized.

- Another study of adults with Type 1 diabetes found cognitive functions (short-term memory, attention and concentration) to be normal the morning after a night with hypoglycaemia (blood glucose 2.2 mmol/L, 40 mg/dl, for 1 hour).

- A British study of adults showed their capacity for exercise was unchanged after an episode of night-time hypoglycaemia (2.6–3.0 mmol/L, 45–55 mg/dl, for 1 hour) even though participants complained of more fatigue and less wellbeing, and felt that they had experienced a bad night's sleep.

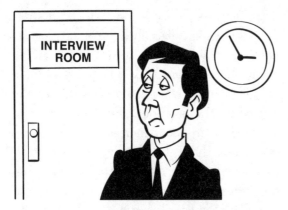

It will be difficult to be as impressive as you should be in a job interview if you have hypoglycaemia, or have had it recently. Usually it will take a couple of hours after a difficult hypoglycaemic episode before you are back on top form.

Learning to recognize the symptoms of hypoglycaemia

Every time your blood glucose measures less than 4.0 mmol/L (70 mg/dl), you should ask yourself: 'Exactly what symptoms caused me to take the blood test now? Did I experience any symptoms 10 or 20 minutes earlier that might have warned me my blood glucose was falling?' If your blood glucose is below 3.5 mmol/L (65 mg/dl) and you have not experienced any symptoms, you should always ask yourself: 'Were there really no symptoms at all warning me that my blood glucose was low?' Ask your friends if they have noticed any change in your behaviour that could have been caused by a drop in your blood glucose.

There are now programmes that train people with diabetes to recognize subtle and variable changes in their behaviour and how they feel while hypoglycaemia is developing. Such programmes include the use of simple cognitive tests, and their success has been demonstrated. To test for bodily symptoms, stand up and walk around. Move your outstretched arm in a circle or hold a pen between your fingers to test for shakiness. To test for symptoms from your brain, repeat your mother's or brother's age and birthday, your friends' phone numbers or your own mobile phone. Whatever test you set yourself should be sufficiently difficult when your blood glucose level is normal for you to notice the difference when doing the same thing while your blood glucose is low.

20

Stress

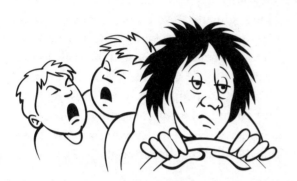

Stress and psychological strain affect your body and will, at times, increase the blood glucose levels as a result of the way different hormones respond to stress. This may vary from individual to individual.

When your body is exposed to stress, the adrenal glands secrete the hormone adrenaline (the 'fight and flight' hormone) which increases the output of glucose from the liver. To explain this, you must understand our Stone Age legacy. During this far-off period, stress was usually associated with danger, for example fighting in battle. The alternatives were to stay and fight or to run away as quickly as possible. Extra fuel in the form of increased glucose in the blood is needed for both these responses.

Today, the same stress reaction can occur in front of the TV if you are watching something exciting, but you will not benefit from the increased blood glucose level. People who do not have diabetes will automatically release insulin from their pancreas to restore the glucose balance. In theory, it is possible for someone who is taking insulin for

their diabetes to take extra insulin in this situation. In practice, this is often hard to accomplish since it is difficult to evaluate one's stress level, and stress (by its very nature) tends to vary from day to day.

In one study, adults with diabetes performed a mental stress test for 20 minutes, causing the blood glucose level to rise after an hour. It continued to be raised by about 2 mmol/L (35 mg/dl) for another 5 hours. The blood pressure was also increased, and the stress induced a resistance to insulin (see page 236) via increased levels of the hormones adrenaline, cortisol and growth hormone. Individuals who were able to produce some of their own insulin found the stress had less influence on their blood glucose level.

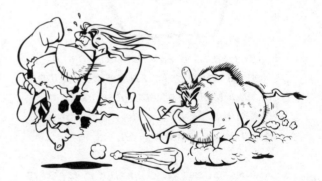

Your body is built to withstand the strenuous life of a Stone Age man or woman. In a stress situation, large amounts of adrenaline are secreted to help prepare the body for fight against, or flight away from, the danger.

Another study used a stress test composed of a 5-minute preparation task, a 5-minute speech task where subjects had to introduce themselves and apply for a job, and a 5-minute mental arithmetic task. Blood glucose levels were raised by approximately 1.0–1.4 mmol/L (18–25mg/dl) with a delay of 30 minutes after the test and lasted for approximately 2 hours. However, the effect of stress on blood glucose was only seen after a meal, and not if the test was performed in a fasting state.

After the earthquake in Kobe, Japan in 1995, HbA_{1c} levels rose in people living in the affected area. The highest increase was found in those who had experienced the death or injury of a close relative, and those whose homes had been severely damaged.

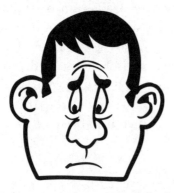

'Negative stress' is experienced when a person cannot change a stressful situation. Insurmountable problems at work, or at home within the family, may contribute to a raised blood glucose level.

Studies of heart attack victims have shown that so-called positive stress is not as dangerous as other forms of stress. Positive stress is defined as the kind of tension that is produced when you have a lot to do, but you choose to do it yourself and you are in control of the situation.

The type of negative stress that increases the risk for heart attack occurs when the person cannot influence the situation, for example if they are having problems at work or at home within the family, such as relationship break-up or divorce. Similar situations may also contribute to an increased blood glucose level. For example, blood glucose readings taken at the hospital are often higher than those taken at home. Raised blood glucose levels have been observed in people with diabetes, in both outpatient and inpatient settings. This is also the case for blood pressure measurements, so called 'white coat hypertension'.

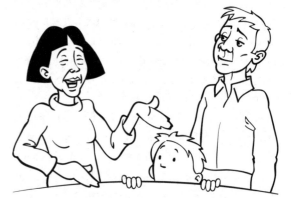

Families who talk to each other, and focus their emotional upset on practical aspects and use problem-solving strategies, are more likely to be better able to deal with stress.

Stress in daily life

Everyday stress factors can cause a higher HbA_{1c}. For example, people who are going for interviews or changing jobs often find that stress leads to a rise in blood sugar levels. Any change to routine makes it more likely that people forget to take medication at the correct time.

Stress

- Stress that cannot be influenced (such as problems in the family or at work) will have the greatest effect on your health.

- Stress can also affect your blood glucose for the simple reason that you will not have as much time to care for your diabetes when life becomes busy and stressful.

- Adrenaline (stress hormone) gives
  1. Increased blood glucose level by:
     (A) Release of glucose from the liver.
     (B) Decreased uptake of glucose into the cells.
  2. Ketones by: Breakdown of fat into fatty acids that are transformed into ketones in the liver.

Learned helplessness is a phenomenon that can occur when you feel unable to keep tight control of a situation, possibly because of unrealistic expectations. One example is when you follow every piece of advice given by the diabetes team and your blood glucose is still remains unstable. This 'teaches' you that it is not possible to control your blood glucose and, after a while, you give up and stop trying. The reason for this is the unrealistic expectation that you can achieve a stable blood glucose level simply by 'trying hard'. An example of a realistic expectation is that your blood glucose will swing between high and low values and that you will have at least one reading above 10 mmol/L (180 mg/dl) every day. It can be realistic to try to achieve a lower average blood glucose (HbA_{1c}) without laying yourself open to an increase in hypoglycaemia-related problems. Realistic expectations for the long term might include being able to manage work or a normal social life without your diabetes getting in the way.

Research findings: stress and HbA_{1c} levels

- One study found that individuals with higher HbA_{1c} levels reported poorer quality of life and more anxiety and depression.

- When the HbA_{1c} value was increased or decreased during the scope of the study, the scores for quality of life, anxiety and depression changed accordingly.

- These results suggest that you will feel better with a lower HbA_{1c}. However, another interpretation is that it is easier to obtain a good HbA_{1c} when you feel well.

- Individuals who had experienced many severe stress factors (unpleasant life events, ongoing long-term problems, conflicts with other people) within the previous 3 months had higher HbA_{1c} in one study.

- Another study showed that stress causes a higher HbA_{1c} but only in individuals who handle the stress in an ineffective way. Anger, impatience and anxiety were examples of ineffective coping mechanisms. Stoicism (not reacting emotionally in stressful situations), pragmatism (handling stress in a problem-oriented way) and denial (disregarding the stress and thereby not letting it affect you) were effective coping mechanisms.

- Denial has also been shown to have a correlation with impaired blood glucose control. This might be explained by the fact that a problem must first be recognized before being solved. Appearing to accept a chronic disease initially, but then refusing to let it affect your daily life negatively, may be an effective form of denial.

- In an analysis of 24 studies (known as a meta-analysis), depression in people with diabetes was associated with a higher HbA_{1c}. However, it is difficult to conclude whether an elevated HbA_{1c} is the result of depression or the other way around.

- Some data indicate that antidepressive medication can improve HbA_{1c} in people with depression.

For more information on psychological aspects of diabetes, see Chapter 29.

21

Coping with sickness

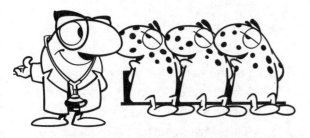

If you have an infection, especially if you are running a temperature, the secretion of blood glucose-raising hormones (particularly cortisol and glucagon) will be increased. So at a time when you are not feeling hungry and eating less, you may be surprised to find your blood sugar rising. If you are treated with diet or tablets, there is not much you can do to correct the high sugar levels. If possible, continue to take your normal tablets and test your blood four times a day if you have the means. You should drink as much fluid as you can when you are ill – up to 3 litres (6 pints) a day, and even more if you have a high temperature and are sweating profusely.

If you are taking insulin, you can deal with the problem of high sugars by taking more insulin than usual. However, it is common to eat less and rest more when you are ill, so these factors usually balance each other out. Start by taking your usual dose. Measure your blood glucose level before each meal and adjust the dose before eating. Correct the high blood sugar using the rule of thumb that 1 unit of insulin reduces the blood glucose by 3 mmol/L.

If your temperature is above 38° C (100° F) you may need to increase your insulin dose by 25% or even more. If you use twice-daily insulin, it can be difficult to meet the changing needs for insulin when you are ill. If you are worried about your blood sugar levels, contact your diabetes nurse to discuss a plan of action. If the problem arises outside working hours you should contact the Out of Hours Service, NHS Direct or, as a last resort, go to A&E.

Good glucose control during illness is important because it increases the body's defence against infections. Document your blood glucose readings (as well as insulin doses) and contact your diabetes healthcare team or the hospital if you are in the least unsure about your condition or how to handle the situation.

What to do if your blood glucose is high

1. If you feel able to eat

   ■ Decide what you want to eat.

   ■ Work out your insulin dose in relation to the size of the meal.

   ■ If your sugar is high, correct it by giving extra insulin.

   ■ Use the formula that 1 unit of insulin will reduce blood glucose by 3 mmol/L.

2. If you feel ill and don't want to eat

- Remember, you may still need insulin.
- Take your usual insulin dose to begin with (unless your blood glucose is low) and try to eat enough to supply the insulin with carbohydrates 'to work with'.
- Aim at preventing your blood glucose level from falling too low by drinking something sugary when necessary.

IMPORTANT RULE

IF YOU START VOMITING, SEEK MEDICAL HELP AND BE PREPARED FOR HOSPITAL ADMISSION. YOU MAY NEED INTRAVENOUS FLUIDS IN A DRIP.

The increased insulin requirements during illness (e.g. a cold with fever) usually last for a few days, but sometimes they can last up to a week after recovery. Sometimes the insulin requirement increases during the incubation period for a few days before the onset of the illness.

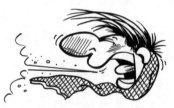

A cold with fever increases your insulin requirements, often up to 25% and sometimes even up to 50%. Begin by increasing your doses if your blood glucose levels are high. Use the rule of an extra unit of insulin for every 3 mmol/L of blood glucose above 10. Increase further if needed, depending on results from blood glucose tests.

Illness and need for insulin

- Fever increases the need for insulin.
- But – decreased appetite and food intake decrease the need for insulin.
- Thus – you will probably have at least the same need for insulin per 24 hours as usual.
- You are likely to need up to 25–50% more insulin when you are feverish.
- It is unusual for people with Type 2 diabetes to develop ketoacidosis. If you are vomiting and unable to keep fluids down, contact your doctor as you will probably need fluids into a vein (a drip).
- But – you may need less insulin if you have gastroenteritis with vomiting and diarrhoea.

Nausea and vomiting

If you feel sick while you are running a temperature, and if you eat less, it is important that the food you do eat contains sugar and carbohydrates, both to give your body nourishment and to lessen the risk of hypoglycaemia. Nausea will usually get worse if you drink large amounts of liquid at one sitting. It is better to drink small amounts frequently, for example a couple of sips every 10 minutes. Oral rehydration solution (ORS), available at the pharmacy, is very useful in this situation, particularly if you are elderly or frail.

Many people don't like the taste of ORS, which is quite salty. Try adding some juice to improve its taste. Sports drinks such as Lucozade can be helpful in this situation as they already contain both glucose and salts, thus helping to prevent dehydration and salt imbalance. A small dose of metoclopramide (Maxolon) can be helpful for preventing vomiting.

If you normally take tablets for your diabetes, it is obviously impossible for them to work if you are vomiting. You may need insulin instead, and for this reason people on tablets for diabetes may need admission to hospital if they are unable to keep fluids or tablets down.

If you are on insulin, it is very important that you keep taking it, even if you cannot eat regular meals. Have something sweet to drink so that your blood glucose level will not fall. Make sure that the drink contains real sugar rather than artificial sweeteners. You could try fruit juice, fruit smoothies or ice cream. Once you have had enough sugary drink to bring your blood glucose level up to a reasonably normal level, do take extra water if you need it, especially if you are running a temperature.

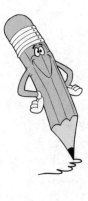

Write down all insulin doses and test results in your notebook. You will find it easier to adjust insulin doses and food intake next time you are faced with the same situation. Make a note of how many units you have taken over 24 hours. This is the best way of measuring how the illness has affected your diabetes.

Insulin treatment while you are ill (excluding gastroenteritis)

- Monitor your blood glucose before each meal and in between if it is high or low.

- Adjust insulin doses according to the results of the blood tests. Increase the pre-meal doses by 1 unit for every 3 mmol/L of glucose above 10.

- Always start out by taking your usual dose (except when you have gastroenteritis, i.e. vomiting with diarrhoea).

- Contact your diabetes healthcare team or the hospital if you start vomiting or if your general condition is worsening.

Gastroenteritis

Gastroenteritis is an infection of the intestinal tract, which usually causes both vomiting and diarrhoea. Very little nourishment will stay in the body and there are generally problems with low blood glucose levels. You may need to lower your insulin doses considerably. Gastroenteritis and food poisoning are therefore exceptions to the rule that the need for insulin will increase during illness. This reduction in need for insulin may go on for some time (possibly 1–2 weeks) after the gastroenteritis has been cured, as the low blood glucose levels cause a drop in insulin resistance (increased insulin sensitivity).

Slower emptying of the stomach contributes to a low blood glucose level when a person has gastroenteritis. You may need to lower the insulin doses by 20–50% in order to avoid hypoglycaemia. Remember to drink plenty of fluids containing sugar, but take small sips at a time as long as you are being or feeling sick. When you are ready to eat, take food with rapidly absorbed carbohydrate as this is easier to digest.

Vomiting without diarrhoea can be a sign that your diabetes is out of control. If it continues, seek medical advice.

How do different illnesses affect blood glucose?

1. **Not much influence at all**
    Illnesses that do not make you feel significantly unwell do not usually affect your insulin requirements either.

2. **Low blood glucose levels**
    These illnesses are characterized by difficulties in retaining nutrients due to nausea, vomiting and/or diarrhoea. Examples are gastroenteritis or a viral infection with abdominal pain.

3. **High blood glucose levels**
    Most illnesses that give obvious distress and fever will increase the blood glucose levels, thereby increasing the need for insulin. Examples are any illness with fever, such as a cold, otitis (inflammation of the ear), urinary infection or pneumonia.

The signs that tell you when to go to hospital

- It is unclear what the underlying problem might be.

- Repeated vomiting.

- Too unwell to check your blood glucose.

- Exhaustion on the part of you or your carer, for example due to repeated night-time waking.

- Blood glucose levels remaining high despite extra insulin.

- Severe or unusual abdominal pain.

- Confusion, or a deterioration of general wellbeing.

Always call if you are in the least bit unsure about how to manage the situation.

Wound healing

There is good evidence that wounds are slower to heal and more susceptible to infection if the blood glucose is high. For this reason, it is important to make sure that diabetes is as well controlled as possible before, during and after any surgical procedure. Foot infections and ulcers are a particular problem for people who have had diabetes for many years, and who may suffer from complications in the form of reduced circulation and loss of feeling in the feet and toes (see also Chapter 32, Problems with feet). If you have any worries at all about your feet, try to see a state registered podiatrist on a regular basis.

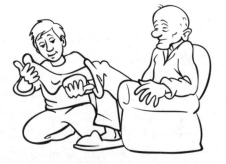

Take care of small wounds and poor friends . . . (Swedish saying)

- Wash the wound with soap and water.

- Apply a clean, dry dressing.

- Signs of infection? See a doctor!
    1. Pain/throbbing from the wound after the first 1–2 days.
    2. Increasing redness of the skin.

3. A red streak in the skin going from the wound towards the body (infection of the lymph vessels).
4. A painful nodule in the groin or armpit (infected or inflamed lymph node).
5. High temperature.

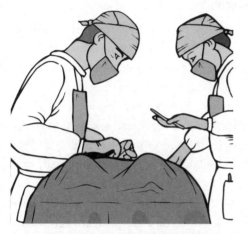

During surgery, it is advisable to administer insulin intravenously. This is a convenient and safe way to obtain a stable blood glucose level without risking hypoglycaemia.

Surgery

People with diabetes should be taken care of in hospital if they need surgery, although many minor procedures are now treated as day cases. The operation should be scheduled for as early in the day as possible. If the surgery is minor and you are only expected to miss one meal, you should be given instructions about how to manage your tablets or insulin so that intravenous insulin can be avoided. However, if the surgery is more major and you are likely to miss more than one meal, you should have intravenous insulin. This is very easy to adjust and ensures that you receive the correct dose of insulin

throughout the operation and during the recovery phase. You should let your diabetes team know if you have to go to hospital for surgery. If you are admitted to hospital in an emergency, you or whoever is with you should try to make sure all staff know about your diabetes.

Drugs that affect blood glucose

Drugs that contain sugar can sometimes affect blood glucose. However, the sugar content is usually low enough not to raise the blood glucose appreciably. If a medication is given with a meal, a small amount of extra sugar is unlikely to make a noticeable difference to the blood glucose level. If it does rise, however, you can give a small extra dose of insulin (½–1 unit/10 g of sugar).

Some drugs which do not contain sugar can still cause a rise in blood glucose. Treatment with cortisol or other steroids (e.g. prednisolone, dexamethasone) causes a marked increase in the blood glucose level, often to above 20 mmol/L (360 mg/dl). This can happen even when the steroid is given as a single dose, for example to treat asthma. When taking cortisol medication for several days or longer, the insulin doses need to be increased considerably. The total dose for a 24-hour period often needs to be doubled, increasing both the pre-meal doses and the intermediate- or long-acting insulin. Steroid inhalers affect glucose levels far less but at times, a slight increase in glucose levels may be seen as a small amount of the drug is absorbed into the bloodstream. You should try to find the lowest possible dose of steroid that is effective to control the asthma. This will make it easier for you to increase your insulin if necessary to counteract the effect of the steroids.

Teeth

It is a good idea to see your dentist regularly, and ask for advice about your dental hygiene so that you can minimize any risk of damage. Be sure to tell your dentist that you have diabetes!

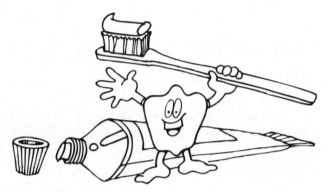

Even if you do not eat too many sweet things, you are at risk of tooth decay. This is caused by glucose in the saliva when your blood glucose level is high. Don't forget to brush your teeth at least twice a day.

Glucose is excreted into the saliva when the blood glucose level is high, and this may contribute further to cavities. The saliva would not normally contain glucose but, if the blood glucose level is above a certain threshold, increased amounts of glucose will be found in the saliva. In this sense, a person with very high or variable blood glucose level has a higher risk of tooth decay. Unfortunately, the agreement between the glucose level, in blood and saliva is not very good, so it not possible to use tests on saliva to estimate the blood glucose level.

A study on adults with diabetes found that they had the same amount of caries as those in the control group who did not have diabetes. This may be because they tended to be more careful about their diet than members of the control group. It may also be that they paid better attention to oral hygiene than the group without diabetes. Either way, it is encouraging for anyone with diabetes to know that they can be proactive in looking after their teeth.

Gingivitis

Gingivitis is an inflammation of the gums caused by bacteria accumulating in the tooth sockets. The bacterial deposits on the teeth harden into tartar. The gums go red and bleed when you brush your teeth. Gingivitis and periodontal disease are slightly more common in people who have diabetes than in people who don't, even in young people. They are also more common when the blood glucose level is high. People with diabetes may also find their gingivitis progresses more rapidly and causes more damage than it does in people who don't have diabetes. Periodontal disease is also more common in smokers.

Having a tooth out

Dental extraction is a common procedure, particularly as people get older. If the person concerned has diabetes, however, the dentist will need to take special precautions. The procedure is usually carried out on a 'walk in' outpatient basis or 'in the dentist's chair'. The dentist or oral surgeon should have a formal protocol to follow when treating a person with diabetes. However, if you are likely to need intravenous insulin, your dentist will refer you to hospital so that this can be carried out safely. If you need to have a tooth extracted, it is essential that you ensure everyone involved in treating you knows well in advance that you have diabetes.

Vaccinations

Just because you have diabetes, this does not mean you shouldn't have the same vaccinations as other other people if you are travelling, for example. See page 207 for more information about vaccinations when travelling abroad.

In addition, everyone with diabetes is entitled to receive an annual influenza vaccination from their GP or health centre free of charge. This is because people with diabetes (along with certain other groups such as people with asthma or people over the age of 65) are more likely to develop complications as a result of a bout of 'flu. Do be sure to take up your opportunity for regular 'flu vaccinations and remind your surgery if you are not called to the 'flu clinic.

22

Type 2 diabetes and younger people

Type 2 diabetes used to be called Maturity Onset diabetes and has traditionally been regarded as a condition which affects older people. In recent years, however, the age of onset of Type 2 diabetes has been falling and now it can be found in teenagers and even in children. In some American centres, half the children have Type 2 rather than Type 1 diabetes at diagnosis. However, in the UK, it is still unusual to meet young people with Type 2 diabetes in children's clinics, although the numbers are definitely increasing. You may be a teenager picking up this book, or the parent of a younger child looking for answers to your questions about Type 2 diabetes.

Why me?

If you have family members with Type 2 diabetes, being overweight may bring on the disease, particularly if you carry excess fat around the abdomen (central obesity). This stops insulin from lowering the blood sugar effectively, a condition known as 'insulin resistance', which is the underlying cause of Type 2 diabetes. With the worldwide increase in obesity in younger people as well as the more mature, Type 2 diabetes is becoming increasingly common. In the UK, young people who originate from South-Asian countries

such as India, Pakistan or Bangladesh are at particular risk of having Type 2 diabetes.

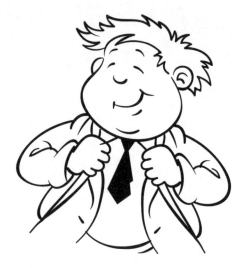

Because it is quite unusual in childhood, you may feel as if you're completely alone and that no one else in the world could possibly have Type 2 diabetes at your age. Try asking the nurses at your clinic if there are other people with the same problem who might like to meet up so you can help and support each other.

Another way to contact other young people with Type 2 diabetes is through social media – many American clinics run websites for their patients. These usually provide information as well as the opportunity for social interaction between patients.

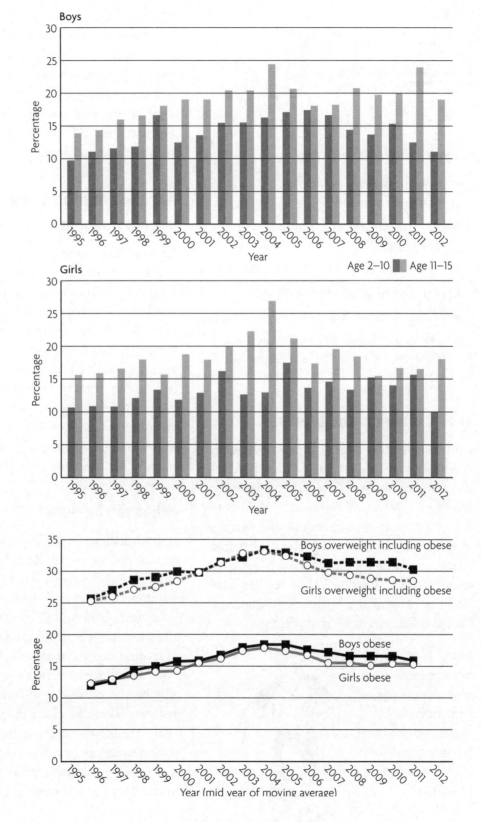

Overweight and obesity prevalence for children aged 2–15, 1995–2012, by sex.

Prevalence of obesity from 1995 to 2012.

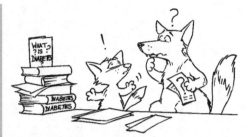

Type 2 diabetes: why me?

- Was it because I ate too much, or because I'm overweight?
- Are the symptoms different because I'm younger?
- What can I do about having diabetes?
- Will I need insulin eventually?
- What does the future hold?
- Are you always overweight when you develop Type 2 diabetes at a young age?

Type 2 diabetes and lifestyle

Unfortunately, the rates of Type 2 diabetes in younger people are increasing rapidly. Over the past few years, less sport is played in schools, and other activities like football after school are being replaced with online games or watching television. Fast food has become cheap, easily available and very high in calories, so most people eat more than they really need with the obvious consequence. (See also Chapter 9, Weight control.)

Many people enjoy playing football. It is also an activity involving lots of people so you may be able to persuade brothers and sisters to join in too.

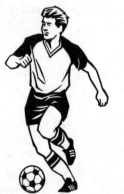

If you have put on excess weight, you will become resistant to insulin and have to produce more insulin to keep your blood sugar normal. Over the course of a few years, your pancreas will be unable to keep up with the excess requirements and your sugar levels will rise. At this stage, you will become aware of symptoms such as thirst and frequent passing of urine.

Are the symptoms any different in younger people?

Like adults, young people with Type 2 diabetes can develop symptoms slowly over a long period. These might include thirst and tiredness, frequent trips to the bathroom, blurred vision and recurring infections. Other symptoms can include yeast infections of the vagina or penis (thrush), which cause itching or burning, particularly when passing urine. On the other hand, you may have no symptoms at all; your diabetes may be picked up by chance when you visit the doctor or nurse about something completely unrelated.

What can be done?

Type 2 diabetes in teenagers is treated in the same way as in adults. The mainstay of therapy is education, where you and your parents, brothers and sisters can talk about your fears and worries, learn about what diabetes means and what you can do about it. It is important to involve the whole family. If you have all been overeating a little, you may not be the only one at risk of developing diabetes. This also allows the whole family to make the lifestyle changes by eating less and taking more exercise. You could choose to do something as a group activity, which will help you keep going and reach your goal. Your GP should refer you to a specialist dietitian who is expert at working with young people. You may find it useful to measure your blood sugar and discover for yourself the effect of exercise, and of particular foods. This will allow you to confirm for yourself that the information from the dietitian actually applies to you.

As well as changes in your diet and exercise, you may need medication to reduce your blood glucose. You will probably be asked to take metformin, which has the advantage of causing a little bit of weight loss as well as lowering the glucose levels. Metformin may cause gastric side effects, such as wind, diarrhoea and indigestion. If so, you should start with a very small dose and increase it gradually. There is also a slow-release form which you may be able to take without problems. There are other tablets you can take as an alternative to metformin; however, they are not approved for use in people under the age of 18. (For more information about tablet treatment for Type 2 diabetes, see Chapter 13.)

Is treatment with insulin inevitable in time?

Unfortunately, your blood sugar levels are likely to rise over time, even if you stick to a good diet, take exercise and take all the recommended tablets. However, if you are very overweight and can manage to lose a lot of weight, the diabetes may go away for several years. If you lose weight this will reduce insulin resistance and make the insulin you produce more effective. It is likely to return at some time in the future as the pancreas finds it more and more difficult to

keep up with insulin production. The stage at which this happens depends on whether you can keep your weight down.

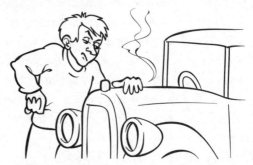

Like an old car, the pancreas will wear out in time and find it increasingly hard to do what it is designed to do. This tends to happen through no fault of the owner. However, you can make your pancreas, like your car, function better for longer if you treat it with care and respect.

What does the future hold?

Unfortunately, all the complications which occur in adult Type 2 diabetes may also occur in young people. Eye problems due to diabetes are extremely rare in young people. The American Diabetes Association plays safe and recommends screening at 10 years old and every year after that. In England, the National Screening Committee recommends that eye screening starts at the age of 12 years. Photographs of the back of the eye (retina) are taken with a special camera. (See page 222 for more information about eye problems.)

Nephropathy or kidney disease can also occur in young people, and you should make sure that your urine is tested for any leaks of protein (microalbuminuria). You should have your blood pressure measured, and some people need a tablet to control blood pressure and protect their kidneys.

Many people with Type 2 diabetes have problems with control of blood fats, and your doctor may want to start tablets to reduce them. High cholesterol, coupled with high blood pressure and insulin resistance, increases the risk of heart disease so it's important to keep this under control even if you think you're too young to run into any problems. Your treatment, though, may be different from that recommended for an older person.

One American study looked at how frequently risk factors for heart disease occurred in groups of young people aged 12–19 years. These included high cholesterol, triglycerides, blood pressure and increased waist circumference. In the general population of American children, 6.4% in this age range had two or more of these risk factors. In young people with Type 1 diabetes, the frequency was 14%, while in those with Type 2 diabetes it was greater than 90%.

Some tablets used to treat diabetes, blood pressure and blood fats should not be taken in pregnancy. If pregnancy is a possibility, it is vital that you do not take a statin (for cholesterol) or an ACE inhibitor (for blood pressure). Indeed, if there is any possibility of an unplanned pregnancy, it is safer not to take this type of medication. You should also take folic acid in the run up to pregnancy. The dose is 5 mg a day and it needs to be prescribed by your GP. The dose of folic acid bought over the counter is not enough to prevent abnormalities in the baby. Folic acid taken in the first three months of pregnancy reduces the risk of the baby developing spina bifida.

Most people with diabetes worry about passing it onto their children and there is an increased risk of this happening. However, the best way to reduce the risk of Type 2 diabetes for your children is to work as hard as you can at a healthy lifestyle for the whole family.

Type 2 diabetes in young people who are not overweight

One special form of diabetes which affects young people is called maturity onset diabetes of the young or MODY (as mentioned at the beginning of this chapter, 'maturity onset diabetes' is an earlier name for Type 2 diabetes). In the 1970s, it was noticed that, in a handful of families, half the members developed diabetes in their teens or 20s (about 50% of family members were affected). These young people developing diabetes were usually not overweight, and the pattern of diabetes suggested a certain sort of inheritance (autosomal dominant). Family members with diabetes have a specific defect in the cells that produce insulin. Research into these patients has increased our understanding of the causes of diabetes. Individuals with MODY can be accurately identified by special genetic blood tests, and the condition turns out to be more common than was originally believed.

There are several distinct types of MODY. One type (MODY 2) involves a modest increase in blood glucose levels, and often does not need any treatment at all apart from care with the diet. People with MODY 2 seldom get complications from their diabetes. Some forms of MODY can be treated successfully with drugs (sulphonylureas), while others may need insulin.

MODY is inherited so if you or your partner have MODY, each of your children has a one in two chance of being affected. You should be referred for genetic counselling and a genetic test if diabetes has occurred in several generations of your family.

Finding out more

Developing Type 2 diabetes at such a young age might seem very daunting with your whole life ahead of you. You can make giant strides in reducing your blood sugar by making simple changes to your diet and exercise regime. If you continue to lose weight, you should be able to put off treatment with insulin for several years. By controlling your sugar, blood pressure and blood fats, you can effectively reduce the risk of any complications from your diabetes. See also the Useful resources box on the next page.

> *Useful resources if you are a young person with Type 2 diabetes, or the parent of a young person with Type 2 diabetes*

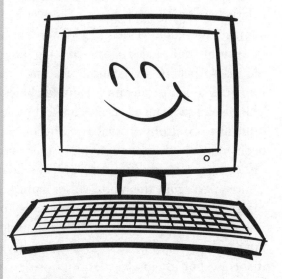

1. **MODY**
   To find out more about this unusual form of diabetes, visit this website: www.diabetesgenes.org
   You will find advice here as well as information.

2. **National Diabetes Education Program (NDEP) www.ndep.nih.gov**
   This website deals with education for patients and carers of those with Type 2 diabetes and is run by the American government. It is an excellent resource and has a number of downloadable fact sheets which you can use for reference.

3. **Royal Children's Hospital, Melbourne http://www.rch.org.au/ diabetesmanual**
   This is another useful information website from Australia.

4. **American Diabetes Association www.diabetes.org**
   The ADA website has a user-friendly Youth Zone, which contains downloadable fact sheets, advice and recipes for foods you might like to try at home.

23

Smoking

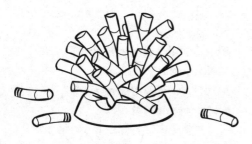

Everyone knows that smoking is bad for you, and the majority of long-term smokers want to stop because the increased risk of death from smoking is well publicised. Out of 1000 people who smoke for 20 years, around 500 will die from a smoking-related disease. The problem is that by the time most people are first diagnosed with Type 2 diabetes, the habit has become a part of their life. This chapter examines the risks presented by smoking in diabetes and what you might be able to do to 'kick the habit'. Your chances of succeeding can be affected by many different factors, some of which are explored below.

The risks

The combination of smoking in conjunction with Type 2 diabetes speeds up the rate at which complications develop, especially those caused by damage to large blood vessels. This includes heart attacks, strokes and problems with circulation to the legs. If you smoke, you can expect to die earlier than someone who doesn't smoke. So if you have

diabetes and you smoke, you reduce your chances of living a long life.

There is plenty of evidence that smoking in conjunction with diabetes is linked to increased risk of stroke, heart attack, peripheral vascular disease, kidney failure and diabetic eye disease. Smoking also leads to narrowing of the blood vessels, and damages blood vessel walls. Nicotine causes constriction of the blood vessels and the release of hormones such as catecholamines which increase blood pressure. Research shows that blood pressure in Type 2 diabetes is particularly hard to control because of accelerated damage to blood vessels. Evidence from long-term studies also shows that smoking increases insulin resistance, leading to impaired glucose tolerance or prediabetes. This insulin resistance may also make it more difficult to control your diabetes after it has been diagnosed, although this is more difficult to demonstrate in a clinical study. Quite apart from the blood vessel damage, high blood pressure and contribution to raised blood glucose, smoking affects the lungs. All smokers, whether or not they have diabetes, put themselves at high risk of chronic lung damage which will limit the capacity to exercise and lose weight. It also makes people more likely to develop cancer – not only lung cancer, but a range of other cancers, such as pancreas, bladder, mouth and larynx.

How do I stop?

Some people think that if they switch from smoking cigarettes to smoking a pipe, they will get rid of the problem. But evidence suggests that even though pipe smoking may be marginally less dangerous than cigarette smoking, this is really only for people who have never smoked cigarettes. Switching your method of smoking will not make any difference. Some people feel that there is no point in stopping smoking because they have been smoking for so long already that the damage must have been done. However, if you stop smoking, your body will gradually repair some of the damage that has been done, and your health will improve. Giving up smoking is a really positive way of increasing your chances of good health and a longer life.

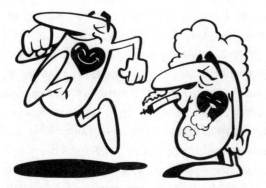

You will stay much more healthy if you give up smoking!

Willpower

It is important to face facts. The chances of giving up smoking by willpower alone are tiny. Over the course of a year, fewer than 5% of people attempting to quit without help actually manage it. They are most definitely the exception rather than the rule.

Counselling services

Your GP will be happy to help by referring you to a 'quit smoking' service. In the UK, as in most developed countries, the health service offers its own smoking cessation service. This is usually managed by a mixture of nurses and counsellors, and sessions are often conducted in a group setting to encourage people to support each other and thus increase their chances of quitting. Without the addition of nicotine replacement or other medication, counselling probably doubles the chances of giving up smoking at one year, but the chances are still probably less than 10%.

Complementary therapies

Although we can offer you little or no scientific evidence that complementary therapies such as hypnotherapy and acupuncture are effective in helping smoking cessation, we know a few people who state that these methods were highly effective for them. The idea of treating you as a whole person, rather than as someone who has diabetes or even just someone who is trying to stop smoking, is an important part of any complementary therapy. This is a view we strongly support. Hypnosis in particular may help by improving relaxation and reducing stress. It is very important though that you seek a qualified, registered practitioner. Some NHS smoking cessation services offer these therapies free of charge. Others may be able to recommend a trusted therapist.

Nicotine replacement therapy

Nicotine, the major habit-forming component of cigarette smoke, is highly addictive. It causes physiological symptoms (changes in body function) which stimulate cravings during the first few days after stopping smoking. Later on, there is a psychological addiction to overcome where you still feel a compulsion to smoke during stressful situations – at work for instance or during a social occasion like a party or going out to the pub.

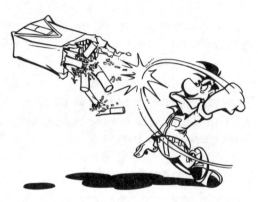

It is never too late to give up smoking. For every day without a cigarette, the damaging effects of tobacco in your body are reduced.

Replacing nicotine from cigarettes using another method of delivery helps with both immediate physiological addiction and later psychological addiction to cigarettes. A number of methods of delivering nicotine have been developed by the pharmaceutical companies. They all increase your chance of being able to give up cigarettes. Methods available from the pharmacy now include gum, patches, lozenges and a nicotine inhaler. Consult your doctor first before trying these products.

Nicotine replacement therapy works best when used in conjunction with support, usually from the NHS Stop Smoking service or similar groups. It is encouraging to see that, depending on which study you look at, people who make use of counselling at the same time as using a nicotine replacement raise their chances of giving up successfully to between 15 and 35%.

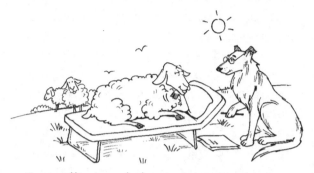

Counselling can help motivate you to give up smoking completely, especially if it used in conjunction with nicotine replacement therapy.

Buproprion

Buproprion (trade name Zyban) was originally developed as an antidepressant medication, but quite soon doctors began to notice that patients who were using it for depressive illnesses began to give up smoking.

Studies using special techniques in animals showed that buproprion affects the addiction and reward centres in the brain. For this reason it can help people to stop a number of forms of addictive behaviour, including cigarette smoking, pathological gambling and excessive eating. In total, the quit rates for studies involving buproprion are around 30–40% at the one-year stage. It appears that buproprion is the most effective add-in to counselling for helping patients to stop using cigarettes.

Buproprion is not without problems however. Like all antidepressant type drugs, it increases your chances of suffering a seizure or epileptic fit. The chance of suffering a fit if you take bupropion is around 1%. This is increased if you suffer from frequent low blood sugars or if you have a lifestyle which itself increases the chance of epileptic fits (e.g. if you drink too much alcohol).

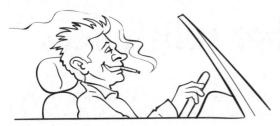

Stopping smoking is difficult but crucial if you are to do your best to avoid future problems and complications associated with your diabetes. Type 2 diabetes accelerates the passage of your life, prematurely shortening it. Smoking also presses harder on the accelerator and cuts further years off your life expectancy.

A number of drugs also interfere with the way in which bupropion is broken down by the body. This can lead to increased levels of the drug in the blood, which can increase the risk of fits. This problem has led to a number of cases of problems with bupropion being featured in the press where patients have used it and been taking drugs such as anti-malarials which interfere with the way the body can rid of it. This means that it is crucial, particularly when you have Type 2 diabetes, that if your GP is considering prescribing bupropion, he or she makes a thorough examination of the other drugs that you are taking, and looks for any which might lead to increased levels of bupropion. You can look for any drugs that may interfere – on the Internet. Your doctor will also want to hear about your lifestyle, particularly with regard to such aspects as the amount of alcohol you drink.

Passive smoking

Passive smoking can damage your prospects with respect to diabetes complications. Although the increased risks are not as great as when you are smoking yourself, they are still considerable. If your partner smokes, encourage him or her to stop.

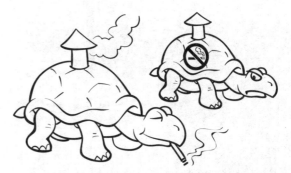

If your partner smokes, encourage them to stop.

Snuff

While snuff is no longer in general use in the UK, it is still quite popular in other countries, particularly in Northern Europe and Scandinavia. Although using snuff doesn't result in long-term respiratory damage, nicotine is absorbed in a highly effective way through the buccal mucosa, is just as addictive, and still causes hypertension and damage to the arterial wall.

24

Alcohol and other substances

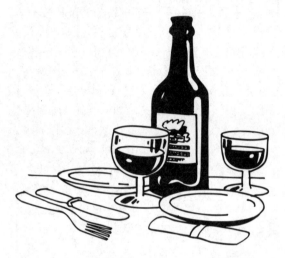

There is no reason why you should not drink alcohol if you have diabetes. However, it is important to know how alcohol works and how it might interact with your diabetes.

Alcohol and the liver

Alcohol counteracts the ability of the liver to produce glucose in response to a low blood glucose. Your liver can release glucose from its glycogen stores (see page 28). If this store is depleted or inaccessible, you will be at greater risk of hypoglycaemia. This alcohol effect on the liver may last for several hours, depending on the amount of alcohol you have consumed. The liver will metabolise 0.1 grams of alcohol/kg body weight per hour. Therefore, if you drink during the evening you may be at risk of hypoglycaemia all night as well as part of the next morning. For example, if you weigh 70 kg it will take 1

hour to break down the alcohol in a bottle of light beer, 2 hours for 40 ml of liqueur and 10 hours to break down the alcohol in a bottle of wine.

Why is it dangerous to drink too much if you have diabetes?

If you are taking insulin for your diabetes, you need to be able to think clearly in many situations so you can take corrective action, for example if you feel yourself becoming hypoglycaemic. You won't be able to do this if you have had too much to drink, in exactly the same way as you cannot drive a car safely after taking more than a small amount of alcohol.

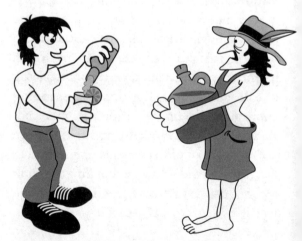

Drinking too much can impede your judgement and cause you to think less clearly.

Scientific studies show the role of alcohol in causing hypoglycaemia has more to do with losing the ability to recognize the signs of impending hypoglycaemia than with reducing the liver's ability to produce glucose. In one study, people, who took insulin for diabetes, drank either white wine (approximately 600 ml, three average-sized glasses) or water 2–3 hours after the evening snack. The morning blood glucose was 3–4 mmol/L (55–70 mg/dl) lower after drinking wine, and five of the six individuals experienced symptomatic hypoglycaemia 2–4 hours after breakfast. If you are on insulin, you need to be aware of this possibility and be prepared to check your blood glucose both at bedtime and before breakfast.

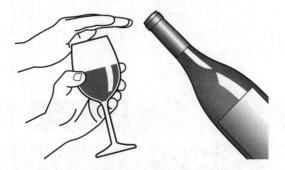

Your doctor and diabetes nurse can tell you how alcohol affects your body, and what the risks might be of drinking too much if you have diabetes. But it is down to you to decide how much alcohol you have, and when it is appropriate to refuse another drink.

Basic rules for people taking insulin

The recommended safe level of alcohol for people with Type 2 diabetes is no different from those without diabetes, which is 2 units of alcohol for women and 3 units for men in one day. If you take insulin, make sure that your friends know you have diabetes and

consider wearing some kind of diabetes ID (necklace or Medic-Alert bracelet). If you are drinking alcohol containing no carbohydrate (e.g. spirits with low-calorie mixers), you should eat something while drinking this sort of alcohol. If there is carbohydrate in your drink – beer or lager – you may find that your blood glucose rises immediately but there is a risk of hypoglycaemia later in the evening or the following morning. Research has shown that the glucose-lowering effect of alcohol may be delayed till the following morning. So, if possible, you should have a good breakfast the next morning and perhaps reduce your morning dose of insulin. Your liver breaks down alcohol slowly, which increases the risk of severe and delayed hypoglycaemia.

If you have also been especially active, playing team games or dancing at a club for example, the combined risks of extra activity with alcohol intake could put you at risk of severe hypoglycaemia.

Everyone is different and there are no hard and fast rules in Type 2 diabetes. You need to learn from experience by checking your blood glucose frequently to discover what happens in your situation.

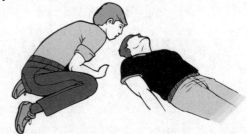

If you develop severe hypoglycaemia after drinking alcohol, the person finding you is likely to assume that you are simply drunk. It is essential that you wear a Medic-Alert necklace/bracelet. (You can also carry an ID card, but this may not be found as readily.)

Units of alcohol (Department of Health information)

Using units is a simpler way of representing a drink's alcohol content, which is usually expressed by the standard measure ABV, which stands for alcohol by volume.

ABV is a measure of the amount of pure alcohol as a percentage of the total volume of liquid in a drink.

The NHS recommends:
- Men should not regularly drink more than 3–4 units of alcohol a day.
- Women should not regularly drink more than 2–3 units a day.
- If you've had a heavy drinking session, avoid alcohol for 48 hours.

'Regularly' means drinking this amount every day or most days of the week.

You can find the ABV on the labels of cans and bottles, sometimes written as "vol" or "alcohol volume" or you can ask bar staff about particular drinks.

Drinks and units

A 750 ml bottle of wine (ABV 13.5%) contains 10 units.

See the guide below to find out how many units are in your favourite tipple.

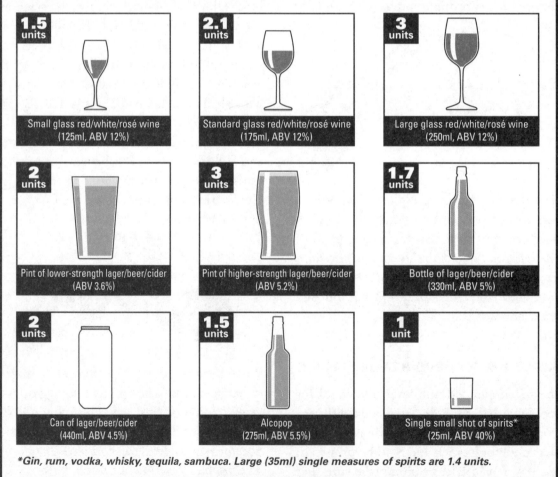

1.5 units	2.1 units	3 units
Small glass red/white/rosé wine (125ml, ABV 12%)	Standard glass red/white/rosé wine (175ml, ABV 12%)	Large glass red/white/rosé wine (250ml, ABV 12%)

2 units	3 units	1.7 units
Pint of lower-strength lager/beer/cider (ABV 3.6%)	Pint of higher-strength lager/beer/cider (ABV 5.2%)	Bottle of lager/beer/cider (330ml, ABV 5%)

2 units	1.5 units	1 unit
Can of lager/beer/cider (440ml, ABV 4.5%)	Alcopop (275ml, ABV 5.5%)	Single small shot of spirits* (25ml, ABV 40%)

Gin, rum, vodka, whisky, tequila, sambuca. Large (35ml) single measures of spirits are 1.4 units.

Source: http://www.nhs.uk/Livewell/alcohol

Tablets and alcohol

Most of the tablets prescribed for diabetes do not lead to hypoglycaemia and will not be affected significantly by drinking alcohol. However, if you are taking a sulphonylurea, this can to lead to hypoglycaemia and this risk will be increased if you drink a significant amount of alcohol. You will need to monitor your blood glucose to make sure it is not too low and you may need to eat some carbohydrate containing food before going to bed.

Dieting and weight loss

As discussed above, alcohol contains a significant number of calories and may lead to weight increase. A beer gut is a good description of central obesity resulting from overindulgence in beer. A pint of beer contains up to 200 calories and certain lagers (e.g. Fosters) contain as much as 220 calories per pint. So drinking 10 pints of beer over a weekend would add 2000 calories to your food intake. A bottle of wine contains about 500 calories. (See also Chapter 9, Weight control.)

Illegal drugs

Drugs affect the brain and nervous system, and will make it much more difficult to maintain motivation to control your diabetes carefully. Drugs make you forgetful and can lead to missed meals or medication, leading to high or low blood sugars. Wear a diabetes ID, which may help you receive the right sort of help if you become confused.

The whole problem with recreational drugs is the obvious fact that they are addictive, and having experimented with them in a casual way, some people soon become dependent to the extent that drugs begin to control their lives.

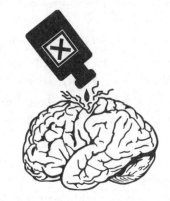

Illegal drugs act as poisons on your brain and are likely to be extremely addictive.

Certain drugs may have specific extra risks associated with the blood vessels. These include amphetamines, which are known to damage the linings of blood vessels thereby increasing the risks of diabetes complications in both the short and the longer term. Many people who are drug users would find it extremely difficult to take good care of themselves and their diabetes while continuing their drug use because of the behavioural aspects of drug use. Casual drug users would have the same problems as those of other medications that interfere with rational self-care at the time.

Benzodiazepines

These are a group of drugs that are used in a controlled way by doctors, prescribing them to people who have difficulty sleeping or suffer from anxiety. But there is a 'black market' for them too, and they are used illegally as 'recreational' drugs.

The best known drug in this group is temazepam. This can make you feel relaxed and sleepy, but if you take a larger dose it can have similar effects to a large amount of alcohol. It can make you talkative or over excited and sometimes aggressive. It also gives you a false sense of confidence and undermines your judgement. It would certainly be very difficult for you to be aware that your blood glucose level was too high or too low, and it may well cause you to forget to take your medication, including insulin.

Cannabis

Use of cannabis is often viewed as less harmful than the use of 'hard drugs' such as heroin, cocaine or amphetamines. In terms of making rational decisions about complex activities such as driving or diabetes self-management, marijuana is likely to be at least as risky as alcohol. Combining cannabis with alcohol (as often happens) adds special risks for making diabetes-related decisions about, for example, when to wake up the next day. Many people who take cannabis find themselves becoming especially hungry and want

to eat everything in sight, especially junk food (the 'munchies') which will raise the blood glucose level considerably and lead to weight gain.

Smoking cannabis has also been shown to be associated both with accelerated cardiovascular disease and increased risk of lung cancer. In addition, studies have shown increased risk of psychological disorders such as schizophrenia.

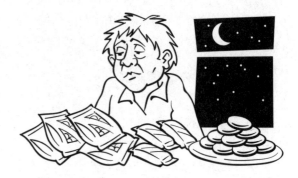

Cannabis can give you the 'munchies', making you want to eat everything you can lay your hands on.

25

Sexual problems and Type 2 diabetes

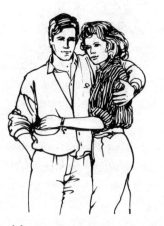

Sexual problems are very common, and are often associated with Type 2 diabetes. However, it is important to be aware that they affect many people who don't have diabetes, both men and women, especially as we get older. Both men and women frequently consult their doctor about problems with their libido and sexual performance.

This chapter examines the impact of mood and depression on sexual difficulties, some of the symptoms that men and women with Type 2 diabetes might suffer because of microvascular problems (see also Chapter 31), and a number of strategies to solve these.

Problems with your erection

Many men both with and without diabetes suffer erectile dysfunction. The severity may range from minor softening which makes penetration of your partner difficult, to problems with ejaculation or complete failure of erection. The underlying cause may not be physical but could be related to depression or problems with your relationship. It can also relate to underlying cardiovascular disease, anatomical problems with the penis itself, or a range of other disorders.

Depression

Many people with diabetes are depressed about their diagnosis, changes in their life, alterations they have to make to their routine to keep good glucose control, disagreements with their partner, problems at work and implications for the future, to name a handful of possible reasons. Whatever the cause, depression is strongly associated with erectile dysfunction. If you have issues in your life which need to be sorted out, medical treatments for erectile dysfunction are less likely to be successful. It is important to talk to your doctor and be properly assessed so that treatment can be tailored to your individual needs. Your GP will be able to direct you to an appropriate person for counselling or advice, whether it be specifically about your diabetes or about your relationship. A number of the tablet treatments for depression can make erection problems worse, so it is worth persevering with counselling advice rather than taking medication. Try to persuade your partner to come with you to counselling sessions, but if this isn't practical share your problems with your partner if at all possible.

Adequate investigation of any medical problems

Erectile dysfunction can be a symptom of disease of the blood vessels (see page 217). Achieving an erection depends on two things:

1. Adequate function of the nerves which can be damaged by microvascular disease (See Chapter 31).

2. A circulation which can provide enough blood to the penis.

A proportion of men with erectile dysfunction also have cardiovascular disease. It is important to identify this because the most widely used treatment for erectile dysfunction (Viagra) cannot be used by men who take a certain treatment for angina, namely nitrates. If you have cardiovascular disease, it is important to make sure that any risk factors are identified and treated. Your GP will be alerted to look for signs of cardiovascular disease if your blood pressure is difficult to control, if you are overweight, if your lipid (blood fat) levels are too high or if you have microalbuminuria (traces of protein in your urine; see page 225). There are a number of ways that health professionals can examine your condition in more detail. These might include a resting ECG, an exercise ECG or specialist referral to a heart doctor to do an ultrasound of your heart under conditions mimicking exercise (a stress ECHO).

You may also have other problems associated with disease of the nerves (neuropathy). These might include a drop in blood pressure when you stand up (postural hypotension).

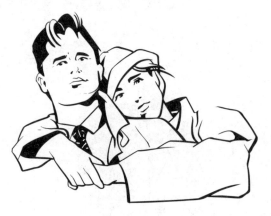

It is a good thing if your partner can come along to counselling sessions with you, as this will help you approach the problem as a shared one.

Medical treatment of erectile dysfunction

It is important to seek specialist advice – your GP will be able to make a referral for you. There are a number of nurse specialists with a particular interest in erectile dysfunction. Before you visit your GP, however, it is worth finding out about potential treatment options. Websites are a good source of information: the Sexual Dysfunction Association (www.sda. uk.net) contains question and answer sections and a range of downloadable pieces of information about diseases and treatments associated with erection problems.

A specialist nurse should be able to help you choose the most suitable approach for managing your needs, and talk to you about all options and their implications.

Tablets

Three products are available at the moment. They belong to the class of drugs known as PDE-5 inhibitors, and go by the brand names of Viagra, Cialis and Levitra. The first drug to be developed, Viagra, was originally intended to be used for treating angina, but it soon became apparent in male users that the main effect was on the arteries supplying blood to the penis, not the arteries of the heart. PDE-5 inhibitors work by dilating the smooth muscle which lines small arteries, leading to increased blood flow. Each of the three drugs has a slightly different profile in terms of how long it takes to work and how long the effects last. They are also available at varying strengths. People with diabetes often require the higher dose, so don't despair if you don't respond adequately to the starting dose. Side effects of these drugs are mainly headache and a fall in blood pressure; sometimes nausea and indigestion can also occur. The fall in blood pressure can be particularly noticeable in individuals taking nitrate tablets for angina. For these reasons, it is a good thing if your partner can come along to counselling sessions with you, as this will help you approach the problem as a shared one. PDE-5 inhibitors should be not be used by people who are taking nitrate tablets.

Local agents

There are three local treatments that you may encounter. These are described in the table overleaf.

Mechanical devices

Various pump or constriction devices can also help you to achieve an erection. They can be very effective but require a sense of humour in both partners.

A rigid prosthesis can be inserted by a surgical operation but this is a last resort.

What happens if nothing works?

Of course it is very reassuring to discover a range of possible treatments. It is possible, however, that none of them will work for you. In this case, you can still achieve physical intimacy with your partner in many other ways. A good source of information is the Sexual Dysfunction Association website – see previous page.

What about women?

Sexual problems in women are similar to those in men with diabetes. Just because there isn't a visible sign which requires intervention, this doesn't mean that troubles don't exist. The same problems which lead to depression in men with diabetes also affect women, and this can lead to reduced libido and decreased arousal during the times when lovemaking is attempted. Counselling and advice about specific problems can help.

Neuropathy in women may cause decreased lubrication on intercourse and make it more difficult to reach orgasm. Adequate lubrication with a suitable water-based personal lubricant can help with this difficulty. A range of water-based lubricants exist, from the standard KY jelly, to exotic varieties that you can have fun choosing with your partner! It isn't an admission of failure to use additional lubrication; many couples with no sexual problems at all find the extra slipperiness adds to their sense of enjoyment.

High levels of sugar in the urine may also lead to increased risk of infection, particularly with Candida ('thrush', a yeast infection) which may lead to problems with vaginal

Name	What does it involve?	Disadvantages	Side effects
Caverject (prostaglandin E)	Caverject involves an injection into the penis which encourages local changes in the blood vessels to promote an erection.	The dose needs to be adjusted, depending on individual response.	Can lead to a persistent erection (priapism) which may need hospital treatment if it persists. Other side effects include pain in the penis or a haematoma (collection of blood).
MUSE (prostaglandin E)	Muse is another preparation of prostaglandin E, administered by pushing the tablet using an applicator down the middle of the penis via the urethra.	This requires some degree of dexterity to administer.	Can be associated with persistent erection, as for Caverject.
Papaverine	In rare cases, this drug can also be used as a local injection for erection problems.	This can also be associated with persistent erection.	If the erection lasts longer than 4 hours, it is important to consult your doctor urgently.

soreness and irritation. Thrush can usually be treated by an antifungal cream or pessary, or a tablet to act upon your entire body. These treatments are available with a prescription from your doctor. For acute infection, topical treatments such as clotrimazole exist. These can be given as a cream pessary to treat infection deep in the vagina, with additional cream to treat itching and soreness of the labia. These local treatments are normally used in conjunction with oral therapy such as fluconazole, 'Canesten oral'.

The best way of eliminating Candida permanently is to maintain good blood glucose control. Apart from this a number of effective treatments exist. Regular washing with a lactic acid based feminine wash such as Lactacyd may reduce recurrent Candida.

Menstruation

Many women who take insulin find that their blood sugar levels increase in the days before their period starts. In a Hungarian study, the premenstrual doses were approximately 3 units higher than they were mid-cycle. However, during the first couple of days of menstruation, the insulin requirements may fall, increasing the risk of hypoglycaemia. If you notice that you have this type of problem, check your blood glucose level especially carefully on the days close to your period. This will enable you to adjust your insulin doses upwards just before it starts and lower them just after it finishes. If your HbA_{1c} is high, this may make your periods irregular or cause you to miss periods altogether.

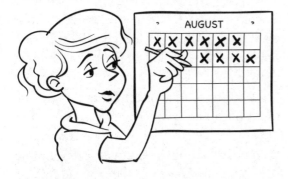

Fertility

Men with diabetes do not appear to be any less fertile than men who do not have diabetes. In addition, women with average diabetes control have much the same chances of getting pregnant as women without diabetes. However, it does appear that women with consistently high blood glucose readings may find it difficult to conceive. This may be a good thing as high blood glucose levels can harm a developing baby and lead to developmental abnormalities. It does make it particularly important, however, that you plan your pregnancy and talk to your doctor or diabetes nurse about the best way to ensure you have a consistently low HbA_{1c} before you start trying for a baby.

Contraception
The Pill

In the past, the 'minipill', containing only progesterone, was usually recommended to all women with diabetes. However, this increases

the risk of 'spotting' between periods and has a narrower time margin for taking the pills (not more than 30 hours between pills in most cases, though new versions such as Cerazette, which suppress ovulation, have a slightly longer potential 'window' between pills.

Combined contraceptives ('ordinary' pills) are more effective in preventing pregnancy, especially in younger women. Combined pills contain two types of female sex hormone. Oestrogen prevents the egg from developing and being released from the ovary. Progesterone prevents the sperm from passing through the mucus at the neck of the womb (cervix). The use of oral contraceptives does not appear to increase the risk of later complications with the eyes or kidneys.

At one time, combined contraceptive pills were thought to raise the blood glucose levels slightly, but more recent studies show no adverse effects on glucose control. If you find it difficult to adjust your glucose control in the week without pills, it might be appropriate to wait longer before having a break, for example taking 3 months-worth of pills without interruption. Today, combined pills are recommended for younger women who have no other complicating factors (such as migraine). In addition, combined pills are not recommended if you smoke (due to an increased risk of thrombosis and heart attack), or if you have high blood pressure or complications with your eyes or kidneys.

Intrauterine devices and implants
An intrauterine device (IUD, coil) is a safe contraceptive for women with diabetes according to recent studies. Problems with infections or spotting are no more common than they are in women without diabetes.

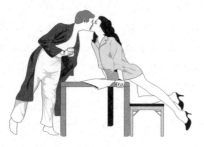

Contraceptive methods

Condom	*The only contraceptive that protects against sexually transmitted diseases.*
Diaphragm and spermicidal jelly Combined Pill	*Not easy to use. Risk of itching as side effect. Sometimes result in a slight increase in blood glucose levels.*
Minipill	*Risk of spotting. Smaller margin for error if a tablet is missed. Carries a higher risk of pregnancy than the combined Pill.*
Intrauterine device (IUD, coil)	*Risk of pelvic infection is low, but an IUD is not recommended for use before the first pregnancy.*
Depot injection	*Can affect metabolic control. Sometimes troublesome side effects.*
Implant	*Same as depot injection but easy to remove if side effects are not acceptable.*
'Morning-after' pills	*For 'emergency' situations. Needs to be taken within 72 hours of unprotected intercourse.*

However, they are not recommended for women who have heavy or irregular menstrual periods. As there is a small risk of infection of the womb or ovary (and thus a risk of becoming infertile), intrauterine devices are not recommended for women who have never been pregnant. However, for a woman who has diabetes complications affecting the eyes or kidneys, intrauterine devices may be a good alternative to contraceptive pills.

Depot injections or implants contain the same hormone (progesterone) as minipills. They will give a higher hormone concentration and affect the blood glucose level more than minipills, however. Common side effects include nausea, increased appetite and irritability, all of which make it more difficult to control the blood glucose levels. The contraceptive depot injection is not considered suitable for women with diabetes as the effects of one injection last for many months. A contraceptive implant contains the same hormone as a depot injection. It is implanted under the skin using local anaesthesia. The advantage is that it can be removed if the woman experiences side effects. This makes it more suitable than the depot injection for women who have diabetes.

Staying healthy

Remember that most contraceptive methods only prevent unwanted pregnancy. It is as important to protect yourself against sexually transmitted diseases. Some of these diseases can be life threatening; others can have a serious effect on a woman's fertility. A condom is the only contraceptive that offers full protection from sexually transmitted diseases.

Talk to your GP, family planning nurse or pregnancy advice service about which type of contraceptive would be best for you. Women using oral contraceptive pills should have regular blood pressure monitoring and gynaecological check-ups.

26

Pregnancy and diabetes

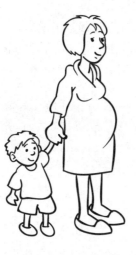

Pregnancy used to be unusual in women with Type 2 diabetes, but many younger people are now developing the condition. The Confidential Enquiry into Maternal and Child Health (CEMACH) published in 2007 found that Type 2 dibetes accounted for around 30% of pregnancies in the UK. One of the first questions a younger woman who is diagnosed with Type 2 diabetes is likely to ask, is whether she will still be able to have babies. Being pregnant exerts a certain strain on every woman, but there is no reason to discourage women with diabetes from having children. The mother's risk of developing diabetes complications in later life is not affected by pregnancy.

Preparing for pregnancy

If you are hoping to start a family, it is really important that you talk it through with your doctor first so that you can learn about and discuss the issues involved. Really good management of blood pressure and blood glucose is crucial to ensure that the strain that having a baby places on your body systems doesn't worsen the complications associated with your diabetes. In addition, the insulin resistance associated with Type 2 diabetes can both make it difficult to get pregnant and increase the chances of suffering a miscarriage.

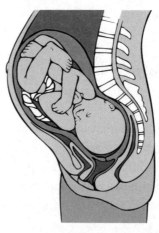

If you make up your mind to sort out your general health and nutrition, as well as your diabetes control, before you get pregnant, you will give your developing baby a better start in life.

All women trying for a baby, no matter what their state of health, need to be careful about their diet in the weeks before conception. Folic acid is an essential vitamin supplement, and you should take a daily supplement of 5 mg. This has been shown to reduce the risk of nervous system abnormalities such as spina bifida. Try to eat balanced meals containing a good range of nutrients (see Chapter 8 for more information about a good diet).

Pre-existing complications such as kidney failure and eye problems can worsen during pregnancy and can increase the risk of pre-eclampsia and premature delivery. If you have any complications of diabetes, you should see a diabetes specialist to discuss how these might affect you and your pregnancy, so you must discuss any significant health problems with your doctor before deciding to become pregnant. If you are taken by surprise by an unplanned pregnancy, you should see your doctor as soon as possible.

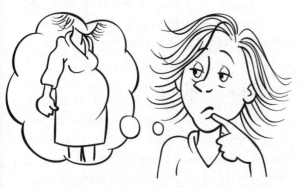

If you have diabetes, it is particularly important that your pregnancy be planned. You must discuss contraception with your doctor.

Glucose Control

A number of drugs used in the treatment of Type 2 diabetes are not recommended for use in pregnancy and may have to be stopped before conception takes place. Glibenclamide, a sulphonylurea, can be used to manage Type 2 diabetes in pregnancy, but is not usually recommended. Insulin treatment is the best way of controlling blood glucose levels, and your diabetes team will encourage you to start insulin treatment. Metformin may be helpful in some circumstances, particularly if you have insulin resistance and polycystic ovary syndrome (PCOS; see page 58). Glitazones, gliptins and GLP-1 agonists should not be used in pregnancy. However, metformin and glitazones may increase your chances of getting pregnant so, if you are taking either of these, you should use reliable contraception. If you become pregnant while taking a glitazone, you should stop taking it immediately and consult your doctor as soon as possible.

Throughout pregnancy it is crucial that glucose control is perfect. You should use insulin injections to respond to your food intake as closely as possible. Poor blood sugar control in the first 3 months may increase the chance of miscarriage and also the chance of the baby suffering from a malformation. The most common malformations occur in the heart, nervous system and skeleton.

Research findings: diabetes and pregnancy

- Women with long-standing diabetes have around a 44% chance of miscarriage. This can be reduced to the general population level by good glycaemic control.

- Birth defects are between 4 and 8 times more likely to occur in patients with diabetes mellitus but the risk is reduced if control is good.

- Most developmental abnormalities occur 3–6 weeks after conception, meaning that good control in the run up to pregnancy is crucial.

- Babies born to mothers with diabetes are at significantly increased risk of excessive size (macrosomia). This may lead to birth trauma to mother and baby. Caesarean section may be advised if the baby is large.

- Good blood glucose control helps to reduce macrosomia.

- Serial ultrasound may be useful in determining timing of intervention for early delivery.

Blood pressure control

Many of the commonly used drugs for blood pressure in diabetes, such as the ACE inhibitors, must not be used in pregnancy as they may harm the unborn baby. For this reason you may need to change your blood pressure medication before you get pregnant. You should remind your GP about changing your blood pressure tablets before you become pregnant.

If you have significant kidney problems, you should speak to your diabetes specialist before attempting to become pregnant. Women with kidney failure are at a higher risk of miscarriage, pregnancy-induced hypertension and premature delivery. Kidney function may worsen during pregnancy but usually returns to the previous level afterwards.

Cholesterol

Your doctor may have advised you to take a tablet known as a statin to reduce your cholesterol level. It is very important that you stop this before attempting to become pregnant. Omitting the statin throughout your pregnancy will not cause you any harm.

During the pregnancy

Most centres have a combined clinic where you can be seen by both the obstetric team and the diabetes specialists, both nurses and doctor. This means that, at the same visit, you can discuss your blood sugar results and also receive detailed care of your pregnancy. It is important that your baby's development and growth are carefully monitored by ultrasound.

Perfect blood glucose control is essential for your own and your baby's health. As well as the risk of abnormalities in your baby, raised blood sugar levels can cause your baby to grow too large. Other problems you may encounter as a result of diabetes include worsening of retinopathy, and increased risk of pre-eclampsia. Although women with kidney complications can have successful pregnancies, they need close monitoring and it is important to discuss all the issues before deciding whether to go ahead.

Gestational diabetes

A woman who develops diabetes during pregnancy has a condition known as 'gestational diabetes' or diabetes of pregnancy. This condition is related to the fact that a hormone produced by the placenta has made you more resistant to insulin. Before becoming pregnant, the insulin you produced was just enough to satisfy your requirements, and your body was able to use it effectively. But as the pregnancy progresses, your body is no longer able to use the insulin effectively, which leads to a rise in blood glucose and the diagnosis of diabetes.

In this condition, the blood glucose is raised and the high blood glucose crosses the placenta to the unborn baby. The baby has its own pancreas, which responds by producing extra insulin. The combination of excess glucose and excess insulin makes the unborn baby grow fat and bloated, so he or she is likely to have a high birth weight. After the birth, the baby is cut off from the high glucose input and then runs the risk of a low blood glucose level (hypoglycaemia) for a day or so after delivery.

Most women who develop gestational diabetes find the condition goes away after the baby's birth, but a small number continue to have diabetes. Once gestational diabetes has been identified, it is likely to recur during subsequent pregnancies. Provided that glucose levels are kept within normal limits (insulin may be needed to achieve this), the baby will be a normal weight and will not be at risk.

Women who have had gestational diabetes have a 40–60% chance of developing Type 2 diabetes later in life. This is because, although the pancreas can produce enough insulin to cope with everyday life, its reserves are low. The extra demands of pregnancy are more than it can manage, hence the need for insulin injections during pregnancy and the increased risk of 'running out' of insulin in the future. You can reduce your long-term risk of diabetes by making changes to your lifestyle. If you can lose weight so that you are in the ideal weight range, this will help, as will a regular programme of exercise such as swimming, walking or jogging. Both losing weight and regular exercise will reduce your insulin resistance, and this in turn reduces the extra strain on your pancreas to produce insulin.

Drug treatments that reduce insulin resistance may also have a role to play in reducing future risk of Type 2 diabetes. Three agents, metformin, troglitazone and rosiglitazone, all have robust study evidence that they do reduce risk of future diabetes in those who are insulin resistant. The TRIPOD study with troglitazone (now no longer available) looked specifically at reducing future Type 2 diabetes in women with previous diabetes in pregnancy. All three drugs reduce the incidence of future diabetes by around 50–70%. At present, none of these agents is licensed for use in people at risk of developing diabetes.

Delivery

The raised levels of sugar in your blood are likely to lead to an increase in your baby's size and weight. For many women, larger babies are more difficult to deliver, and carrying a big fetus can lead to other problems toward the end of your pregnancy. This means that the majority of maternity units in the UK will now recommend strongly that you come in a week or two before your due date to have your labour induced, or arrange for you to have a planned caesarean section. Full-term, large babies born to mothers with Type 2 diabetes are at increased risk of birth trauma, such as damage to the shoulders, during the later stages of delivery.

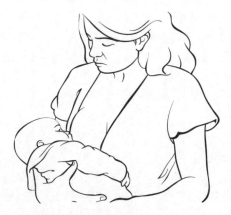

Feeding your baby

Breastfeeding is a good idea for mothers with diabetes mellitus. It is very beneficial for babies and has been shown to reduce their risk of future diabetes. Studies have shown that blood glucose control may improve while you are breastfeeding, although there is an increased risk of hypoglycaemia in women who choose to breastfeed. Unfortunately, most of the oral treatments for diabetes are secreted in breast milk and may cause levels of blood sugar to drop in the baby. For this reason, you may well have to stay on insulin therapy while breastfeeding.

Breast milk contains a significant amount of calories. Coupled with the birth of the baby, breastfeeding will be associated with a significant decrease in your insulin requirements. During your inpatient stay it is worth discussing with one of the diabetes specialist nurses how much you should reduce your insulin by.

Eventually, when the baby is weaned, you may be able to restart tablet treatment for your diabetes. If you have breastfed for a number of months, you may well be lighter and have less body fat than when you became pregnant. For this reason, you might need less diabetes treatment as you will be less insulin resistant.

Do not try to breastfeed while you are hypoglycaemic: feed yourself first so that you can feed and look after your baby safely. Always seek medical advice if you are in any doubt. If you find breastfeeding too difficult, there is no reason why you should not bottle-feed.

27

Social and employment issues

If you have been diagnosed with Type 2 diabetes recently, there is no reason why this should have a negative impact on your life. People with Type 1 and Type 2 diabetes are able to carry out most occupations and any sporting activity. The only job which can theoretically be a problem with diabetes is if you are an HGV driver and need insulin treatment. Even this is becoming a possibility nowadays as there is a move to have fewer restrictions as a result of the movement for equal opportunities. You may be disappointed at the increased cost of life and health insurance; this is caused by the additional risk of heart disease in people with diabetes. If you need treatment with insulin, you will have to inform the DVLA if you hold a driving licence.

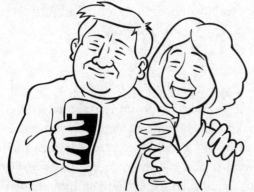

You need to be aware, however, that your doctor cannot communicate anything about your diabetes, or any other aspect of your health, to a third party without your permission.

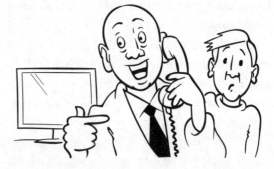

It is important to understand that your doctor cannot talk to anyone else about your health problems without you giving your permission first.

Social life

Diabetes should not interfere with a normal social life, though this may require a bit of extra planning depending on the treatment you take.

Eating out

Eating out with friends is an important part of many people's social life, and there is no reason why you should feel you need to give it up. As an appropriate diet for someone with diabetes is, to all intents and purposes, a really healthy diet, there should be no problem preparing food for others. Chapter 8 gives you more information about what makes for a healthy diet.

If you are invited to a meal at someone's house, it would be a good idea to talk to them first. You should explain that, because of diabetes, you have to be careful about the amount of sugar and fat you eat. If you are on insulin, you would also like to know if there is going to be a major delay in the timing of the meal. Most people would far rather know your situation and be involved in helping you manage it for an evening than find themselves entertaining a guest with a low blood sugar!

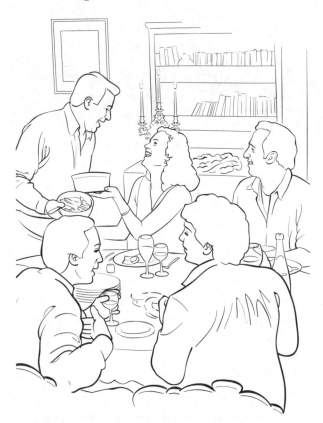

There is no reason why your diabetes should stop you enjoying meals with friends.

Eating in a restaurant or having a take-away should be less of a problem as you can choose from a range of dishes. Many people using a basal bolus regime choose to take extra short-acting insulin to cover the additional food they eat. Estimating the amount of carbohydrates in the food and deciding how much insulin you need is a skill that develops with experience, but you will find some guidelines in Chapter 8, Nutrition. If you are not sure how large a portion you will be given (in a restaurant, for example), you should wait until you see the plate before deciding what dose of insulin to take. Modern insulin pens allow people to give themselves their insulin discreetly at the table if necessary, without anyone noticing. Do not take your insulin dose before leaving home in case the meal is delayed.

If you are not on insulin but taking tablets, you will find the advice on page 86 more helpful.

Diabetes ID

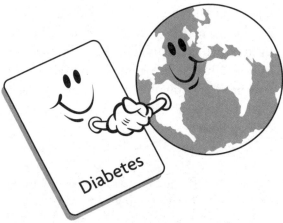

If you take insulin or a sulphonylurea (e.g. gliclazide) to control your diabetes, there is a risk of you becoming hypo. It is therefore a sensible precaution to carry something on your person showing that you have diabetes, such as a special necklace or bracelet (Medic-Alert or something similar). It is not uncommon for a person with diabetes to be mistaken for being drunk when in fact he or she is hypoglycaemic.

If you take insulin and are travelling abroad, it is a good idea to have some kind of identification stating that you have diabetes and therefore need to carry insulin and accessories. Insulin companies and diabetes associations often have special cards with text in different languages explaining what help you will need if you become hypoglycaemic.

An insulin passport was introduced in England in 2012 on the recommendation of the National Patient Safety Agency. This was to address the worrying frequency of errors in prescribing and dispensing insulin. All patients taking insulin should now be provided with an information leaflet and plastic cards which indicate the type(s) of insulin they are using.

Being a parent with diabetes

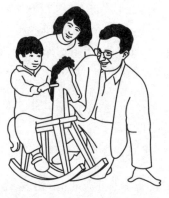

Many people worry about how their diabetes will affect their children, especially if those children are still young. After all, parenting is both an important part of a person's social role and a job of work in itself (and a very important one). For many people, their role as 'parent' is the most important role they fill. In general, maintaining a balanced, healthy lifestyle, and taking as good care of your diabetes as you possibly can, will benefit your children. It is best to be honest and 'up-front'

with your children about the fact that you have diabetes. They are likely to benefit from a healthy eating plan aimed at the whole family.

Whatever age they are, your children will probably want to know (at some stage) whether they are likely to develop Type 2 diabetes too. Of course, no one knows for sure, but they do have a higher risk than someone with no Type 2 diabetes in their immediate family. However, there are things they can do to make the development of diabetes less likely, such as eating well, taking regular exercise and keeping their weight at a healthy level. If they do go on to develop diabetes at some stage, however, they will benefit from the example you give to them now.

Adoption

Some countries have restrictions on adoption by a parent with diabetes. Such restrictions are usually due to outdated information about life with diabetes, but you may be required to get medical clearance indicating your ability to manage your diabetes and provide appropriate self-care.

Diabetes and work

In general, people with Type 2 diabetes can do whatever work they want. Those treated with diet and tablets with no risk of hypoglycaemia do not have any restrictions on their employment. Sulphonylureas carry a theoretical risk of causing hypoglycaemia, but this is more likely in a frail elderly person than someone who is holding down a job. People starting insulin therapy will be under restriction if they drive Large Goods or Public Service vehicles (i.e. HGVs or buses).

In a survey of employment among a sample of 200 people attending a hospital diabetic clinic in London (in 1999), the rate of unemployment was 12% compared with an average rate in Greater London of 4%. However, those individuals attending the hospital clinic were more likely to have significant problems which might prevent work. Of those not working, 50% had retired on medical grounds and were receiving disability allowances, while 37% were in receipt of a Disability Living Allowance.

The Disability Discrimination Act was passed in 1995 and revised in 2005. It aims to prevent discrimination against people who are disabled, specifically mentioning diabetes as being covered by the Act. Changes are about to be made to the DLA process and many people are worried that it will be more difficult to qualify for this allowance. It may, for instance, provide the money for a disabled person to have their own car and thus be able to get to work.

The Disability Discrimination Act

Describes 'discrimination' as occurring when:

- A disabled person is treated less favourably than someone else.

- The treatment is for a reason relating to the person's disability.

- There is a failure to make a reasonable adjustment for a disabled person.

Diabetes UK offers sensible advice on what to say to a (prospective) employer. The organization points out that while there is no legal requirement to tell your employer or potential employer that you have diabetes, by doing so it will make it easier to look after your diabetes and you will, for instance, be able to arrange clinic appointments without embarrassment. Diabetes UK advises you to be honest about your condition and if diabetes is brought up at interview, try to accentuate the positive: having diabetes means that you lead a healthy lifestyle and will have a thorough medical check-up every year.

So while an employer, or potential employer, cannot demand to know facts about your health without your consent, it is often in your interest to be as open as possible. This will be easier if you are in a stable position, where your colleagues and managers know and trust you already. It is understandable that you might feel more vulnerable when applying for a new job. If an employer needs information, you should provide this as fully as possible at the beginning, so you won't need to go back to answer more questions later.

Whether you are employable in a particular job is based on three key questions, regardless of whether or not you have diabetes:

1. Are you fit to carry out tasks with an acceptable level of risk?
2. Will doing the job make your health worse?
3. Will this job mean you are likely to be a risk to people you come into contact with (particularly hypoglycaemia risk)?

What is an occupational role that involves significant risk? Most people whose work falls into this category would be involved with driving (e.g. buses, trains, taxis, heavy goods vehicles), with operating machinery, with climbing ladders, or with taking responsibility for others. More unusual and exotic occupations such as deep-sea diving would also come under this definition.

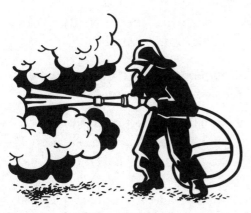

Policemen, firefighters and pilots are examples of professionals who might be putting their own or other people's lives at risk if they develop severe hypoglycaemia. In most countries, you are not allowed to work as a pilot or policeman if you have diabetes. But being a firefighter or driving an ambulance may be possible if you do not have problems with hypoglycaemia.

If your job doesn't involve significant hazard, and your performance in a particular role is satisfactory, your employer can't penalise you for having time off to attend review appointments for your diabetes. Indeed, a responsible employer should welcome the fact that you are proactive in looking after yourself.

Fitness for employment

The following points should be considered when assessing a person's suitability for employment, where there is a risk of injury to self or to others connected with the work in question:

- Where the job involves driving or any other particular hazard, such as operating dangerous machinery, potential employees should be evaluated according to the same criteria as a person without diabetes.

- The Disability Discrimination Act will apply and is in place to protect the rights of people with diabetes.
- The person's health should be under regular review by their GP and nurse or hospital clinic.
- Control of blood glucose should be reasonably stable.
- If the potential employee is on insulin therapy, he or she should be confident in self-monitoring blood glucose levels.
- The person should have a normal awareness of approaching hypoglycaemia, and not be subject to disabling attacks of hypoglycaemia.
- Annual reviews should be carried out by an appropriate diabetes specialist.

Telling your colleagues

A common reaction when someone is first diagnosed with Type 2 diabetes is, 'Do I really have to tell the people I work with?' It is never easy to give personal information to colleagues, but if you are at risk of a hypo you should warn the people you work with on a daily basis that if you start behaving in a peculiar way they should persuade you to take some sugar. Warn them too that you are likely to be pretty uncooperative if this happens and may even resist their attempts to help you – but could they please persevere anyway.

It can be difficult to admit to your workmates that you are taking insulin but, if you keep it secret, you run the risk of causing a scare by having a bad hypo. The natural response of anyone who doesn't know what is going on will be to dial 999 and if this happens you are likely to be taken to hospital by ambulance for treatment. If you get your colleagues onside before a problem arises, however, it is very likely they will be able to help you to avoid getting into such a situation.

Discrimination, and what to do about it

Unfortunately, there is still too much ignorant prejudice against people with diabetes and you can come up against this when you are looking for work, changing job, or at a point where you are vulnerable (such as a contract coming up for renewal). Unfortunately, this sort of discrimination does happen, especially in large organizations, although it can be difficult to prove. The Disability Discrimination Act covers people with diabetes, but taking a company to court can be difficult. You will need the support of your own diabetes team if you wish to take proceedings against an employer under the Disability Discrimination Act.

Diabetes UK has had discussions with medical officers responsible for occupational health in several large organizations. There is useful information on the Diabetes UK website, although it does date back to 2001.

The IRFD (International Register of Firefighters with Diabetes) is a UK organization that works to prevent diabetes discrimination in employment.

Shift work

People whose diabetes is controlled with diet and tablets should not be faced with difficult decisions if they have to work shifts. It should be easy to take once a day tablets around the same time each day and fit other tablets in with meals, which may of course be eaten in the middle of the night.

Guidelines for safe shift-working for people on insulin

- Aim for an injection of short- and intermediate-acting insulin every 12–16 hours, or use a basal bolus regimen. This way of giving insulin makes it much simpler to plan for shift work.

- Try to eat a good meal after each injection.

- If there is a gap of 6–8 hours when you are changing from one shift to another, take some short-acting insulin followed by a meal.

- Because your pattern of insulin and food intake is constantly changing, you will have to test your blood glucose more frequently than usual. You cannot assume that one day is just like another.

- If your blood glucose results are not good, be prepared to make changes in your dose of insulin. You will soon become an expert in managing your own diabetes.

Many people taking insulin are able to combine shift work with good control of their blood glucose. They do have to be organized about it, however, as most insulin regimens are designed around a 24-hour day. Shift workers often find that, just as they are settling into one routine, everything changes and they have to start again. It is hard to generalize about shift work as there are so many different possible patterns, but the guidelines above give some basic rules which should be helpful for anyone in this situation.

Many people work irregular hours, even if they are not doing shift work, and many of the same principles apply here too. People with an erratic lifestyle often find that a basal bolus regime gives them more freedom and flexibility. A basal bolus regime is usually easier to deliver using an insulin pen (see page 121).

Diabetes and the Armed Forces

Although military service is no longer compulsory in the UK, it is still obligatory in many other countries. However, young people in many parts of the world will automatically be exempt from mandatory service if they have diabetes.

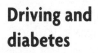

If you have Type 2 diabetes and want to become a soldier, sailor or airman, you will find that the Armed Forces are exempt from the Disability Discrimination Act and, therefore, they are able to refuse you entry. Diabetes UK is working to try and reverse this situation and are looking for examples of discrimination, which they can use to fight for this cause. It is likely that if you take tablets which carry no risk of hypoglycaemia, you should be able to argue for admission.

However, they may turn you down on the grounds that, in the course of time, you are likely to need insulin treatment. If you are already in the Forces and develop Type 2 diabetes, you may be asked to take on a desk job on the grounds that you may come to harm if you have a hypo while engaged in active soldiering.

Driving and diabetes

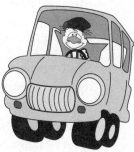

Diabetes can have an impact on your ability to drive safely in two ways. Firstly, it puts you at risk of hypoglycaemia, which will affect your concentration, may impair your judgement and, in severe cases, it may even lead to loss of consciousness. Secondly, diabetes can affect your eyesight, either because of high blood glucose levels leading to lens distortion and blurred vision, or because of damage to the retina or cataracts, which can be longer-term complications of diabetes. When actuaries calculate the increased risk that diabetes brings to driving, it is similar to that of epilepsy, at around 25%.

For the purposes of advice about driving and diabetes, the Driver and Vehicle Licensing Authority (DVLA) makes specific recommendations as to whether the licence you carry is a Group 1 or Group 2 licence. A Group 1 licence is a standard car or motorcycle licence that also allows you to drive a private minibus. A Group 2 licence is for passenger-carrying vehicles like coaches, and heavy goods vehicles. If you hold a Group 2 licence, you need to inform the DVLA that you have diabetes regardless of the treatment you are taking.

The DVLA changed the rules in 2011 and anyone driving a normal car or motorcycle (Group 1) with Type 2 diabetes controlled by diet or tablets (apart from sulphonylureas) or GLP-1 agonists does not have to inform the DVLA. However, anyone taking insulin or a sulphonylurea, who wants to hold a normal licence for car or motorbike:

- Must not have had more than one episode of severe hypoglycaemia within the preceding 12 months.

- Must not have impaired awareness of hypoglycaemia which has been defined by the Diabetes Panel for Group 1 vehicles as 'an inability to detect the onset of hypoglycaemia because of a total absence of warning symptoms'.

A severe hypo is one where help is needed from a third party. The most serious cases are those where the ambulance service or paramedics have been involved. In a nutshell, the new rules do not distinguish between hypos that occur during the night or the day. It is simply a case of 'two strikes and you're out'. These rules are new but it appears that people who lose their licence as result of a hypo can only re-apply after disqualification for a year.

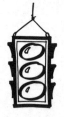

To consider while driving

1. Check your blood glucose level before you drive and every 2 hours when on a long journey. It should not be below 4.5 mmol/L (80 mg/dl) when you set out. Your driving performance will be impaired if your blood glucose level falls below 4 mmol/L.

2. Eat before driving or riding a bicycle. Keep dextrose tablets or rapid-acting glucose drinks in the glove compartment of your car.

3. Pull over and stop the car if you have hypoglycaemia. Wait until your glucose is >5.5 mmol/L before continuing. Remember that your thinking and judgement may take up to an hour to return to normal.

4. Be extra careful when the risk of hypoglycaemia is increased – for example, after playing sport or when you have recently adjusted your insulin doses.

5. Alcohol in the previous 12 or more hours increases the risk of hypoglycaemia.

6. Changes in your blood glucose level can cause blurred vision.

7. Try to avoid driving if you make major changes in your insulin regime. Wait until you are confident about the effects of the change.

8. If you have hypoglycaemic unawareness (no warning signs when your blood glucose is low), driving will always be risky. See page 146 for advice on how to treat this problem.

For people driving Group 2 vehicles (lorries or buses), there is no need to inform the DVLA if your diabetes is controlled by diet alone. If you are on any tablets (apart from sulphonylureas) or GLP-1 agonists, you should inform the DVLA who will allow you to drive, provided there are no problems with your eyesight. If you take a sulphonylurea (which could lead to a hypo), you can only apply for a licence if the following conditions are met:

- There has not been any severe hypoglycaemic event in the previous 12 months.

- The driver has full hypoglycaemic awareness.

- The driver must show adequate control of the condition by regular blood glucose monitoring, at least twice daily and at times relevant to driving.

- The driver must demonstrate an understanding of the risks of hypoglycaemia and there are no other debarring complications of diabetes.

The same rules apply to people who take insulin but, in order to prove that they do not have low sugars without warning, they have to use a blood glucose meter with a memory function to measure and record blood glucose levels for at least three months prior to submitting their application.

28

Travelling with diabetes

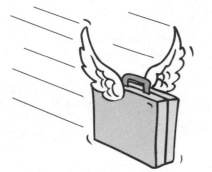

Travelling is an important part of life for many people, and you should not avoid this activity just because you have diabetes. If you think things over and plan ahead, no destination or mode of travel is impossible. However, travel across time zones, unaccustomed periods of heavy exercise and risk of infections all mean you need to be prepared when you go on holiday.

Diabetes should not interfere with any travel plans you have. If your diabetes is controlled by diet, tablets or GLP-1 injections, there are really no problems, though you may consider blood testing in case your diabetes goes out of control while you are away from your familiar surroundings. If you take a sulphonylurea, such as gliclazide or glimepiride, hypoglycaemia becomes a possibility so it is essential to be able to test your blood glucose. One of the features of air travel is that meals do not always arrive when expected so you need access to biscuits or glucose-containing sweets in case your blood glucose drops at an awkward time.

Travelling with insulin

If you take insulin to control your diabetes, travel needs a bit of extra planning. Ask your doctor for additional insulin supplies, in case some equipment gets lost or damaged. If you need insulin from a doctor in a foreign country, it should be possible to get identical or very similar insulins to your own anywhere in the world. However, the newer analogue insulins will be much more expensive than the older types of insulin (soluble or isophane). If you are going through airport security, bring with you an open letter from your doctor confirming that you have diabetes and need to carry insulin, needles and blood testing equipment. An official letter is worth a thousand words when you are stopped at customs! Bring along the box of insulin from the pharmacy where your name is printed (especially important if you are flying to the US).

While you are away, you should test your blood glucose more frequently than usual as changes in food and activity levels may lead to unexpectedly high or low readings. Always take spare insulin, at least twice the amount you expect to use. Keep insulin and pens/syringes in your hand luggage but make sure that you have an extra supply in another bag in case you lose one bag. Don't put insulin in the check-in luggage as there is a risk of it freezing in the aeroplane luggage hold at high altitudes. Besides, there is always the risk of your luggage being lost or arriving late.

You should have no problem obtaining insulin from a pharmacy abroad if you can prove that you have diabetes. Take a card on which your doses, concentration and brand of insulin are documented, or bring the original box with the pharmacy's label. It may be difficult to store your insulin in a refrigerator all the time, but it will usually not be wasted during a short trip, as long as you avoid temperatures above 25–30°C (77–86°F). Remember that it can be extremely hot (up to 50°C, 122°F) in a closed car on a sunny day. Bring a thermos flask or similar with you, containing cold water (cool it with ice before putting insulin into it) on hot days. Cool storage bags suitable for carrying insulin are available (try Amazon.com or www.frio.co.uk). Insulin is absorbed more quickly from the injection site if you are very warm and that this can result in unexpected hypoglycaemia.

Names of insulin abroad

Type	UK	US
Rapid-acting analogue	NovoRapid Humalog	NovoLog Humalog
Regular insulin	Actrapid Humulin S Insuman Rapid	Novolin R Humulin R
NPH insulin	Insulatard Humulin I	Novolin Humulin N
Basal analogue	Lantus Levemir	Lantus Levemir
Mixed insulin (70% NPH)	Mixtard 30 Humulin M3	Novolin 70/30 Humulin 70/30
Mixed analogue	NovoMix 30	NovoLog 70/30
(75% basal)	Humalog Mix 25	Humalog Mix 75/25

Most insulins can be found under different names in different parts of the world. If you plan a longer trip, have the insulin vial and box available or ask your doctor to write down what types of insulin you use so that you can get them from the local pharmacy if you lose your supplies. Be aware that in the US, pre-mixed insulins have their proportions stated in the opposite ways from the UK!

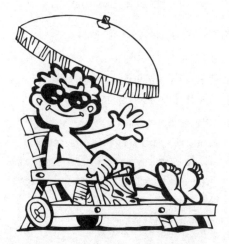

Remember that insulin cannot withstand heat and sunshine as well as you can. The boot of a car or bus will be too hot for insulin in the summer and too cold during the winter.

Insulin that has been frozen loses some of its potency. Don't leave it in the car on a skiing trip, for example. Keep your insulin bottles or pen injector in an inner pocket if it is below freezing outside. Damaged insulin will often turn cloudy or clumpy, sometimes with a brownish colour. Some blood glucose strips can give too high a reading when it is very hot outside and too low a reading when it is very cold. Many glucose meters will give you a warning if the temperature is outside the safe range.

Blood glucose is measured in mmol/L in some countries and mg/dl in others.

1 mmol/L = 18 mg/dl

10 0mg/dl = 5.6 mmol/L

Make sure that you have dextrose and glucagon when travelling, sailing or hiking. With glucagon you can treat a serious hypo-glycaemia even if you are a long way from emergency care. Make sure that your friends know how and when dextrose and glucagon should be used.

Passing through time zones when on insulin

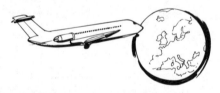

Multiple injection treatment

When you travel to other continents, there will be a time difference. If you go westwards, the day will be longer, and if you go eastwards, it will be shorter. If you are taking short-acting insulin before food and background insulin once a day, you should consider changing to splitting the dose of background insulin so that you take it twice a day. This means that when you cross time zones, you can continue taking long-acting (background) insulin approximately every 12 hours and short-acting insulin before you eat. This system takes most of the uncertainty out of the time zone problem.

Passing through time zones

(Adapted from the work of Kassianos, 1992)

Multiple daily injections

✈ *Going west (longer day):*
- Take mealtime insulin as usual.
- Usual doses of basal and bedtime insulin are adjusted to the 'new' day and night.

✈ *Going east (shorter day):*
- Decreased number of meals.
- Take bedtime dose of insulin as usual.

Two-dose treatment

✈ *Going west (longer day):*
- Extra doses of mealtime insulin with meals.
- Usual dose of pre-mixed insulin before evening meal at destination.

✈ *Going east (shorter day):*
Night-time flight:
- Take the ordinary mealtime insulin with dinner/tea.
- If the night on the plane is shorter than 4–5 hours, miss the second dose of pre-mixed insulin and take instead short-acting insulin before you eat.

Daytime flight:
- Usual insulin dose with breakfast.
- Reduce pre-mixed insulin at dinner/tea time on the plane by 5% for each time shift hour.

Two-dose treatment

If you take twice daily injections of mixed insulin, it is best to stick with the ordinary in-flight menu. Due to the pressure differences in the cabin, air bubbles may accumulate in the pen cartridges. To avoid this, remove the needle immediately after each injection. If you notice air bubbles in the insulin, get rid of them before taking an injection (see page 123). Jet lag may make you feel a bit weary before adjusting to the new time zone, and it will usually take a couple of days before your energy levels and sleeping pattern are back to normal.

Safety rules for flying within the US

✈ Syringes or insulin delivery systems should be accompanied by the insulin in its original pharmaceutically labelled box.

✈ Capped lancets should be accompanied by a glucose meter that has the manufacturer's name embossed on the meter.

✈ An intact glucagon kit should be kept in its original preprinted, pharmaceutically labelled container.

✈ No exceptions will be made. Prescriptions and letters of medical necessity will not be accepted.

✈ A passenger encountering any diabetes-related difficulty because of security measures should ask to speak with a Complaints Resolution Officer (CRO) for the airline.

Vaccinations

You should have the same immunization and malaria prophylaxis as travellers without diabetes. Indeed, it is particularly important that you do this, as illness can lead to difficult consequences which make your blood glucose more difficult than usual to control. Vaccination for hepatitis A, typhoid and other diarrhoeal diseases is a sensible precaution if you travel to areas where these may be a problem. It is sensible to have the vaccinations well ahead of the trip, as some cause an episode of fever that can affect the blood glucose for a few days.

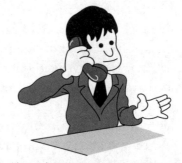

Remember that you are never more than a phone call away from your diabetes healthcare team when on holiday or a business trip.

Ill while abroad?

When you buy travel insurance, check the small print on the policy to find out whether it only covers acute illness, or whether it also covers any problem related to your diabetes. If you are a citizen of the UK or another EU country, you should acquire a European Health Insurance Card (EHIC). Apply online at www.dh.gov.uk/travellers – it is a very efficient service.

Always say that you have diabetes if you need to see a doctor abroad. In some third world countries, precautions against cross infection are not as stringent as we expect in the UK. You may need to be wary of injections and blood transfusions. If you are travelling to less developed parts of the world, you should take advice about the standard of medical care before you set off.

Diarrhoea

Since you may have difficulty with blood glucose levels and insulin adjustments if you are ill, you should take some antibiotics with you in case you need them. Ciprofloxacin 500 mg twice daily, for 5–10 days, is recommended only if you have severe or prolonged symptoms. In cases of resistance, you may be offered a single (1000 mg) dose of azithromycin or a three-day course of 500 mg per day. Sulphametazole or trimethoprim are recommended as alternatives for women who are or might be pregnant.

Since this treatment is not really covered under the NHS, you should be prepared to pay. This is safer than waiting till you develop diarrhoea while abroad, when you may have difficulty obtaining reliable supplies of the correct antibiotic.

Considering the risks of gastroenteritis, you should avoid drinking water in some countries if you cannot be sure it is entirely clean. Avoid all tap water (even frozen, i.e. ice cubes!) Bottled water and fizzy drinks (cola, fizzy lemonade or similar) are usually safe. Oral rehydration solution (e.g. Dioralyte) is a good alternative if you feel sick or are vomiting (see 'Nausea and vomiting' on page 162).

If you travel in primitive conditions, water should be disinfected by boiling it briefly or by using purifying tablets (Chlorine, Puritabs, Aqua Care or similar). If you do not drink enough while you are outdoors in the heat,

you will risk dehydration, which causes insulin to be absorbed more slowly. A high blood glucose level above the renal threshold (see Chapter 7, High blood glucose levels) will also cause you to lose extra fluid as you will be passing more urine.

Problems with travel sickness?

- Take medication: depot adhesives (e.g. scopolamine) or travel pills.
- You will be less likely to feel sick if you eat 'little and often' rather than large helpings several hours apart.
- Avoid fizzy drinks.
- If possible, sit in the front if you are in a car or bus, so you can see the road.

Extra documentation

Remember to get a letter signed by a nurse or doctor to authorise you to carry blood testing equipment, finger prickers and, if you are taking injections of GLP-1 agonists or insulin, pens and needles.

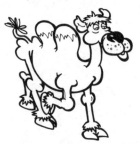

A camel can survive many days in the desert without drinking on account of its hump. Diabetes makes you more sensitive to dehydration. Be sure always to drink plenty of fluid when you are in a hot country, especially if you have problems with diarrhoea or vomiting. If you find yourself feeling or being sick, you should drink often, but only a few sips at a time.

Diabetes equipment you may need on the trip

- ID and necklace or bracelet indicating that you have diabetes.
- Any tablets you are taking to control your diabetes, with spares in case some get lost or you are delayed.
- Finger-pricking device, and lancets if you want to test your blood sugar.
- Test strips for blood glucose, and meter.
- Extra insulin pen and/or syringes if you are being treated with insulin (prefilled pens are handy for this).
- Dextrose/glucose tablets and gel.
- Glucagon, if you are taking insulin.
- Anti-diarrhoeal medication (such as Immodium).
- Oral rehydration solution (such as Dioralyte).
- Travel sickness medication.
- Paracetamol or aspirin (whichever suits you best) for suppressing fever.
- Clinical thermometer.
- Telephone and fax numbers for your diabetes healthcare team at home.
- Insurance documents and EHIC card.

29

Psychological aspects of Type 2 diabetes

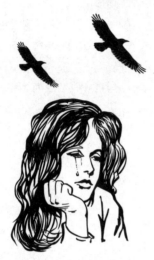

'You cannot stop the birds of sorrow from flying over your head – but you can stop them from building a nest there.'

Chinese saying

This account of the psychological consequences of Type 2 diabetes starts with practical observations which should apply to most people with the condition. At the end of the chapter, there is a description of some research findings in greater detail.

No two people respond in the same way on being told that they have Type 2 diabetes. Responses range from quiet acceptance to intense anger. If you are lucky, your health professionals will take time to discover what perceptions about diabetes you had at the outset and take a detailed family history about diabetes and cardiovascular disease. You may find you have a great deal to 'unlearn' before you can move on.

The different ways people respond to being told they have diabetes will be due in part to differences in personality. But the way they are told, and the extent to which their health professionals give them time to take in the information will also be factors. So, too, will the extent to which individuals feel supported by their doctor and diabetes nurses. If you leave the clinic feeling that your fears have not been addressed and your questions have not been answered, you may find yourself becoming angry and upset. These negative emotions can lead to depression and a (false) belief that you can do nothing to help yourself, so it is really important to try to ensure this situation does not develop. You can ask to see a different doctor or nurse if one is available. If not, you do have a perfect right to say that you feel you are not being listened to properly. Your health professional may not realize the extent to which his or her communication skills are falling short.

Common responses to the diagnosis of Type 2 diabetes

- Relief that symptoms are not due to a more serious condition.

- Anxiety about future complications.

- Early lack of concern followed by indignation, when the need for lifestyle changes becomes apparent.

- Demands for detailed information about the next move.

- Self-blame about body weight, lifestyle, etc.

- Anger about the loss of health, impact on occupation (e.g. HGV drivers) or delayed diagnosis.

- Bewilderment about the lifestyle changes required.

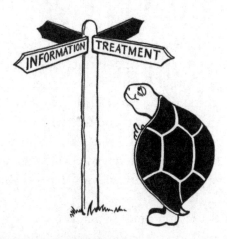

Need for information

Not only do people vary in their response to hearing the diagnosis of diabetes, they also vary in how and when they need to be given information about the condition. Some people want to be told all the details about the causes of diabetes and the likely treatment, while others are too numbed by the diagnosis to take on board anything but the basics. Just because your response is different from someone else's, doesn't mean it is any the less 'normal'.

If you find you have a strong emotional reaction, it is important you are given the time to deal with this before starting to learn about your diabetes and how to manage it. If you are not given a chance to adjust, you will simply not be able to absorb much, or even any, of the information you are given. Don't forget, your partner and other family members may also be in a state of shock, particularly if they too know little about diabetes. As a family, you may find it takes quite a long time for you all to get to grips with the implications of this complex condition.

Your doctor or diabetes nurse may approach the whole subject of information by asking you directly how much you want to be told. People often complain later that they were told too much, too quickly. A lot of time and effort goes into producing information leaflets, but these are not an effective way of providing education about diabetes unless a sympathetic health professional takes the time to talk you through the contents. It is all too easy never to get around to reading something that is simply handed to you when you are upset.

Psychological support

Anyone attending a diabetes clinic run by a GP or practice nurse will have an expectation of receiving some degree of psychological support. At the very least, this should include an acknowledgement of the emotional response to the diagnosis and an exploration of any fears they may have about diabetes. This process should be repeated at subsequent consultations, when people have had time to consider the problem and feel ready to express deep-seated anxieties. Some people are unable to accept the diagnosis and need specialized psychological help.

Handling the diagnosis of diabetes: what your health professional should do

- Tell you that you have diabetes, after first asking whether you would like a partner or other close companion present.

- Ask you what you already know about diabetes.

- Take a detailed family history from you, paying particular attention to whether either of your parents or other close relatives have/had diabetes or cardiovascular disease (e.g. high blood pressure, stroke).

- Ask whether you have any friends or workmates with diabetes.

- Ask whether you know anything about how they reacted to their diagnosis.

- Give you basic information, including a brief explanation of the differences between Type 1 and Type 2 diabetes.

- Arrange further education sessions for you with the practice nurse.

- Arrange for you to take part in group sessions (e.g. as part of the DESMOND programme) if possible.

- Make all necessary medical and screening appointments, e.g. for retinal screening or biochemistry tests, and teach you how to test your own blood and urine for glucose levels.

Group/peer support

The most effective and least complicated form of psychological support comes from other people with diabetes, preferably those with a similar experience of Type 2 diabetes.

This is incorporated into most structured group education packages, and several programmes are in place in the UK. One such programme, called DESMOND, is based on recognized principles of adult learning and is promoted by the Department of Health. For more information, see the section on patient support programmes in Chapter 35.

Support from partners and other family members

Diabetes is a condition that is with you for 24 hours of every day, so those who live with you will also be living with your diabetes. You will make life easier for those you love if you talk to them about how you are feeling and, wherever possible, encourage them to come with you to clinic appointments. If there is diabetes in your family, you may already have been through the experience of watching a parent or a sibling come to terms with the diagnosis. What can you learn from what they have already shown you? Will you react the way they did, or will you try to behave differently?

It is also important that anyone you spend time with on a regular basis (friends, colleagues, etc.) knows that you have diabetes so that if you have a hypo, for example, they are not taken by surprise. Enlist their help rather than risk embarrassing yourself by putting them in a situation where they don't understand what is happening to you.

Anxiety and Type 2 diabetes

One might assume that people with Type 2 diabetes would be less anxious about their condition than those with Type 1 diabetes. The onset of their disease is less dramatic, and their life is not turned upside down by the immediate need for insulin accompanied by other major lifestyle disturbances. However, there are many changes that people with both forms of diabetes have to come to terms with, as indicated in the box overleaf.

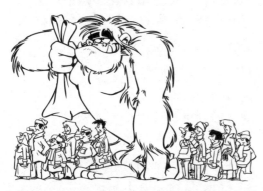

Diabetes is an invisible handicap and can't be seen from the outside. You may sometimes feel better if nobody knows. However, both you and your friends will find it easier in the long run if you let everyone know. If, for instance, you become hypoglycaemic, everyone will understand what is going on and what to do if you have informed them beforehand. Many people have described how embarrassing and troublesome they found it, having to explain their diabetes for the first time when they became hypoglycaemic and needed help.

Sadly, many young people with Type 1 diabetes are still threatened by parents, relatives and even healthcare professionals that they risk blindness, kidney failure and loss of limbs if they fail to meet the intrusive demands of diabetes and keep their blood sugar under control. In contrast, the onset of Type 2 diabetes is often a gradual process which at the beginning involves changing to a healthy eating pattern. The menace of insulin injections is several years ahead, and

the main health risks of Type 2 diabetes, namely heart attacks and strokes, are faced by all individuals in an affluent middle-aged population, whether or not they have diabetes. Given these observations, it is perhaps surprising that most formal research studies suggest that anxiety is at least as common in Type 2 as in Type 1 diabetes.

Research findings: anxiety and Type 2 diabetes

- A research group from Germany studied 420 people with diabetes using a questionnaire to screen for anxiety. Those who screened positive were invited to a diagnostic interview. In this group, minor anxiety was more common in Type 2 diabetes (21%) than in Type 1 diabetes (15%). However, the risk of severe anxiety was only increased in patients with Type 2 diabetes on insulin (6.7%), while patients with either Type 1 or Type 2 diabetes not on insulin had the same risk of severe anxiety as the nondiabetic population (5.2–5.7%).

- Similar results were reported in an American study, which investigated emotional distress in 815 primary care patients with Type 2 diabetes. Using a 20-item self-report measure of diabetes related emotional distress, they found significantly higher levels of distress among patients treated with insulin (24.6%) compared with those taking tablets (17.8%) or diet alone (14.7%). The greater distress in patients on insulin was attributed to disease severity and the burdens of self-care.

- These two studies suggest a relationship between insulin therapy and increased anxiety. However, these findings should be taken seriously by doctors and nurses in view of the widespread pressure to introduce insulin therapy early in the course of Type 2 diabetes.

- A review of 18 studies from the US and Europe looked at 2584 patients with diabetes and showed that generalized anxiety disorder was present in 14% of those with diabetes compared with 3–4% of the general population. In this study, there were no differences between Type 1 and Type 2 diabetes.

Depression and Type 2 diabetes

Once you have been diagnosed with diabetes, it will be with you for life. This is a situation which many people will find upsetting. However, many research studies have shown that the majority of people with diabetes have a normal quality of life unless they are affected by complications which interfere with daily living.

On the other hand, depression is a very common problem and so is diabetes. So there are many people with a tendency to suffer from depression or anxiety, who go on to develop diabetes quite independently. Whatever the cause of their depression, people who feel negative about themselves find it difficult to summon up the energy to look after their diabetes properly. This makes it more difficult for them to maintain good control.

The DESMOND education programme mentioned above appears to reduce the risk of depression among people with newly diagnosed diabetes. Depression scores were lower in those patients who took part in

DESMOND than in a matched control group. This improvement was statistically significant one year after the course was delivered.

Issues to come to terms with following a diagnosis of diabetes

- Frequent blood testing.
- Dietary changes.
- Driving regulations.
- Embarrassment about hypos.
- Feeling socially different.
- Impact on employment.
- Fear of complications.
- Realization that it is for life.

Diabetes and underlying psychiatric illness

Diabetes is more common in patients with psychoses, such as schizophrenia. An analysis of medical insurance claims in people with schizophrenia showed that the risk of having diabetes with complications was twice that of the population as a whole.

Schizophrenia

It has emerged that some of the newer anti-psychotic drugs which are now used to treat conditions such as schizophrenia may actually cause diabetes. A recent survey of patients with schizophrenia in the US examined 15,767 patients who had been treated for psychosis over several years with one of four drugs: olanzapine, risperidone, quetiapine, or halo-peridol. Compared with the older drug haloperidol, all three newer agents increased the risk of diabetes by over 60%. The risk was higher in people over 50 years.

Research findings: depression and Type 2 diabetes

- A review of 42 studies showed that diabetes increased the odds of having depression by two to threefold. The wealth of data in this article makes it hard to single out a headline result. However, in controlled studies, the frequency of major depression was 9.0% in patients with diabetes compared with 5.0% in controls, while the risk of less severe depression using self-report scales was 26.1% in diabetes and 14.4% in controls. The increased risk of depression was identical in Type 1 and Type 2 diabetes (2.9 versus 2.9).

- A survey of 8 studies looking at the lifetime frequency of major depression found it to be significantly higher in those with diabetes than in control subjects: 17.5% versus 6.8% respectively.

- The increased chance of depression in adults with Type 2 diabetes was confirmed in a survey of 10 controlled studies, comprising 51,331 patients, which showed a frequency of 17.6% in people with Type 2 diabetes compared with 9.8% in control subjects.

- The 1999 National Health Interview Survey uncovered some interesting observations about the relationship between diabetes, depression and functional disability in a representative sample of the adult US population. Over 30,000 individuals were interviewed to identify the presence of diabetes, depression and functional disability, which was defined as difficulty in performing activities of daily living and routine social activities. Depression without diabetes increased the risk of functional disability threefold, while diabetes on its own increased the risk by 2½ times. The combination of depression and diabetes led to a sevenfold increase in the risk of disability.

- A recent study from Norway further examined the relationship between diabetes and depression. A huge population of 65,000 were included in the study, which came up with the following conclusions:

  (i) The presence of other conditions (mainly heart disease) was associated with depression in Type 2 diabetes but not in Type 1 diabetes.

  (ii) Individuals with Type 2 diabetes without other medical conditions had the same risk of depression as the healthy non-diabetic population.

  (iii) Depression itself appears to increase the risk of developing both Type 2 diabetes and heart disease. Factors normally associated with depression, namely low education and physical inactivity, are also linked to depression in people with diabetes.

Diabetes and severe psychosis

People with a psychosis that reduces their grasp of reality cannot make the connection between good blood glucose control and the risk of future complications and therefore have no motivation to maintain a disciplined way of life. Anecdotally, some of the most damaged and deformed feet are seen in patients with schizophrenia who have developed neuropathic sensory loss due to diabetes.

Type 2 diabetes and eating disorders

It would be easy to assume that the overweight, overeating person who develops Type 2 diabetes would be a likely candidate to have an eating disorder. The literature is ambivalent. A study from Italy compared three groups of patients: a group of 156 obese patients with Type 2 diabetes, a group of 192 obese individuals who did not have diabetes but who were keen to lose weight, and a control group of 48 obese patients (who did not necessarily have diabetes) selected at random. Using a score to identify people with eating disorders, these turned out to be almost twice as common in the non-diabetic groups. Thus, in this population, the presence of diabetes did not lead to an increased risk of developing an eating disorder.

An Australian study found that in a group of 215 women with Type 2 diabetes, 22% had an eating disorder of some description. The problem was more common in those women who were diagnosed at a younger age and who were heavier. As a group, those with an eating disorder could not motivate themselves to control their food intake or to increase their exercise.

Can psychological interventions help?

The same Australian group went on to investigate whether psychological treatment could help patients who had Type 2 diabetes and an eating disorder. They found that CBT (cognitive behavioural therapy) and NPT (non-prescriptive therapy) were both helpful and also improved control of their diabetes.

A systematic review was carried out of randomized controlled trials comparing psychological interventions for improving control of diabetes with a control group receiving the usual care. In an analysis of 12 of these trials, psychological therapies resulted in significantly better glycaemic control, with a difference in HbA_{1c} of 0.76%. More intensive psychological therapies appeared to be even more effective, with a 1% reduction in HbA_{1c}. Psychological therapy, usually a variant of CBT, was associated with a reduction in psychological distress but did not appear to affect weight control.

Taking control

Emotional factors have a major influence on the way people cope with the demands of Type 2 diabetes. Clinicians should address the anxieties and guilt that many people experience and should try to help patients accept the diagnosis and clarify their treatment goals.

As a rule of thumb, anxiety and depression are twice as common in people with diabetes as those without, and the presence of cardiovascular complications magnifies the risk.

As time passes, most people are able to face up to the diagnosis of Type 2 diabetes and take control of their lives. It is worth trying to be positive about living with this intrusive condition.

30

Complications of the cardiovascular system

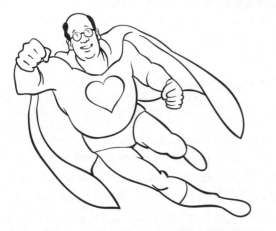

If you have Type 2 diabetes, much of the emphasis on good blood glucose control and many of the tablets you are prescribed will be designed to reduce the risk to your heart and blood vessels. These are known as macrovascular (i.e. large vessel) complications as opposed to microvascular (small vessel) complications, which are described in the next chapter.

What are macrovascular complications?

Macrovascular complications affect the large arteries in your body which supply blood to your heart, legs, kidneys and brain, among other parts of the body. If these become clogged up (the medical term is 'thrombosed'), you will be at risk of developing heart

disease (often leading to heart attacks), kidney failure, foot ulcers and strokes. Unfortunately, heart attack and stroke represent the major cause of death (up to 75%) in patients with Type 2 diabetes. Thus, it is important to do everything possible to reduce your risk of large vessel complications.

Blood glucose levels

What is the evidence for a link between high blood glucose and macrovascular complications?

A number of studies have shown that the relationship between blood glucose and cardiovascular risk is a continuum. In other words, even before diabetes is diagnosed, while the blood sugar is slightly raised, there is a small increased risk of heart disease. As the sugar becomes even higher and diabetes becomes apparent, so the risk becomes greater. Type 2 diabetes is also associated with a number of other risk factors for heart disease, such as hypertension, abnormal blood fats (cholesterol) and increased fat around the waist.

The link between lowering blood sugar and reducing the rate of heart attack in diabetes has been shown in the UKPDS (see Chapter 36, Outcome studies). This study looked at the effect of reducing blood sugar and blood pressure on the rate of complications and found that, in the group who had intensive lowering of their blood sugar, there was a strong trend to a reduced risk of heart attack. After the UKPDS was completed (the initial study took 20 years), patients who had taken part were contacted annually for a further 10 years. This showed that the effect of tight blood glucose control soon after diagnosis had a very prolonged protective effect on the heart. This 10-year follow-up (extending the total study time to 30 years) also confirmed the effect of metformin in reducing the risk of future heart attack.

What can I do about it?

The important message is that you should try to follow the advice you are given about your diet and blood glucose-lowering treatment. While controlling sugar is only part of the answer to reducing heart disease, strokes and other macrovascular complications, it does play an important role.

Blood pressure

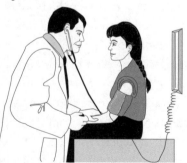

Control of blood pressure is very important in reducing your likelihood of developing complications of diabetes. Your blood pressure should be checked routinely at every clinic visit.

What is the evidence for a link between high blood pressure and macrovascular complications?

Raised blood pressure (hypertension) is very common in people who have diabetes. You have twice the risk of hypertension if you have Type 2 diabetes compared with a person of similar age with no diabetes. The combination of uncontrolled blood pressure and diabetes more than doubles the risk of macrovascular complications. The best research evidence comes from the UKPDS (see Chapter 36, Outcome studies). In this study, intensive, relatively small reductions in blood pressure of 10/5 mmHg caused a reduction in the risk of stroke by 44% and of heart attack by 21%. Larger trials, conducted across the whole population but including people with diabetes, also showed a reduction in a combined outcome of death, heart failure, stroke and heart attack if blood pressure was treated effectively. National and international guidelines now recommend a lower target for blood pressure in Type 2 diabetes of 140/80 mmHg. This is because the UKPDS showed that the lower the blood pressure, the lower the risk of these complications. In the case of kidney damage from diabetes, the target blood pressure should be less than 130 mmHg.

What can I do about it?

The key is to follow lifestyle advice and take the tablets your doctor prescribes for you. It goes against the grain for most people to take up to 10 different tablets a day, but each tablet will have a specific action either to improve blood glucose, reduce blood pressure or to control cholesterol. We know from the UKPDS that most people need three or more different tablets to achieve tight blood pressure control, especially now the target blood pressure is so stringent. The UKPDS also showed that the lower the blood pressure, the greater the protection, so the normal target is 140/80 mmHg. If there is any evidence of kidney damage, this target is lowered to 130/80 mmHg. Research studies have shown that a specific type of drug called an ACE (angiotensin-converting) inhibitor (drugs with names that end in '-pril', such as ramipril, perindopril, etc.) or an angiotensin II receptor blocker (with names that end in '-sartan', such as valsartan, losartan, etc.) may be particularly useful in diabetes because they protect the kidneys from the effects of diabetes and hypertension. If you are not already taking this type of medication, perhaps you could ask your doctor about this. There are at least four different classes of drug which control blood pressure, and it is worth experimenting till you find a combination that controls your blood pressure without causing side effects.

Cholesterol levels

What is the evidence for a link between blood fats and macrovascular complications?

High blood fats (cholesterol) can lead to deposits being laid down within the blood vessels, particularly the arteries, causing them to become narrow and less efficient. This leads to a greater risk of heart attack or stroke than in someone whose arteries are normal.

Until recently, all of the evidence for treating blood fats in patients with diabetes came from subsets of trials across the whole population. All showed a substantial benefit for patients with diabetes who already have cardiovascular problems. The CARDS study

used a statin (atorvastatin) to investigate its effect in preventing heart disease in people with diabetes who had not had previous heart problems. It showed a reduction of 37% in a combined outcome of stroke, acute coronary events, or the need for a coronary bypass operation. There is good evidence that people with Type 2 diabetes should take a statin to reduce their cholesterol level.

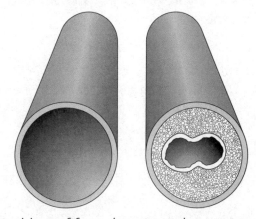

Build-up of fatty deposits in the arteries gradually blocks the flow of blood.

What can I do about it?

Unfortunately, dietary changes alone are not very effective in reducing your cholesterol in Type 2 diabetes, although of course you should try to reduce saturated fats and total calories. Based on the available evidence, medical scientific bodies such as the Joint British Societies (JBS) now recommend that all patients above the age of 40 years who have diabetes should take a statin. In addition, if you have microvascular complications, poor blood glucose control, a raised total cholesterol of more than 6.0 mmol/L, high blood pressure, low good cholesterol or high triglycerides (energy fats in the blood), they recommend that people with diabetes should start a statin any time above the age of

18 years. However, statins are not safe in pregnancy and should never be prescribed if there is a real possibility of pregnancy. If you suffer any sort of cardiovascular event such as a stroke, TIA (ministroke), angina or heart attack, and have diabetes, you should take lipid-lowering medication such as a statin without any question.

Heart and large blood vessel diseases
Diagnosis

1. Blood pressure measurements.
2. Examination of pulses in the feet and lower legs, with a Doppler device if necessary.
3. Analysis of cholesterol and triglycerides in the blood.

Treatment

1. Stop smoking.
2. Increase the amount of physical exercise or physiotherapy.
3. Avoid putting on weight.
4. Avoid undue stress (see Chapter 20).
5. Don't drink too much alcohol.
6. Control high blood pressure.
7. Eat foods high in fibre and low in fat. Increase fruit and vegetable intake.

Insulin resistance

What is the evidence for a link between insulin resistance and macrovascular complications?

Insulin resistance is a condition where extra insulin is needed to maintain normal levels of blood glucose. Insulin resistance in fat cells leads to the breakdown of stored triglycerides to release fatty acids into the blood. Resistance to insulin means that higher levels of insulin are needed to bring about storage of glucose in muscle and liver, which both cause higher levels of glucose in the blood. Insulin resistance is the underlying cause of the metabolic syndrome (see Chapter 33, Associated diseases). It is not easy to measure the degree of insulin resistance by means of a blood test. However, people with central obesity and a high waist circumference are likely to be resistant to insulin. In practice, the amount of insulin that people need to control their sugar levels is a good guide to the degree of insulin resistance.

The problem is that insulin resistance occurs many years before diabetes is diagnosed and of course plays a major part in the causation of diabetes. In the time before diabetes comes to light, insulin resistance increases the risk of cardiovascular disease, which is why many people are diagnosed with diabetes at the time of a heart attack.

What can I do about it?

The most effective way of lowering insulin resistance is to lose weight and take exercise, which may be easier said than done! Even a small increase in your exercise regime will have a positive effect on your weight, blood pressure, blood glucose and blood fats. If you lose 10% of your body weight, the effect on your level of insulin resistance (and hence your cardiac risk factors) would be substantial.

There is evidence from the UKPDS study (see page 256) that metformin, a drug which reduces insulin resistance and lowers blood glucose has positive effects on cardiovascular outcomes. Metformin is therefore seen as the glucose-lowering therapy of choice for patients with Type 2 diabetes. Pioglitazone is a potent reducer of insulin resistance and affects a range of cardiovascular risk factors such as blood pressure. A study using pioglitazone has shown a reduction in the number of cardiovascular events over a 3-year period in patients with diabetes at high risk of vascular disease.

Who needs aspirin treatment?

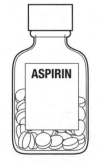

Scare stories about increased risk of bleeding or newly discovered side effects may make it difficult for patients to see why they would be helped by anti-platelet, 'blood-thinning' medication such as aspirin. In reality, aspirin treatment is recommended for all patients with diabetes over 50 years of age. The National Institute for Health and Clinical Excellence (NICE) recommends aspirin in Type 2 diabetes if the 10-year risk of heart disease is greater than 15%. However, NICE advises caution in using aspirin if the blood pressure is higher than 145 mmHg. So control your blood pressure below this level before starting aspirin at a standard small dose of 75 mg daily. This is the equivalent of ¼ of a standard aspirin tablet, or one junior aspirin.

Some recent studies have cast doubt on whether people with no previous history of heart attack or stroke derive any extra protection from taking aspirin. We suggest you discuss this with your GP.

There are a few conditions (such as a history of problems with bleeding stomach ulcers) which mean that a person should not take aspirin. Your doctor will be able to tell you whether or not you are at risk in this way and it is important you talk to him or her before you start taking aspirin. For those people who do not have one of these conditions, the advantages of taking aspirin outweigh the disadvantages. However, it is really important that you consult your doctor first, to make sure there are no reasons for you not to take aspirin.

New cardiovascular risk markers

Scarcely a day goes by without a new marker for cardiovascular risk being reported in the tabloid press. Those in vogue recently include CRP (C-reactive protein – a marker of the amount of inflammation in your blood) and a number of other inflammatory chemicals in the blood, and homocysteine (an amino acid, one of the building blocks of proteins). There are good population studies which all support an association between these chemicals and increased cardiovascular risk. However, there is no evidence that intervening by trying to change the blood levels of these markers has any effect on the risk of a cardiovascular event.

Helping yourself

In essence the message for reducing the risk of heart attacks, strokes or similar problems is simple. If you can lose weight and take regular exercise, you will cut your risk of heart attack. In addition, your doctor may prescribe for you a large number of different medications, and you may feel it is too much. But you need to take them. A heart attack or a stroke is an all or nothing event, and there is good evidence that taking medication for high blood glucose, high blood pressure and high cholesterol can stave off the risk of a heart attack or a stroke.

31

Microvascular complications

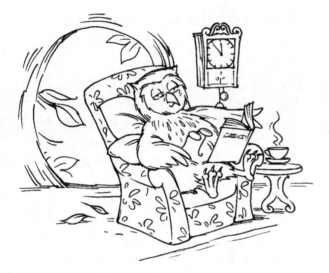

Microvascular complications are those which affect the small blood vessels of the body, specifically those supplying the eyes the kidneys, and the nerves. Damage to these small vessels can result in the following:

- Retinopathy (changes in the retina at the back of the eye) which may lead to blindness if left untreated;

- Nephropathy (damage to the kidneys) which causes leakage of protein and may lead to kidney failure;

- Neuropathy (nerve damage) resulting in loss of sensation in the feet and more rarely the hands or problems with the functions of the body controlled by the internal (autonomic) nervous system. These include sexual problems (see Chapter 25).

In Type 1 diabetes, the risk of microvascular complications is largely governed by the degree of blood glucose control and the length of time the person has had diabetes. In Type 2 diabetes, the picture is a bit more complicated. The reason for this is that some people with newly diagnosed Type 2 diabetes have actually had the condition for up to 10 years without it being discovered. During this time, a great deal of damage may already have been done to small and large blood vessels. The UKPDS (see Chapter 36, Outcome studies) found that over 25% of newly diagnosed patients already had some sign of retinopathy. We also know that sometimes people with Type 2 diabetes are diagnosed after developing a foot ulcer or infection as a result of nerve damage (neuropathy), and these people usually have some degree of retinopathy of which they have been unaware. Keeping the blood glucose and blood pressure under good control will minimize the risk of developing small vessel problems and will reduce the risk of further damage in people who have already developed some complications before they discover they have diabetes.

Complications affecting the eyes (retinopathy)

The risk of eye damage has decreased considerably as a result of better diabetes care, regular screening to detect changes before they cause damage to vision and improved treatments if eye problems arise. Good control of blood glucose and blood pressure help to protect against retinal changes and delay progression of any changes that may have developed already. Most people who have had diabetes for 15–20 years are likely to have some retinal changes, although they may be very minor. If the changes are severe enough to threaten sight, laser treatment may be necessary to preserve vision. Treatment for retinopathy can be very effective if used promptly but is less effective if delayed until visual damage has occurred. Approximately 1 in 1000 people will suffer serious visual loss as a result of diabetes each year.

Early changes (known as background retinopathy) do not affect sight. The first changes are small swellings on the fine blood capillaries in the retina (known as micro-aneurysms). These may be followed by small haemorrhages or leakage of fluid (exudates) in areas of the retina which are not important for vision. Such changes may get better if blood glucose control improves. If they occur in the central area of vision, known as the macula, which is responsible for detailed vision such as reading, recognizing people's faces and driving, there is a risk that vision may be damaged and laser treatment is required before significant visual changes occur. This condition is known as maculo-pathy.

In some people with severe retinal damage, new blood vessels develop at the back of the eye. These new vessels are fragile and may rupture, leading to a bleed into the eye which will seriously affect vision. This is known as proliferative retinopathy and requires laser treatment to preserve vision.

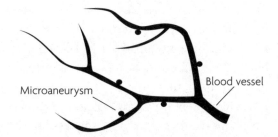

After many years of high blood glucose levels, the blood vessels of the retina will become brittle, and small bubbles (called microaneurysms) can form. They do not affect your vision, but can be seen on a photograph of the retina.

It is important to treat both maculopathy and proliferative retinopathy promptly, before any significant visual loss occurs. For this reason annual retinal screening is recommended for all people with diabetes so that changes can be detected at an early stage, before vision is damaged. In the UK, national screening programmes using digital photographs of the retina are in place to ensure that every person with diabetes is offered annual screening (unless they are already under follow-up by an eye clinic.) It is very important to make sure that you have annual retinal screening – if you do not receive an appointment you should ask the doctor or nurse at your surgery to make sure you are offered one

Treatment

The most important preventative treatment is good control of blood glucose and blood pressure.

If the changes reach the stage where they threaten to reduce vision, laser treatment is used. Maculopathy is usually treated by a small number of laser shots around the macular area.

This is called 'focal' laser treatment and takes only a few minutes to perform. Laser treatment for proliferative retinopathy is equally effective but requires many applications of laser to the back of the affected eye. This is a longer procedure and may take 20–30 minutes. Sometimes this requires more than one session with up to a thousand applications of laser at each sitting. Once the retina has been widely treated with laser, the new vessels will recede along with the risk of bleeding. In some circumstances the laser treatment may be only partially effective and additional treatments may be recommended. Maculopathy may respond to injections into the eye, similar to those used to treat macular degeneration. If proliferative retinopathy leads to bleeding into the jelly (vitreous) in the middle of the eye, removal of the jelly and replacement with clear fluid (vitrectomy) may restore vision.

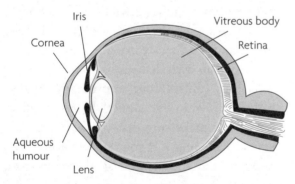

The eye seen in cross-section. Eye damage is first noted in the retina. At check-ups, the retina is photographed after dilatation of the pupil. An eye specialist will have a close look at the pictures.

Disturbed vision at unstable blood glucose levels

Blurred vision is a common symptom of unstable diabetes. This is due to the changes in glucose which affect the shape of the lens and hence make focusing difficult. It is not in any way dangerous for your vision, nor is it associated with future visual impairment.

Sometimes the disturbed vision can continue for several weeks and you may find that a pair of cheap reading glasses will resolve the problem. In any case, your vision will return to normal in time.

Glasses

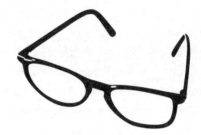

Your blood glucose levels should be stable when you are tested for new glasses. Otherwise, your vision will be affected by temporary changes in blood glucose. After the onset of diabetes, it may take 2–3 months of normal blood glucose levels before the lens returns to its usual shape, and you should obviously not be tested for new glasses during this time.

Contact lenses

People with diabetes can wear contact lenses. However, you should avoid long-term lenses (that are replaced every second or third week) as the protecting cell layer of the cornea tends to be more brittle if you have diabetes.

Complications affecting the kidneys (nephropathy)

The process of developing kidney failure is a gradual one. Only a small number of people with evidence of minor kidney damage go on to develop kidney failure. There are several distinct stages and each stage may last many years before progression to the next. There are well recognized ways of slowing down this process.

Stages of kidney damage

1. Microalbuminuria

The blood vessels of the kidneys are formed into small clusters where waste products in the blood are filtered into the urine. Damage to the walls of these blood vessels causes leakage of protein into the urine. A technique has been developed to detect tiny amounts of protein (known as microalbuminuria) in the urine.

Microalbuminuria is measured on a small sample of urine and is expressed as a ratio of albumin to creatinine. The creatinine ratio corrects for the fact that the flow rate of urine varies greatly. The threshold for defining microalbuminuria is an albumin–creatinine ratio greater than 2.5 mg/mmol in men and 3.5 in women. It is a very sensitive test, and false positives can occur as a result of physical exercise, smoking and infection in the urine. If the test is positive, it should be repeated and a specimen of urine should be sent for testing to rule out an infection. Persistent micro-albuminuria is the first sign that there is a problem with the kidneys. However, it can be treated and often reversed by controlling blood glucose and blood pressure. There is also evidence that particular blood pressure tablets, called ACE inhibitors or angiotensin receptor blockers (ARBs, sometimes known as sartans) have a protective effect on kidneys at this early stage of damage.

2. Proteinuria

If the protein leakage progresses, this may cause high blood pressure, which then increases leakage of protein into the urine to levels that can be detected by a simple urine dipstick method. This is known as proteinuria and the urine test strip is called Albustix. Albumin is the most basic protein in the blood and is manufactured by the liver in response to the needs of the body. If the leakage of protein (albumin) becomes very severe (more than 5 g in 24 hours), it exceeds the amount that can be replaced by the liver even though it is working at full stretch. At this point, the level of albumin in the blood falls below normal, and this in turn leads to fluid retention. This condition is called the nephrotic syndrome, and once this has developed, it is difficult to reverse the leakage of protein. The fluid retention can only be treated by removing the excess fluid by diuretics – known as 'water tablets'. Its progression can be slowed by the usual measures of controlling blood glucose and blood pressure to tight targets.

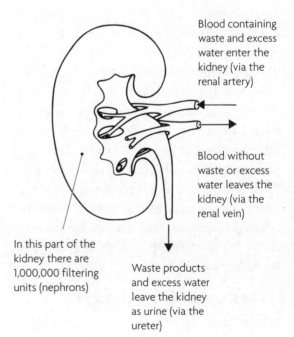

Blood containing waste and excess water enter the kidney (via the renal artery)

Blood without waste or excess water leaves the kidney (via the renal vein)

In this part of the kidney there are 1,000,000 filtering units (nephrons)

Waste products and excess water leave the kidney as urine (via the ureter)

3. Abnormal kidney function

A number of people may drift quietly into kidney failure without feeling particularly unwell. Indeed, it is often picked up by chance on a random blood test. However, kidney failure does have a number of consequences which affect the general working of the body. It is a slow, progressive process which takes place over years but, as the kidneys deteriorate, more metabolic problems arise and the person feels increasingly unwell. Because the body is unable to remove waste products, there is a build-up of acid in the blood. People with kidney failure also become anaemic and have problems with the calcium levels in their blood. This form of anaemia can be treated by EPO (erythropoietin) injections to stimulate the bone marrow. The calcium defect is treated with vitamin D tablets.

4. Established (or end-stage) kidney failure

At this stage the kidneys can no longer remove waste products from the body, which puts the individual at risk of coma. The first line of treatment is peritoneal or haemodialysis. Peritoneal dialysis is usually done by the patient in his or her own home three times a day. This avoids the need for high-tech equipment and allows a little more independence. It is quite intrusive, however, and can interfere with normal daily activities. Haemodialysis is usually carried out three times a week in a specialist kidney centre. Most people who have dialysis are keen to receive a kidney transplant, which gives them back their freedom.

The stages of kidney damage

1. Microalbuminuria.
2. Proteinuria.
3. Abnormal kidney function.
4. End-stage kidney failure.

Treatment to delay end-stage renal failure and maintain wellbeing

1. Good glucose control (HbA_{1c}).
2. Stop smoking.
3. Microalbuminuria is treated with an ACE-inhibitor or angiotensin receptor blocker (ARB) to protect the kidneys.
4. Maintain blood pressure target of less than 130/75.
5. Treat urinary tract infections.
6. Anaemia is treated with EPO injections.
7. Calcium abnormalities are treated with vitamin D.

Treatment of end-stage renal failure

Peritoneal or haemodialysis or renal transplant.

Complications affecting the nerves (neuropathy)

Nerve fibres are made of very long and thin cells, which can be affected after many years of diabetes. Damage to the blood vessels supplying the nerve fibres results in a decreased supply of oxygen. This causes injury to the insulating covering (myelin sheath) of the nerve and ultimately results in poorer nerve impulses. This can lead to loss of sensation and/or pain. The longest nerves are the most vulnerable, so problems arise primarily in the feet. Later on, this loss of sensation can progress up the legs. The fingers may eventually be affected by numbness, and people with this problem find difficulty in picking up small objects and doing up buttons.

Treatment: loss of sensation

This condition is painless and may only come to light when the feet are examined at the annual review. In other words, people are not usually aware that they have lost sensation. However, it is a potentially serious condition since it removes the warning that people receive when their feet are being damaged, for example if a new pair of shoes is causing a blister. People with loss of sensation in their feet must have regular foot checks and follow the specialist advice they are given regarding footwear.

Treatment: pain due to nerve damage

Unlike loss of sensation, this can be a very distressing condition. The type of pain people describe is very variable but tends to be like the effect of stinging nettles. It normally affects both feet or legs symmetrically, and is typically worse when resting – especially when you are trying to get to sleep at night.

There are a number of drugs which can ease neuropathic pain. The first tablets your doctor will probably try are duloxetine or amitriptyline. These were both developed as anti-depressants but were found to have pain-relieving properties. If these fail or cause unacceptable side effects, your doctor could try gabapentin or pregabalin. These were originally developed to treat epilepsy, but can often help to relieve this unpleasant neuropathic pain.

The autonomic nervous system

The autonomic nervous system controls those parts of the body which are not under our direct control and which tend to work automatically without us being aware of them – until something goes wrong. The autonomic nerves control the digestive system, bladder and sexual functions, the heart and blood vessels, the sweat glands and the eyes. Because the autonomic nervous system normally does its work without us even being aware of it, it is usually very hard to cope when it fails to work normally. Any item on the above list may be present to a minor or severe degree, and sometimes the severity may vary from one day to the next. For instance, a mild degree of indigestion can be helped with an antacid purchased over the counter. However, if the nerves to the stomach are completely destroyed, the stomach becomes paralysed and behaves like a floppy bag. This prevents the normal passage of food into the gut, causing a delay in absorption, which slows conversion of food to glucose. This condition (called gastroparesis) can make it impossible to control diabetes, especially in those who have an injection of insulin before each meal. Because the absorption of food is completely unpredictable, it is impossible to make the normal calculations about the type of food and the dose of insulin.

Various forms of treatment, such as antibiotics, have been tried for gastroparesis with variable results. In the last few years, specialist centres have treated this problem by injecting botulinum toxin into the muscles at the outlet of the stomach. Early results of this procedure are promising. If you have this rare complication, you may be advised to delay your mealtime insulin injection until 30–60 minutes after your meal.

Other consequences of autonomic neuropathy are listed in the box on the next page. They are very rarely a problem in Type 2 diabetes, apart from sexual problems, which are discussed in Chapter 25.

Problems with the autonomic nervous system

Organ	Problem
Digestive system	Indigestion, heartburn, feeling bloated. Food sits in the stomach undigested and leads to vomiting later (gastroparesis). Diarrhoea, constipation, loss of control of the bowels.
Urinary system	Passing small amounts of urine frequently. Leaking urine. Loss of urge to pass urine when the bladder is full.
Sexual function	Inability to maintain an erection (men). Vaginal dryness (women).
Heart and blood vessels	Feeling dizzy with low blood pressure on standing up. Feeling faint on changing position. Heart beating rapidly at rest.
Sweat glands	Increased sweating, especially at night or when eating. Reduced sweating, even when hot. Dry skin on the feet.
Eyes	Hard to adjust when going from bright to dark. Difficulty night driving.

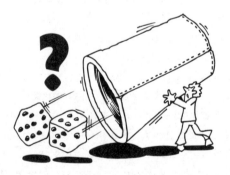

Many people believe that complications strike randomly among the population with diabetes. Others feel that it will not matter whether or not you 'manage well', complications will strike anyway. In fact, modern research has clearly shown that the degree of long-term complications depends directly upon the blood glucose levels over the course of the years that a person has diabetes.

Other consequences of autonomic neuropathy are listed in the box above. They are very rarely a problem in Type 2 diabetes, apart from sexual problems, which are discussed in Chapter 25.

Avoiding complications: the evidence

There is good evidence from the UKPDS that controlling both blood pressure and blood glucose has profound effects on the risk of developing microvascular complications. This study showed that for every 1% reduction in HbA_{1c}, there was a 37% fall in the risk of microvascular complication. Blood pressure control also helped microvascular complications – with a 13% reduction for every 10 mmHg fall in blood pressure.

The Steno-2 study from Denmark investigated the effect of controlling risk factors to the best possible extent in patients with Type 2 diabetes. By working hard to improve HbA_{1c}, blood pressure, cholesterol and lifestyle, patients in this study reduced their risk of microvascular complications by 60%.

A number of studies have shown that a particular class of drugs, the renin–angiotensin system drugs, ACE inhibitors and ARBs, are particularly valuable at protecting the kidneys from microvascular complications. Most clinicians now recommend ACE inhibitors or ARBs as the first-choice blood pressure-lowering drugs.

32

Problems with feet

With the onset of Type 2 diabetes, you can no longer take your feet for granted. In the past, you could do whatever you wanted on or to your feet and be confident that they would recover with a bit of rest. Diabetes, however, may cause changes to your feet which put them at risk of permanent damage and, in particular, ulceration. It is effective, simple and cheap to check your feet every day, and to follow the advice laid out in this chapter.

Why do foot problems happen?

You need to be particularly careful if the sensation of your feet is reduced. Up to 80% of people with foot ulcers have a previous history of peripheral neuropathy. This causes loss of sensation, predominantly in the feet, due to damage to the nerve endings responsible for light touch, pain and other sensations. Autonomic neuropathy affects nerves that operate automatically outside our direct control. This includes regulation of the blood supply to the skin and control of sweating. Damage to the autonomic nerves results in reduced sweating which can lead to dry and cracked skin, providing an entry route for infection.

Nerves which control the way our muscles work (motor nerves) can also be affected by diabetes, leading to motor neuropathy. This can lead to abnormalities in the shape of the feet, clawing of the toes and problems with callus (hard skin) formation under areas of increased pressure. Ill-fitting shoes may add to the pressure and increase the risk of ulceration.

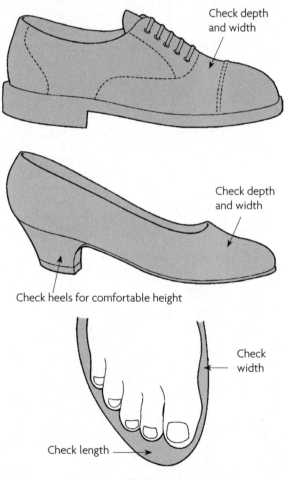

Check depth and width

Check depth and width

Check heels for comfortable height

Check width

Check length

Always check the fitting of your shoes very carefully. Ill-fitting shoes can damage your feet.

Foot problems can also occur as a result of poor blood supply to the feet because of narrowing of the arteries. This is called peripheral vascular disease. Around 45% of patients with foot ulcers have problems with the arteries in their legs. This is why the blood supply to the feet should be assessed at the annual physical check for people with diabetes.

Minimizing the risk of foot problems

Even if you have no nerve damage and a normal blood supply to the feet, you must take care of your feet. Neuropathy is related to poor control of blood glucose so by keeping your diabetes under good control, you can reduce the likelihood of developing neuropathy in the future. Vascular disease is

The major complications of diabetes causing foot problems

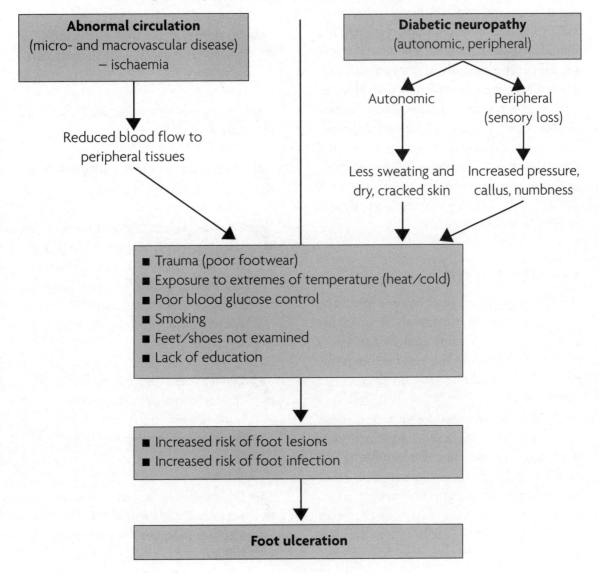

related to the cluster of risk factors: insulin resistance, blood pressure, high cholesterol and to a lesser extent blood glucose. Smoking forms a deadly duo with diabetes to accelerate and accentuate the risk of a number of complications (see Chapters 30 and 31) so you should try to give this up. You should follow medical advice concerning treatment with a statin and for blood pressure.

If your doctor or diabetes nurse tells you that your feet are at risk, what should you do? You should find out why they think your feet are at extra risk, which is likely to be either reduced sensation or poor blood supply. You should be under the care of a podiatrist, a foot specialist who can advise on care of nails, general foot hygiene and help with appropriate footwear. Your podiatrist should see you regularly, and you should follow his or her advice about footwear, foot inspection and general foot care. The podiatrist will probably give you a contact number so you can seek advice if you have any worries, such as pain or discoloration in your feet.

Treating foot ulcers

If you develop a foot ulcer, no time should be wasted in starting treatment. A specialist podiatrist must examine your feet to assess the depth of the ulcer. You may need an X-ray of your foot to rule out any involvement of the bone. If there are signs of infection, a swab will be sent to identify the exact bacterium responsible. This will help your doctor to choose the best antibiotic for treating you. If there is a serious foot infection, you may need antibiotics given into a drip (intravenously), which is the most reliable way of getting antibiotics to the ulcer in the highest concentration. In the past, intravenous antibiotics could only be given in hospital, but many areas now employ specialist nurses who can visit people at home and administer antibiotics by this route.

FOOT CARE RULES
Dos

Do wash your feet daily with soap and warm water. Do not use hot water – check the temperature of the water with your elbow.

Do dry your feet well with a soft towel; be especially gentle between your toes.

Do apply a gentle skin cream, such as E45, if your skin is rough and dry.

Do change your socks or tights daily and keep them in good repair.

Do wear well-fitting shoes. Make sure they are wider, deeper and longer than your foot, with a good firm fastening that you have to undo to get your foot in and out. This will prevent your foot from moving inside the shoe.

Do run your hand around the inside of your shoes each day before putting them on to check that there is nothing that will rub your feet.

Do 'wear in' new shoes for short periods of time and check your feet afterwards to see if the shoe has rubbed or pinched your feet.

Do cut your toenails to follow the shape of the end of your toes, not deep into the corners. This is easier after a bath as your toenails will soften in the warm water.

Do check your feet daily and see your podiatrist or doctor about any problems.

Do see a registered podiatrist if in any doubt about foot care.

FOOT CARE RULES
Don'ts

Do not soak your feet.

Do not put your feet on hot-water bottles or sit too close to a fire or radiator. Avoid extremes of cold and heat.

Do not use corn paints or plasters or attempt to cut your own corns with knives or razors in any circumstances.

Do not neglect even slight injuries to your feet.

Do not walk barefoot.

Do not let your feet get dry and cracked. Use E45 or hand lotion to keep the skin soft. Avoid putting moisturiser between the toes.

Do not cut your toenails too short or dig down the sides of your nails.

Do not smoke.

Seek advice immediately if you notice any of the following:

- Any colour change in your legs or feet.

- Any discharge from a break or crack in the skin, from a corn or from beneath a toenail.

- Any swelling, throbbing or signs of inflammation (redness or heat) in any part of your foot.

Any infection is likely to cause blood glucose levels to rise, and it is important to try and control them as high sugars will promote the infection. Swelling should be kept under control, usually by resting the foot and keeping it up as much as possible. Even when there is a serious foot infection involving the bone, there may be very little pain because of nerve damage.

Any dead tissue around the ulcer will interfere with the healing process, and the podiatrist will remove as much of this as possible – a process called debridement. Occasionally, an infection may be too deep and entrenched to be eradicated by antibiotic treatment and debridement. In such severe cases, some degree of amputation may be necessary and the surgeon will only remove part of your foot if there is absolutely no hope of recovery. An amputation is a frightening experience. Your doctor or surgeon should discuss this with you honestly and supportively.

If the ulcer is partly or entirely due to poor circulation, you will have tests to identify the exact cause. The first test will be a colour Doppler, which will provide information about the site and degree of the narrowing of the blood vessels. If the results are positive, the next test will be an angiogram, where a small tube is threaded into the artery.

Depending on the findings, it may be possible to reduce the block by mechanically widening the artery. This procedure is called an angioplasty. Alternatively, the surgeon may decide to carry out a bypass operation, using a graft to restore the blood supply to your foot.

Looking after your feet: first aid measures

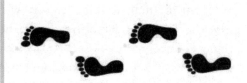

- Minor injuries can be treated at home provided that professional help is sought if the injury does not improve quickly.

- Minor cuts and abrasions should be cleaned gently with cotton wool or gauze and warm salt water. A clean dressing should be lightly bandaged in place.

- If blisters occur, do not prick them. If they burst, dress them as for minor cuts.

- Never use strong medicaments such as iodine.

- Never place adhesive strapping directly over a wound: always apply a dressing first.

Charcot foot

Charcot foot is a rare complication of Type 2 diabetes. It only occurs in people who already have a significant degree of nerve damage.

The symptoms normally arise following minor trauma. The foot is often painful and is always swollen, warm and red. It is a serious condition, which if diagnosed late and not treated properly will lead to severe deformity of the foot. This in turn causes disability and the likelihood of future ulceration.

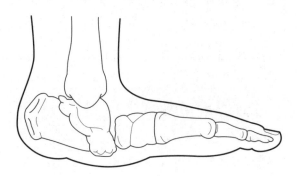

Deformity in a Charcot foot.

Because it is a rare condition, many doctors are unaware that this is the likely diagnosis if someone with diabetes comes to see them with a warm, swollen, red and painful foot. A podiatrist specialising in diabetes will be able to make the diagnosis and start the correct treatment. First, there should be a careful examination of the foot, with measurement of the temperature difference between the feet. The Charcot process can only develop in the presence of a good blood supply and when there is already nerve damage. The foot should be X-rayed, which may reveal a fracture of one or more of the long bones in the foot.

Without proper treatment, the warmth and redness of the foot will return to normal, but with continued walking, the arch will collapse and the foot take on a convex shape giving it a rocker-bottom appearance. This is unsightly, interferes with normal mobility and exposes the foot to risk of ulceration.

Treatment consists of immobilisation of the foot with either a plaster cast or a special boot, designed to provide total support and maintain the normal shape of the foot. The active process lasts from 3 to 9 months, and throughout this period, it is important to rest as much as possible and to retain the normal shape of the foot by immobilization.

33

Associated diseases

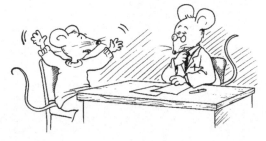

Type 2 diabetes has a different underlying cause from Type 1 diabetes and conditions associated with these two types of diabetes are also very different. Type 1 diabetes is an autoimmune disease, and thus people with this condition are at risk of other auto-immune conditions such as thyroid disease or coeliac disease. Type 2 diabetes is caused by insulin resistance, which is at the root of a number of other conditions all of which are related to Type 2 diabetes. In this chapter, we discuss conditions similar to simple Type 2 diabetes, and diseases in which diabetes occurs as a secondary phenomenon.

- Diseases associated with Type 2 diabetes are very different from those associated with Type 1 diabetes.

- Insulin resistance is associated with cardiovascular disease.

Insulin resistance

Insulin resistance occurs many years before the onset of Type 2 diabetes and indeed does not always progress to diabetes and raised blood sugars. We believe that insulin resistance is caused by increased storage of fat in the central portion of the body, particularly around the gut and the internal organs. This central fat is very poor at storing lipids called triglycerides, which are an energy source, so the level of triglycerides in the blood begins to rise. Central fat also produces a number of chemicals that promote a rise in the blood pressure. Thus, people who carry a lot of weight around their middle tend to have high blood pressure and high levels of fats including cholesterol and triglyeride. The high blood fats lead to insulin resistance, so that more insulin is needed to maintain the normal sugar levels in the body. Chronic inflammation may occur inside the blood vessels, leading to atherosclerosis or narrowing of the arteries. Insulin resistance may cause gout, which supports the view that gout is a 'disease of good living'.

Features of the metabolic syndrome

- Central obesity.
- Raised triglycerides.
- Raised LDL cholesterol.
- Low HDL cholesterol (the protective form).
- High blood pressure.
- Insulin resistance.
- Abnormal glucose metabolism/ Type 2 diabetes.

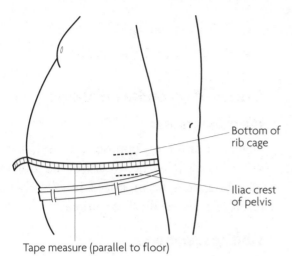

Tape measure (parallel to floor)

Bottom of rib cage

Iliac crest of pelvis

Carrying a lot of fat around your middle can put you at risk of developing the metabolic syndrome. The illustration shows you how to measure your waist. You are at risk of developing metabolic syndrome (and therefore Type 2 diabetes) if your waist is above 102 cm (40 inches) if you are a white man, 88 cm (35 inches) if you are an Asian man or a white woman, or 80 cm (32 inches) if you are an Asian woman.

If, as a result of insulin resistance, the pancreas is unable to produce enough insulin, sugar levels will drift upwards until diabetes develops. This combination of central obesity, high blood pressure, abnormalities of triglycerides and cholesterol and abnormal glucose tolerance is known as 'the metabolic syndrome'.

Problems associated with insulin resistance

In addition to the problems mentioned above, insulin resistance may be related to other important medical conditions, including polycystic ovarian syndrome (PCOS), non-alcoholic steatohepatitis (NASH) and acanthosis nigricans.

The best way to reduce insulin resistance is to lose weight. The glitazone class of drugs lower blood sugar levels by reducing insulin resistance, but unfortunately these also lead to weight increase, which can be very dispiriting to people who are being encouraged to lose weight on medical grounds.

Polycystic ovarian syndrome (PCOS)

PCOS is a condition affecting women, which causes:

- Irregular periods;
- Reduced fertility;
- High testosterone levels;
- Excess body hair.

Most, but not all, women with this condition are overweight with central obesity. Treatment with metformin, which is known to improve insulin resistance, may have a dramatic effect and lead to restoration of normal periods and facilitate pregnancy. Metformin is not particularly effective at reducing body hair.

Non-alcoholic steatohepatitis (NASH)

This is a potentially serious condition, in which excess fat is stored in the liver. This leads to enlargement of the liver and occasionally pain in the right side of the abdomen. Simple liver blood tests are raised and an ultrasound shows the typical appearance of fatty liver. However, the only way of proving the diagnosis is to do a liver biopsy. NASH may progress to cause permanent liver damage (cirrhosis), although this process takes many years. People with NASH usually have central obesity and other markers of insulin resistance.

There is no proven treatment for NASH but pioglitazone, which reduces insulin resistance, may be helpful.

Acanthosis nigricans

In this condition, the skin becomes thickened and dark with a velvety appearance. This is seen mainly at the back of the neck and in the skin folds – armpits and groin. It also affects pressure areas such as the elbows and knuckles. It is found in people with central obesity and indicates insulin resistance and hence an increased risk of Type 2 diabetes. Skin tags are often found in the same patient.

Maturity onset diabetes of the young (MODY)

This condition was first described about 40 years ago and, more recently, has been the subject of research which has taught us a great deal about the causes of Type 2 diabetes. People with MODY develop Type 2 diabetes in their teens or 20s and are not usually overweight. It is a genetic disease and affects many people in the same family. There are at least six different types of MODY, but the most common variant can usually be controlled with sulphonylurea tablets. At the time of diagnosis, many people with MODY are assumed to have Type 1 diabetes because they are young and not overweight. They are therefore started on insulin. Once the true diagnosis has been made, however, they can often be successfully switched to treatment with a sulphonylurea. (More information about MODY can be found in Chapter 22, Type 2 diabetes and younger people.)

Consider MODY if you:

- Are thin;
- Are young;
- Have a strong family history;
- Present with Type 2 diabetes.

Causes of secondary diabetes

Hormonal causes

Several hormones oppose the action of insulin, and two of these (cortisol and growth hormone) may be produced in excess as a result of other medical conditions.

Cushing's syndrome

This is a condition in which the body produces extra amounts of adrenal steroid hormone (cortisol) which is known to have a strong anti-insulin effect. In addition to diabetes, people with untreated Cushing's syndrome have high blood pressure and are overweight with a rounded 'moon' face.

Acromegaly

This is caused by overproduction of growth hormone due to a tumour in the pituitary gland, which lies at the base of the skull. This causes enlargement of the jaw, hands and feet and a number of other medical problems including high blood pressure and arthritis. Diabetes often seems to persist even when the underlying problem has been treated.

Pancreatic disease and pancreatitis

Any condition which causes damage to the pancreas may lead to diabetes. Pancreatitis is an inflammation of the pancreas which leads to a release of digestive juices into the abdomen. The most common causes of pancreatitis are gallstones and excess alcohol consumption. It is not an easy condition to treat and often recurs. Each attack causes further permanent injury to the pancreas, which eventually becomes so damaged that it can produce neither pancreatic juice nor the hormones insulin and glucagon. At this stage, the person will develop diabetes and, in addition to treatment with insulin, they are likely to require replacement of pancreatic enzymes to allow the normal digestion of food.

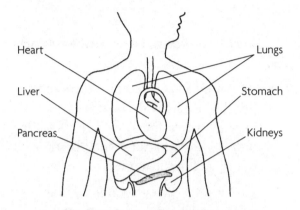

Any condition that damages your pancreas may lead to diabetes.

Haemachromatosis

This inherited condition also causes damage to the pancreas. In haemochromatosis, the body is unable to deal normally with iron, and there are high levels of iron in the blood. This is deposited in various parts of the body including the skin, joints and pancreas. After many years, the pancreas is destroyed by the iron and diabetes occurs. If diagnosed early, haemochromatosis can be treated simply by taking off a pint of blood every few weeks or months. The condition runs in families and it is important to screen family members so those with the condition can be treated early and the unpleasant consequences avoided.

34

Type 2 diabetes in later life

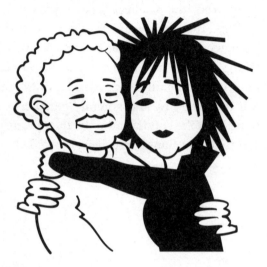

Management of Type 2 diabetes in later life needs to take into account not only the benefits of good diabetes control, but also the overall health of the individual. There is no point striving to achieve good blood glucose levels for long-term benefit if another health problem, for example heart failure or breathing problems, means that life expectancy is reduced and the treatment for diabetes is having an adverse effect on overall wellbeing. For this reason, it is sometimes wise to relax blood glucose targets and aim only to keep the person free of symptoms of either high or low blood glucose levels. Deciding on the level of blood glucose control you want to aim for, and the lengths you are prepared to go to in order to achieve the target can be quite difficult and is something you may want to discuss with your doctor or nurse.

Some questions you may need to consider are:

● Do I want to take several tablets and possibly insulin with the risk of hypoglycaemia and other side effects, in order to protect against complications of diabetes in the future ?

● Do I want to do everything I can to protect myself against diabetes-related ill health in the future?

This chapter examines the treatment targets for an older population, specific drug side effects, and the needs of particular groups such as those older people who are living with special support in a nursing home.

Best possible blood glucose levels

If possible, you should still aim to get your average blood level, as measured by HbA_{1c}, down to around 58 mmol/mol (7.5%). There is some evidence that aiming for lower targets (HbA_{1c} less than 48 mmol/mol or 6.5%) or trying to achieve good control after years of high blood glucose levels, may actually increase the risk of death – possibly as a result of hypoglycaemia (see Chapter 36, Outcome studies for more information.) However, the UKPDS (see page 256) suggested that there was a delay of several years before good glucose control led to a benefit in terms of reduced complications.

Many older people find it very straight-forward to achieve good control without any particular hardship, and there is some evidence from Australia that older people with diabetes tend to have lower HbA_{1c} results. However, some people simply do not wish to make the attempt to achieve good control, especially if this involves giving themselves insulin. Studies have shown that, in older people, high blood sugars or repeated episodes of low blood sugar are associated with a worsening of memory problems. This is clearly an incentive to keep the blood sugar as normal as possible, provided you can do this without risking hypoglycaemia. How-ever, if you have a lot of other medical problems, live alone, don't have easy access to help when needed, you might want to run your blood sugars at a higher level to ensure that you do not become hypoglycaemic. This is perfectly understandable and it is worth discussing your fears and difficulties with your doctor or diabetes nurse.

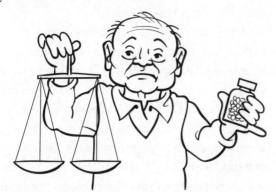

Most older patients find a compromise.

Glucose-lowering drugs: which is best for you?

Metformin

As discussed in Chapter 13, metformin has good data to show it reduces cardiovascular complications. It is now the first-choice drug for treating Type 2 diabetes. There are, however, some problems with metformin. It should not be used if you have kidney failure, which is more likely in older people. It is also associated with side effects particularly nausea, abdominal bloating, flatulence and diarrhoea. If you can take it, metformin is the best choice, but because of side effects, it may not be an option for significant numbers of older patients.

Sulphonylureas

The main difficulty with sulphonylureas is the risk of hypoglycaemia (low blood sugar). This is a particular worry when patients are taking a long-acting sulphonylurea such as gliben-clamide. If you are taking this drug, you should suggest to your GP that your pre-scription is changed to another class of anti-diabetes drug or a short-acting sulpho-nylurea. The likelihood of suffering a low blood sugar is increased if you have kidney failure, as sulphonylureas are eliminated from the body by the kidneys and this process is protracted if the kidneys are not working properly. If you have been found to have this problem, your doctor may need to reduce your daily dose. Your risk of developing hypoglycaemia is increased if you miss a meal or work hard in your garden.

Gliptins and GLP-1 analogues

Both these classes of drug can be used in older people and there are no special concerns. The advantage is that they do not cause hypoglycaemia or lead to weight gain. Gliptins can be considered for anyone who is not achieving the target blood glucose on metformin alone or if metformin is not tolerated. GLP-1 agonists can only be used in patients who are overweight (BMI greater than 35) but can be effective in this group of patients. For more information about these treatments see Chapter 13.

Pioglitazone

Pioglitazone can be useful in older people as it reduces insulin resistance and does not cause hypoglycaemia. However, it does cause fluid retention and increased risk of heart failure. As heart failure is more common in older people, pioglitazone should be used with great caution. There is also a suggestion that there may be an increased risk of bladder cancer with pioglitazone but this is still being assessed.

Insulins

Many older patients are scared of the idea of going on to insulin therapy, and no one enjoys the prospect of injecting themselves and doing regular blood tests. However, with modern blood testing devices and pens for injection, most people find this acceptable. The important thing to realise is that high blood glucose levels can have a significant impact on how you feel and many people who decide to make the change to insulin because of high glucose levels say they did not realise how much better they would feel if their blood glucose were lower. A high blood glucose can make you feel tired and lacking in energy, something which may be attributed to age rather than uncontrolled diabetes. Thirst and frequent passing of urine can disturb sleep and contribute to fatigue. Infections are more common and can be more difficult to shake off. There are good reasons for making sure that the blood glucose is not high enough to lead to symptoms, and if insulin is the best way of achieving control, age should not be a barrier to using it.

The major concern with insulin in the older patient – as with younger people – is hypoglycaemia. Severe hypoglycaemia, defined as needing help from a third party, occurs in less than 1% of patients per year, and a low blood glucose which the patient can correct on their own occurs in less than 5% per year. However, there is no doubt that these risks are higher in older people. Studies have shown that knowledge of the symptoms of hypoglycaemia is very poor in old people. There is also evidence that the symptoms themselves are different in the elderly. The usual complaint is lightheadedness and unsteadiness and they may not realise that they are hypo. This means that the main aim of blood glucose control in older people should be to keep the sugar levels within a reasonable range – often between 5-15 mmol/L – so that both high and low blood sugar levels can be avoided. If the HbA_{1c} is below 58–64 mmol/mol, this may mean that the risk of hypos is too high.

If you live alone and are becoming frail, hypoglycaemia can represent a real threat to your independence. It is worth talking to your GP or diabetes nurse about ways of avoiding the dangers of a low blood glucose, such as making sure a snack is near to hand, and identifying what support is available. Inevitably, to avoid the risk of low blood sugar, many patients allow their blood glucose targets to float upwards. Newer insulins may be used to reduce the risk of low blood sugars. In particular, the long-acting analogues (Lantus and Levemir) reduce the risk of night-time hypos.

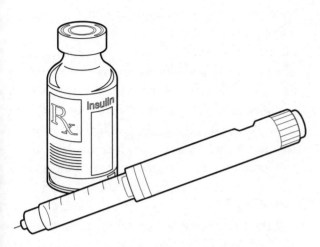

Management of other risk factors if you are older

Aspirin therapy

As discussed on page 221, there is good evidence for the use of aspirin treatment in older patients. A number of large studies have proven the benefit of using aspirin. These include the HOT study, the Early Treatment Diabetic Retinopathy study and a big meta-analysis (where researchers lump a number of trials together) called the Anti-Platelet Trialists Collaboration, all of which have shown positive benefits in the aspirin treated group. There are of course risks of bleeding which may be higher in the older patient, so if you have uncontrolled high blood pressure or a history of stomach ulcers or persistent indigestion, you should discuss the question of aspirin with your doctor or diabetes nurse. In most cases, the benefits of aspirin in reducing cardiovascular events outweigh the risks.

You should also talk to your diabetes nurse or doctor about the number of insulin injections that would be the best for you. As a rule, the more frequently you inject insulin, the easier it is to tailor the dose to your needs and adjust the dose in response to your blood glucose level, your food intake, your energy levels and the timing of meals. However, many older people find constant adjustment of the insulin dose difficult and confusing and may even forget to take the insulin. It might be more attractive just to give a fixed dose of insulin once or twice a day and try to live your life round this. This is a decision you have to make yourself, and your diabetes nurse or doctor should be keen to have this debate with you.

Finally, you may be partially sighted, have arthritis, have had a previous stroke or have another disability which affects your ability to do glucose monitoring or manage the insulin injections. A number of aids do now exist, including a 'speaking' glucose monitor and devices which help you fix the pen or injector to a particular spot. A district nurse may be able to visit to give your insulin injections if you are unable to manage this yourself.

Blood pressure control

It is important not to over treat high blood pressure as this will lead to dizziness and make walking a problem. As a general rule, older patients are less tolerant of tablets used to reduce blood pressure and usually do better with small doses. However, several studies have shown that controlling blood pressure in the elderly reduces the risk of heart attack and stroke.

Reducing cholesterol in older adults

Very few clinical trials have been carried out in patients over 80 years of age and there is some disagreement among experts about the value of treating older people with statins. The few studies that have recruited octogenarians have shown that statins are of benefit in lowering the risk of heart attack, although an observational study showed that statin therapy did not seem to have a positive effect in those over 80 years of age. So the jury's out.

There is some evidence that a low dose of a statin might provide some protection with very little risk of side effects. However, you should of course discuss this with your doctor or practice nurse.

Management of erectile dysfunction if you're older

Unfortunately, it seems that problems with maintaining an erection are associated with both Type 2 diabetes and increasing age. It's estimated that between 50 and 95% of men aged above the age of 60 years have some problems with their erections. Sex may well still be an important part of your life, and problems with performance can be distressing for you and your partner. Before your GP or health professional can arrange treatment for you though, it's important to assess any risk factors for vascular disease. Unfortunately, erectile dysfunction often goes hand in hand with cardiovascular problems, and angina or ischaemic heart disease can restrict access for you to tablet treatments for erection problems such as Viagra or Cialis. The good news is that there are a number of possible treatments which may suit you; these include vacuum constriction devices to help you achieve erection, injections into the side of the penis and administering medication down the urethra to name a few options (see also Chapter 25). The difficult thing is talking about it, and once you've managed that, the rest is a great deal easier.

Diabetes foot care

Unfortunately, foot problems related to diabetes contribute significantly to the tribulations of older people with Type 2 diabetes. Old age is a risk factor for diabetic foot problems and also increases the risk of the main causes of foot ulcers, namely poor blood supply and nerve damage. Other risk factors include limited mobility, smoking, alcohol consumption and bony deformities. It is important that you educate yourself about the factors that lead to foot problems and act upon them. Your feet should be examined every time you consult for your diabetes. If you have any risk factors for diabetic foot problems, you should be looked after by a specialist foot team, either in the hospital clinic or in the community. More information about foot problems in diabetes can be found in Chapter 32.

Diabetes in a care home

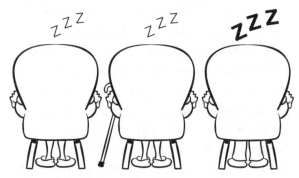

People with diabetes form a significant proportion of the population in most care homes. The average is about 25% and there may be a number of others with diabetes in whom the diagnosis has not been made.

Traditionally, people with Type 2 diabetes who live in a care home have less stringent diabetes care than people in their own home. As people with diabetes become older, they may no longer be able to make self-management decisions and the combination of diabetes and dementia is particularly challenging. This may affect all aspects of diabetes care including food choices and medication. Decision-making naturally falls on care home staff, who may be poorly equipped to take on this role. This is frequently due to a lack of knowledge on the part of staff. Studies have shown that intervention with a diabetes education programme designed for care home staff improves the standard of care. The Institute of Diabetes for Older People (IDOP) has identified the need to train people working in care homes in the combined management of diabetes and dementia and the organization is developing educational programmes to address this need.

IDOP has produced a set of "pocket cards" which provide succinct information about diabetes focused on management in older people. Examples of some of the content of the pocket cards are illustrated here.

General rules

The main reason for satisfaction among people in residential accommodation is that normal human activities are maintained. If residents are engaged in conversation, kept as active as possible, receive good nutrition and are not allowed to become dehydrated, their quality of life will be high. On the other hand, if any or all of these are missing, the resident will become inert, distressed, un-cooperative and generally unhappy.

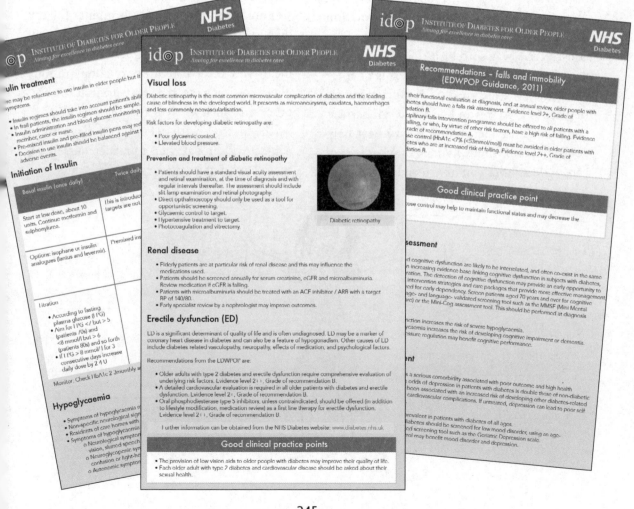

35

Support and information

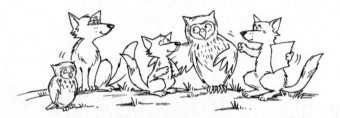

Once you have been told that you have Type 2 diabetes, you will have to take on responsibility for this for the rest of your life. There is plenty of support and information available to help you deal with this in a constructive way so that it does not disrupt your life or cause you distress. This chapter looks at what structures and organizations are in place to help you and how you can harness your time and energy in order to best help yourself. We begin by looking at what sort of care and facilities you have a right to expect.

What care should you be getting from your primary care team?

Your GP and practice nurse will be responsible for your regular care. They should know you as an individual and be well placed to provide the help you need. They will see that you go onto the practice's register of patients with diabetes. This will ensure that you are given regular appointments for the diabetes clinic and appropriate additional screening. Being on this register should also mean you receive reminders about immunizations such as the 'flu vaccination and other care such as eye screening.

The person with whom you have most contact will probably be a practice nurse with special training in diabetes care. This nurse will

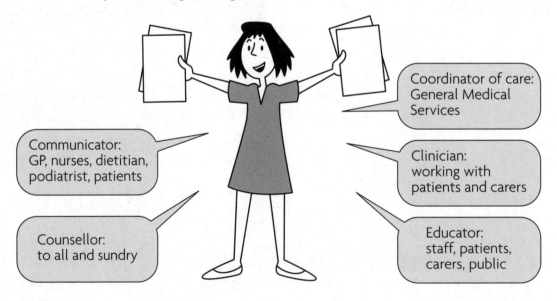

Coordinator of care:
General Medical
Services

Communicator:
GP, nurses, dietitian,
podiatrist, patients

Clinician:
working with
patients and carers

Counsellor:
to all and sundry

Educator:
staff, patients,
carers, public

be your main point of contact should you have any worries about your diabetes or any related issues, so you may find you come to know him or her very well in time. Indeed, the practice nurse with a special knowledge of diabetes will have links with all the other professionals with whom you are likely to come into contact, and will be well placed to provide you with a great deal of support as well as information. You should also be referred to a dietitian, a podiatrist (chiropodist) and a pharmacist as appropriate.

The practice nurse and GP at your health centre will have access to more specialist help if necessary. This will either come from the hospital diabetes team or possibly from a community diabetes team. Unfortunately, the NHS is in the throes of another period of drastic reorganization and different places will have their own ideas on how to provide specialist support for GPs and practice nurses who are working with people with diabetes. There is not meant to be a uniform pattern of care – no "One Size Fits All" and you will have to discover what system has been adopted by your local health commissioning group.

Finding help from other sources

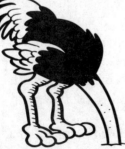

'Ostrich strategy', i.e. not caring about diabetes and not taking any responsibility for its management, is among the most dangerous things a person with diabetes can do. Your diabetes team can contribute with knowledge, tips and advice – but living with your diabetes is something only YOU can do.

People react in different ways to the shock of diabetes: some behave like an ostrich and pretend they don't have diabetes, while others set out to try to find out everything there is to know about diabetes within the first few weeks. Whatever your reaction, you should make contact with your local Diabetes UK group. You will come across people who are living with diabetes and who have learnt to cope with many of the daily problems. These people should provide an extra dimension to the information that you have been given by doctors, nurses, dietitians and other professionals.

Diabetes UK

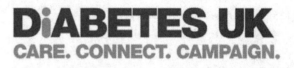

Diabetes UK (formerly the British Diabetic Association) was founded in 1935 by two people with diabetes, the author H.G. Wells, and Dr R.D. Lawrence, who worked at the diabetes clinic of King's College Hospital, London. In a letter to *The Times* dated January 1933, they announced their intention to set up an 'association open to all diabetics, rich or poor, for mutual aid and assistance, and to promote the study, the diffusion of knowledge, and the proper treatment of diabetes in this country'. They proposed that people with diabetes, members of the general public interested in diabetes, and doctors and nurses should be persuaded to join the projected association. Over 70 years later, Diabetes UK is a credit to its founders.

Diabetes UK now has more than 170,000 members and an income in 2011 of £30 million. In many countries, there are separate organizations for people with diabetes and for professionals, but Diabetes UK draws its strength from the fact that both interest groups are united in the same society.

Diabetes UK is the largest organization in the UK working for people with diabetes, funding research, campaigning and helping people to live with the condition. The Careline (0845 120 2960, Monday–Friday, 9am–5pm) offers confidential support and information on all aspects of diabetes. In order to make the Careline accessible to all, there is access to an interpreting service.

Diabetes UK currently supports over 120 research projects in all aspects of diabetes at a cost of nearly £6 million in 2012.

Diabetes UK
10 Parkway, London NW1 7AA
Helpline: 020 7424 1030/1000
Careline: 0845 120 2960
www.diabetes.org.uk

Publications

Up-to-date information and news is published in *Balance*, a magazine that appears every other month. *Diabetes for Beginners* is provided for newly diagnosed people, both Type 1 and Type 2 (insulin dependent and non-insulin dependent). Diabetes UK produces its own handbooks, leaflets and videotapes for teaching purposes and also sells those produced by other publishers. It constantly lobbies for high standards of care for those with diabetes. Diabetes UK also has an excellent website (see above).

Living with diabetes

Diabetes UK organizes 'living with diabetes' days. These are one-day conferences for people with diabetes, their carers, families and friends, giving an opportunity to talk to

healthcare professionals and people living with diabetes and to discover more about Diabetes UK. For more information contact the conference team at Diabetes UK, telephone 020 7424 1000.

Diabetes UK holidays

The first diabetes holidays for children in the UK took place in 1935, and these have grown into a large enterprise. During the summer, at several different sites throughout the UK, 250 children aged between 7 and 18 years enjoy a week away with Diabetes UK. These educational holidays are organized by the care interventions team, and they give the opportunity for children to meet others with diabetes and to become more independent of their parents. They aim to give the children a good time and encourage them to try new activities, while teaching them more about their diabetes and providing a well-earned break for their parents.

Diabetes UK family weekends

The care intervention team also organizes family weekends to include the parents of children with diabetes. These cater for about 200 families each year. While parents have talks and discussions from specialist doctors, nurses and dietitians, there are activities for children throughout the weekend that are supervised by skilled and experienced helpers.

Local Diabetes UK groups (previously called branches)

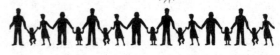

There are over 350 branches and parents' groups throughout the country. These are run entirely by volunteers, and because of their commitment millions of pounds are raised for research into diabetes each year. Diabetes UK groups also aim to increase public awareness of diabetes, and they arrange meetings for local people with diabetes and their families to offer support and information.

Parent support groups

The parents of children with diabetes often feel they have special needs – and that they can offer particular help to other parents in the same boat. Over 80 parent support groups exist throughout the UK, and these have added a sense of urgency to the main aim of Diabetes UK: to improve the lives of people with diabetes and to work towards a future without diabetes.

In addition to self-help, the parents' groups also raise money for research.

The care intervention team now runs a 'Parent-link', which is a network support system for the parents of children with diabetes that aims to put parents in touch via a gradually expanding database. Parent-link sends out a newsletter called *Link-Up* four times a year.

Insurance

Many people with diabetes experience discrimination in terms of increased premiums or restricted terms, and even have policies refused when taking out insurance. Faced with the general lack of understanding within the insurance market, Diabetes UK has negotiated its own exclusive schemes to provide policies suited to the needs of people with diabetes and those living with them. Diabetes UK Services offers competitively priced home and motor, travel and personal finance products. For details of home, travel and motor insurance, as well as personal

finance, telephone 0800 731 7431 (or e-mail diabetes@heathlambert.com).

Joining Diabetes UK

Diabetes UK works to influence the decisions made about living with diabetes, and the more members it has, the greater its influence can be. Diabetes UK cannot continue to provide its services and activities to all people with diabetes without your support. If you would like more information about joining Diabetes UK, contact the Supporter Development department on 0207 323 1531 or write to Diabetes UK at the address shown above.

Other useful organizations

Institute of Diabetes for Older People (IDOP)

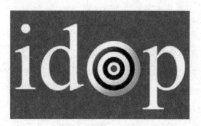

This was founded in 2008 by Professor Alan Sinclair, who is Director of the organization. IDOP has two principal aims:

- To enhance the quality of diabetes care for older people through new initiatives in clinical practice, audit, and research.

- To provide a forum for scientific interchange between health professionals and scientists, and involve people with diabetes and their carers and families, in educational programmes which directly promote their health and well-being.

IDOP has a useful website with an account of its activities. It is currently arranging a national audit of standards of care for diabetes in residential and nursing homes. It is working to set up a training programme for professionals who work in care homes and in domiciliary care about diabetes and dementia.

> **IDOP**
> **Putteridge Bury Campus**
> **Hitchin Road, Luton**
> **Bedfordshire LU2 8LE**
> **Tel: 01582 743285**
> **http://instituteofdiabetes.org**

International Society for Pediatric and Adolescent Diabetes

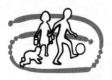

ISPAD is the only global (professional) advocate for children and adolescents with diabetes. It is an association for diabetes teams (doctors, nurses, dietitians, educators, psychologists and all others involved in the care of children with diabetes). The society is committed to promoting the best possible health, social welfare and quality of life for all children and adolescents with diabetes, anywhere in the world.

> **ISPAD**
> **www.ispad.org**

Juvenile Diabetes Research Foundation (JDRF)

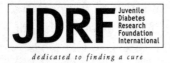

This organization was founded in 1970 by a small group of parents of children with diabetes. The JDRF exists to find a cure for diabetes and its complications. It supports diabetes all over the world and provides research funds at a level comparable to that provided by Diabetes UK.

> **JDRF**
> **19 Angel Gate, City Road,**
> **London EC1V 2PT**
> **Tel: 020 7713 2030**
> **www.jdrf.org.uk**

International Diabetes Federation (IDF)

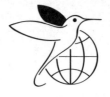

International Diabetes Federation

The IDF is open to members of all countries. It promotes diabetes interests in many different areas. An international conference is held every 3–4 years, with the two most recent being in South Africa (2006) and Montreal (2009). The 2013 conference was held in Melbourne in December 2013.

You can obtain more information about the IDF from your local diabetes association, or from the website at www.idf.org

Diabetes Ireland

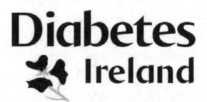

The aims of Diabetes Ireland are:

- To represent people with diabetes.
- To help and provide information for

people with diabetes, their families and the community.

- To create awareness and foster programmes for the early detection and prevention of diabetes.

- To support and encourage advances in diabetes care and research.

- To raise funds which will make the achievement of these aims possible.

The activities of the Federation include the dissemination of non-judgemental advice and information through meetings, its magazine (*Diabetes Ireland*) and by request. The Federation provides support through its telephone helpline and regular public meetings. It raises awareness of diabetes by running campaigns and actively lobbying on behalf of people with diabetes in areas where they are encountering discrimination, as well as for national service development. All the above activities are possible only through the close collaboration of all people concerned with diabetes, whether their interest arises through their work or through living was condition.

Diabetes Ireland
19 Northwood House,
Northwood Business Campus,
Santry, Dublin,
Republic of Ireland
Helpline: 1850 909 909
www.diabetes.ie

British Heart Foundation

This national charity funds research, promotes education and raises money to buy equipment to treat people with heart disease. Increasingly, it also provides information on preventing heart disease and heart attack, and staying as healthy as possible for as long as possible. The helpline HeartstartUK can arrange training in emergency life-saving techniques for lay people.

British Heart Foundation
Greater London House,
180 Hampstead Road,
London NW1 7AW
Helpline: 0300 330 3311
www.bhf.org.uk

National Kidney Federation (NKF)

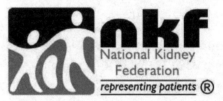

The NKF is a UK-wide charity run by kidney patients for kidney patients. While it used to be concerned almost solely with people with advanced or end-stage renal failure, there is now much more emphasis on people at earlier stages of kidney disease too. If you have even a mild form of kidney disease, the NKF can help you find information and support to keep your kidneys as healthy as possible for as long as possible.

Given the high numbers of people with diabetes who go on to develop some degree of kidney damage, it is important to be aware of this organization and what it has to offer.

National Kidney Federation
The Point, Coach Road, Shireoaks,
Worksop S81 8BW
Helpline: 0845 601 02 09
www.kidney.org.uk

RNIB

 supporting blind and partially sighted people

If you have microvascular complications affecting your eyes, you may want to be aware of this organization. The RNIB (founded as the Royal National Institute for the Blind) offers a range of information and advice on lifestyle changes and practical adaptations for people facing sight loss, and produces a mail order catalogue of useful aids. It also offers support and training in Braille.

RNIB
105 Judd Street, London WC1H 9NE
Helpline: 0303 123 9999
www.rnib.org.uk

The Stroke Association

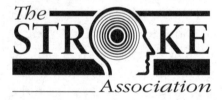

This UK-wide charity works to combat stroke in people of all ages, including people with diabetes. The Stroke Association funds research into prevention, treatment and better methods of rehabilitation. It also helps stroke patients and their families directly through its Rehabilitation and Support Services. These include Communication Support, Family and Carer Support, information services and welfare grants. The Association campaigns on behalf of people who are affected by stroke, and acts as a voice for its members.

The Stroke Association produces a number of publications including patient leaflets, *Stroke News* (a quarterly magazine) and information for health professionals.

The Stroke Association
240 City Road, London EC1V 2PR
Helpline: 0845 303 31 00
www.stroke.org.uk

Practical and financial support
Claiming benefits

Some people with diabetes may be eligible for disability benefits and incapacity benefits, depending on the effect that the condition has on their lives.

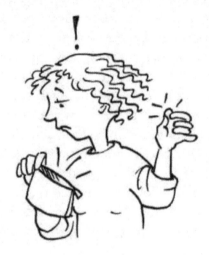

The benefit process is all up in the air at present as the Department of Work and Pensions introduced a new system called Universal Credit in 2013. This replaces the following benefits:

- Income-based Jobseeker's Allowance;
- Income-related Employment and Support Allowance;
- Income Support;
- Child Tax Credits;
- Working Tax Credits;
- Housing Benefit.

Universal Credit is designed to provide a simple system with the hope that it will "help claimants and their families to become more independent and will simplify the benefits system by bringing together a range of working-age benefits into a single stream-lined payment". There are anxieties about the system as it relies on a central IT system which may decide to behave like all large government computers. So far there have been negative comments in the press about this innovation. We will have to wait and see how people with disabilities related to diabetes are treated by the system of Universal Credit.

At the present time, you may be eligible for allowances such as Disability Living Allowance (DLA) and Attendance Allowance if you have a physical or mental disability, or need support from another person. However, the government is in the process of reforming the benefits system and changes are planned to these allowances. The proposals include a benefit cap (i.e. 'a limit on the total amount of benefit that most people aged 16–64 can get').

Disability benefits are mainly for people who need help in their daily lives. They might pay for some of the extra transport costs involved in not being able to drive, a cleaner or home help for a few hours a week, or some aids to help you in activities around the home. Your local Citizens Advice Bureau can check whether you are getting all the benefits to which you are entitled. They, as well as your diabetes specialist team, should also be able to provide advice on filling in the forms. Information on the benefits available can be obtained by calling your local benefits enquiry line or the Disability Benefits enquiry line on Freephone 0800 882 200.

It is very important to remember that you are not alone when it comes to applying for benefits, and these are not separate from your general care. If you are planning to apply for benefits, discuss this with your doctor or other healthcare professionals who look after you. They can often provide important supporting material about your diabetes, care of your condition and complications, all of which may increase your chances of a successful application for financial support.

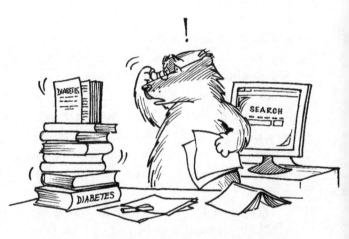

A number of benefits are also available for those affected by loss of vision. Details of these can be obtained from the RNIB. These may include qualification for Disability Living Allowance or reduced price services such as your TV licence. The RNIB website also has contact numbers to talk to an adviser about what further help may be available.

Prescription advice

If you have Type 2 diabetes and are treated with tablets or insulin, you are entitled to free prescriptions. You do need to apply for an exemption certificate though; the nurse, doctor or pharmacist will have a leaflet with details of how to apply.

If you have diabetes, you are entitled to free eye tests. Unfortunately, however, you are not entitled to free dental care. If you are entitled to benefits such as Income Support, you may be able to claim some help with the cost of dental treatment.

Reimbursed accessories

In most countries, insulin is available free of charge for people who need it for their diabetes. Syringes, pen injectors and needles are often either free or reimbursed as well. Other accessories such as indwelling catheters are reimbursed in some countries, though not in all. Sometimes the person with diabetes has to pay for blood glucose meters, while the sticks for testing are free or reimbursed. In the UK, blood testing meters are usually available free, but some funding bodies have insisted on people using a simple basic meter, which allows them to save money.

There have also been restrictions on the use of blood glucose meters by people with Type 2 diabetes. It is generally accepted that for a time after diagnosis, taking blood glucose measurements after eating certain foods and after activities may be a very useful way of learning about your diabetes. You should be able to make a good case for using a meter over a short period of time in order to answer a particular question but the routine use of glucose monitoring in Type 2 diabetes is becoming a thing of the past. If you take sulphonylureas (such as gliclazide) or insulin, it is essential that you can measure your blood glucose, especially when driving, because of the risk of hypoglycaemia.

Diabetes and the internet

There is a vast amount of diabetes information available on the internet. Be aware that information on the internet is often not reviewed by healthcare professionals and may only be the opinion of the person writing it. You need to judge information critically and discuss anything of interest with your diabetes nurse or doctor.

Associations

The associations listed below, can be trusted to produce reliable information.

Diabetes UK
www.diabetes.org.uk

Diabetes Federation of Ireland
www.diabetesireland.ie

American Diabetes Association (ADA)
www.diabetes.org

Diabetes Australia
www.diabetesaustralia.com.au

International Diabetes Federation (IDF)
www.idf.org

Juvenile Diabetes Research Federation (JDRF)
www.jdrf.org

Diabetes Exercise and Sports Association (DESA)
www.diabetes-exercise.org

Government departments

Department of Health
www.dh.gov.uk

National Institute for Health and Clinical Excellence (NICE)
www.nice.org.uk

Using the Internet

Both medical companies and institutions have home pages displaying information and news. Use one of the search services to find the type of information you are looking for.

Over the past few years, there has also been an explosion in interactive sites such as chat rooms, and this may be a way to make new friends who share some of your experiences in adjusting to life with diabetes.

Since internet pages are constantly being updated, and many change their addresses from time to time, we have chosen not to include more links in this book.

36

Outcome studies in Type 2 diabetes

The world of Type 2 diabetes care has evolved rapidly. The main reason for this is that a large number of outcome studies which have been completed over the past few years have provided information about the best way of caring for people with Type 2 diabetes. This chapter looks at some of the key studies and what they tell us. It also looks forward to studies reporting in the near future.

What is an 'outcome study'?

In any medical research project, it is important to define clearly what endpoints are being measured. In the United Kingdom Prospective Diabetes Study (UKPDS), hundreds of thousands of measurements were made during and after the study. Some of these looked at the effect of treatment on the blood glucose and the quality of life, but the most important findings were the actual medical problems (or outcomes) that affected patients in the study, such as heart attacks, laser therapy and, worst of all, death. Each endpoint was carefully checked independently by two separate adjudicators, and any disagreement was referred to a third arbitrator. So an outcome study examines what important events are prevented by a certain form of treatment, rather than just measuring differences in blood values, which do not affect people's lives in the same way.

More than 10,000 articles on diabetes research are produced every year. Many small advances have resulted, but so far these have been in treatment rather than cure.

Outcome studies looking at the effect of controlling blood glucose

UKPDS

This study reported in 1998, and informed us about the importance of keeping both blood sugar and blood pressure under good control. It looked at 3867 patients with newly diagnosed Type 2 diabetes and measured the effects of tight control of blood glucose versus less tight control. It also looked at 1148 patients with newly diagnosed Type 2 diabetes and hypertension, again measuring the effects of tight versus less tight blood pressure control.

What did it show?

After an averge of 15 years of patient follow-up, the study showed that for a difference of 0.9% in HbA_{1c} between the tight and the less tight groups for blood glucose control, there was a reduction in complications related to diabetes of 12%. Most of this was due to a 25% reduction in damage to the eyes and kidneys, known as microvascular events. The study also showed that the individuals taking metformin for lowering of blood glucose appeared to have fewer heart attacks and strokes than those taking other glucose-lowering treatments. The blood pressure study showed that a lowering of the blood pressure by 10/5 mmHg in the intensive blood pressure control group led to a 24% reduction in complications related to diabetes. This included a 32% reduction in deaths and a 44% reduction in strokes, to name just a couple of the benefits.

What does the UKPDS tell us?

The UKPDS established the need for metformin to be used first for the treatment of raised blood glucose as, compared with other treatments used for lowering blood glucose, it showed positive benefits in reducing the risk of cardiovascular disease. The UKPDS also showed that reducing both the blood glucose and blood pressure has a large benefit in reducing complications related to diabetes.

Doctors have responded to the results of the UKPDS by trying to get as many people as possible below the recommended targets for blood glucose and blood pressure.

Over the past few years, the UKPDS has continued to provide a valuable resource to study a number of other risk factors related to Type 2 diabetes and will continue to give us useful insights for many years to come.

Ten year follow-up of survivors of the UKPDS

At the end of the main UKPDS in 1998, it was decided to follow up the patients to discover whether there were any long-term effects of being in either the tight control group or the standard control group of the UKPDS. Within 12 months of the end of the study, the difference in HbA_{1c} between the two groups disappeared. This was because once they were out of the study, the less well controlled group were encouraged to get their HbA_{1c} down to the levels seen in the tight control group. Over the ten years after the patients left the study, the group that originally had tight control continued to have a reduced risk of all complications (by 24%) and fewer heart attacks (15%). This is described as the legacy effect of early tight blood glucose control. The group who were given metformin did even better and had a 33% lower risk of heart attack.

What does the UKPDS follow-up study tell us?

1. That a period of tight control of blood glucose from diagnosis and continued for up 15 years provides a lasting benefit for another 10 years, even if the tight control is relaxed.

2. Metformin protects against heart attacks and people treated with metformin from diagnosis maintain this reduced risk for many years.

Two contrasting studies published in 2008

1. ADVANCE study. This was a truly international study organized from Australia but including centres in

Canada, China, India, Malaysia, Philippines and New Zealand as well as 14 European countries including UK and Ireland. Over 10,000 patients were recruited into the study, which was designed to build on the results of the UKPDS and discover whether intensifying blood glucose with HbA_{1c} down to 6.5% (48 mmol/mol) would provide additional benefits. Like the UKPDS, there was also a blood pressure arm to the study to investigate whether routine blood pressure control carried further benefit. By the end of the study those in the intensive group were taking two tablets for their diabetes and less than 50% were also on insulin.

2. ACCORD study. This study was carried out in Canada and the USA and again more than 10,000 patients took part. The aim in this study was to aim at an even lower HbA_{1c} of 6% (42 mmol/mol) by using a large number of tablets and insulin. At least 75% of those in the intensive group were taking three different tablets and insulin in order to achieve this very low blood glucose.

What did these two studies tell us?

Patients in the intensive group of the ADVANCE had 10% fewer complications of diabetes and in particular, the risk of developing kidney problems was reduced by 21%. This was achieved at the expense of more hypos in the intensive group.

The ACCORD study on the other hand came up with findings which sent shockwaves through the diabetes world. The study was set up in the expectation that the intensive blood glucose control group would have less in the way of complications. In the event the opposite was true and the blood glucose arm of the study had to be stopped prematurely as there was a significantly increased risk of death in the intensive group. The actual numbers were 257 deaths over 3½ years in the intensive group and 203 in the standard treatment group over the same time period. This is a 22% increase and the risk of dying of a heart attack was 35% greater in the intensive group. Further analysis showed that the people at greatest risk of dying during the study were older patients (over rather than under 65 years) and those who entered the study with poor control (HbA_{1c} greater than 8%, 64 mmol/mol).

Effects of the ACCORD study

Once the surprising results of this study percolated through to advisory bodies such as NICE, they reduced the pressure to keep the HbA_{1c} as low as possible. NICE has raised the target HbA_{1c} from 6.5 to 7.5% (48–58 mmol/mol), and there has been an understanding among healthcare professionals that driving down the HbA_{1c} may not always be a good idea, especially in older people.

Veterans Diabetes Trial

The Veterans Diabetes Trial appeared in 2009 and the results come between those of ADVANCE and ACCORD. This was an all American study carried out in military veterans. The study included 1791 patients, much fewer than the 10,000 plus in ADVANCE and ACCORD. They had had diabetes for an average of 11 years and in many cases their control had not been good. The study lasted 5.6 years and during this time the intensive group had HbA_{1c} of 6.9%

(52 mmol/mol) compared with 8.4% (67 mmol/mol) for the standard group.

After this period of over 5 years, the intensive group had a similar risk of heart disease and of diabetic complications. However more people in the intensive group had hypos.

Conclusions from all blood glucose studies

- Tight control of blood glucose soon after diagnosis has a long-term beneficial effect in reducing complications.

- Metformin protects against heart attacks.

- Very tight blood glucose control (HbA$_{1c}$ of 6%) may be dangerous especially in the following groups:
  - those over 65
  - those with previously high HbA$_{1c}$ who are difficult to control
  - those with a long duration of diabetes (more than 10 years).

Outcome studies looking at control of blood pressure

UKPDS

The UKPDS was originally concerned only with blood glucose but a blood pressure arm was introduced and 1148 patients were recruited from the blood glucose part of the study to establish whether tight control of blood pressure reduced the risk of death and diabetic complications. Two different types of treatment for blood pressure were compared with standard treatment. Average blood pressure in the standard group was 154/87 and in both treatment groups was 144/82. The group with lower blood pressure had 32% fewer deaths, 37% less diabetic complications and 44% fewer strokes. Both types of treatment for blood pressure were equally effective.

UKPDS 30-year follow-up study

The UKPDS 30-year study also looked at the long-term effect of tight blood pressure control on the risk of future complications. Unlike the blood glucose study, in which the benefits of tight control during the study were sustained for 10 years after the end of the study, there was no legacy effect from initial tight blood pressure control and the benefits of early tight control were not maintained after the study had ended.

ADVANCE BP

11,140 patients in the ADVANCE study were treated with a particular blood pressure treatment (perindopril and indapamide), aiming at a blood pressure of less than 135 mmHg. The intensive group were followed for 4.3 years and over this time had the following benefits:

- 10% reduction in all diabetic complications.

- 21% reduction in kidney complications.

ACCORD-BP

In parallel with the ACCORD blood glucose which caused such a sensation, there was a study comparing intensive blood pressure control with standard treatment. Average blood pressure in the two groups was 119 and 134 mmHg. Thus the group with standard treatment had a lower blood pressure than the intensive group in the UKPDS which had taken place 20 years earlier. The findings of this blood pressure study were less exciting than the blood glucose arm of ACCORD. Tight blood pressure control had no effect on the overall death rate. However, as in all other studies, the risk of stroke was reduced by 40%.

Swedish National Register blood pressure study

This was an observational study making use of the comprehensive National Diabetes Register which is maintained in Sweden. In this study, 12,677 patients with Type 2 diabetes who were also taking treatment for blood pressure were followed for 5 years. Those with a blood pressure of less than 140 mmHg had a much lower risk of heart disease but there was no obvious benefit for taking the blood pressure below this level.

HOPE

The HOPE study examined the benefits of ramipril, an ACE inhibitor drug used for lowering blood pressure, in a mixed population of patients with and without Type 2 diabetes.

What did it show?

In total, 3577 people with diabetes were included in the study. They were randomized to ramipril 10 mg per day or placebo, and there was a 25% reduction in the risk of major cardiovascular events in the group taking ramipril. The study also showed that ramipril delayed the worsening of kidney disease due to diabetes.

What does this mean?

This study and a number of others using ACE inhibitors and the similar drugs called angiotensin-2 receptor blockers have shown positive effects on both cardiovascular events and a reduction in microalbuminuria – a marker of kidney disease. These drug classes now have a central place in the management of blood pressure and as part of a holistic strategy of managing Type 2 diabetes. As with statins, if you have diabetes you almost have to find a reason not to be taking one rather than look for a reason to start!

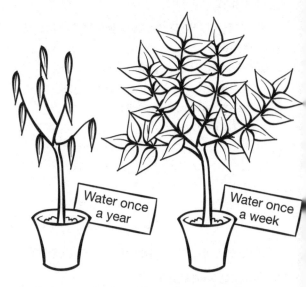

Water once a year

Water once a week

Sometimes the benefits of a particular treatment become evident during the course of a trial, so the trial is stopped early.

ASCOT

ASCOT (the Anglo-Scandinavian Cardiac Outcomes Trial) was an international trial that recruited over 19,000 patients with high blood pressure but no previous heart disease. Approximately 4500 of these people had Type 2 diabetes. There were two 'arms' to the trial, one which confirmed the previous finding that lowering a slightly raised cholesterol level with a statin (this time atorvastatin) reduced the risk of heart attack and stroke. The second arm compared the effects of two different regimes for reducing blood pressure.

What did it show?

The blood pressure-lowering arm reported in 2005. However, it had been stopped early because the benefits of treating patients with a combination of perindopril (an ACE inhibitor drug) and amlodipine (a calcium channel blocking drug), as opposed to a combination of atenolol (a beta-blocker) and bendrofluazide (a diuretic or 'water tablet'), were too clear to be ignored.

Combined results from both arms of the trial indicated the following:

- The risk of heart attacks and strokes was lowered by approximately 46% for patients being treated with amlodipine, perindopril and atorvastatin.

- Patients without diabetes who were being treated with amlodipine and perindopril appeared to be 29% less likely than those being treated with atenolol and bendrofluazide to develop Type 2 diabetes. This may be due in part to the withdrawal of bendrofluazide, to a protective effect of perindopril or to a combination of the two.

What does this mean?

The clear benefits enjoyed by those patients taking the combination of amlodipine and perindopril have prompted the British Hypertension Society to review its guidelines on prescribing. A combination of an ACE inhibitor drug with a calcium channel blocker is now the first treatment of choice for patients with heart disease.

Studies looking at the effect of reducing cholesterol levels

Heart Protection Study

The Heart Protection Study was one of the biggest studies of a cholesterol-lowering drug (simvastatin). It studied patients with and without diabetes.

What did it show?

There were 20,536 patients in the study, 5963 of whom had diabetes. These people were allocated randomly either to the group being given simvastatin 40 mg daily or to the group being given a placebo (dummy) tablet. Patients were followed up for a period of 5 years. Over that time, the simvastatin treatment group had cholesterol levels that were on average about 1 mmol/L less than those in the placebo group. In this study, the risk of major cardiovascular events such as stroke or heart attack was reduced by 33%. People with diabetes who had LDL (bad cholesterol; see page 63) levels lower than 3 mmol/L, and who would not have been treated in the past, benefitted with a 27% reduction in the risk of cardiovascular events.

This study also showed that simvastatin is an extremely safe drug with a low risk of side effects. There have been worries that simvastatin might cause liver problems, but less than 0.5% (five out of a thousand) of patients in this very large study had evidence of liver damage, and this risk was the same in both the simvastatin and the placebo group.

What does this mean?

If all the cholesterol-lowering studies with drugs of the statin family are taken together, there is now strong evidence that the vast majority of patients with Type 2 diabetes should be given a statin tablet to reduce their cholesterol and hence their cardiovascular risk. We know that Type 2 diabetes greatly increases the risk of cardiovascular events. So where we can demonstrate reductions in risk with a tried and tested drug, it is important to encourage its use.

Women who are pregnant or planning a pregnancy should avoid taking a statin.

CARDS

CARDS, the Collaborative Atorvastatin Diabetes Study, is the largest study of a statin (atorvastatin) to be carried out in people with Type 2 diabetes. The study involved an important collaboration between a number of key researchers in diabetes from across universities in the UK and Ireland.

What did it show?

A group of 2838 patients between the ages of 40 and 75 years with fairly average cholesterol levels (total cholesterol was 5.4 mmol/L of which LDL level was 3.1 mmol/L) were randomized to receive the lowest dose of atorvastatin (10 mg) or a placebo tablet. As well as Type 2 diabetes, they also had to have another risk factor, such as cigarette smoking, high blood pressure, diabetic eye disease or proteinuria (indicative of diabetic kidney disease). These patients were followed up for about 4½ years. The number of patients who had at least one cardiovascular event such as a stroke or heart attack was reduced by 37%, and stroke reduction was greatest, at 48%. The

people who joined this study would not have been considered a high-risk group, so the results are very impressive.

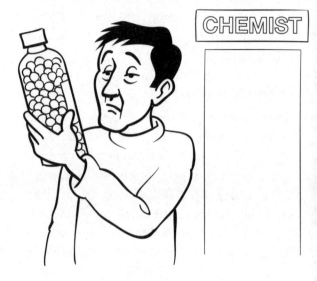

Statins have been found to be very effective in reducing the risk of strokes and heart attacks. If you have Type 2 diabetes, it is likely your doctor will put you on them at some stage.

What does this mean?

Taken together with other studies looking at the use of statins in patients with Type 2 diabetes, this study has provided the final piece of the jigsaw to support the use of statin-type drugs in most patients with Type 2 diabetes. Since the publication of the CARDS study, an evidence review has taken place carried out by the joint British Societies (the specialist bodies for cardiovascular and diabetes care). These bodies recommend statin treatment for all people with Type 2 diabetes and a cholesterol level above 4.0 mmol/L, unless there is a contraindication which means they are unable to take them.

A study which tries to correct all risk factors: the Steno-2 study

For years, it was accepted that if you managed one risk factor aggressively, there would be little to be gained by managing other risk factors to similar stringent targets. The Steno-2 study was designed to test the hypothesis that reducing all possible risk factors to tight targets would have a synergistic effect in reducing heart attacks, strokes and other cardiovascular problems.

What did it show?

The study looked at 160 people with diabetes who also had microalbuminuria, which put them at risk of heart disease. These were entered into either an intensive or a conventional management group. The conventional group were managed to standard Danish guidelines, whereas the intensive group were given very tight targets for glucose, blood pressure, lipids and microalbuminuria and treated with aggressive drug intervention and lifestyle advice. The greatest reductions were seen in blood pressure, lipids and micro-albuminuria in the intensive group, with a much smaller fall in glucose, representing the fact that blood glucose targets are much harder to achieve. Over a period of 8 years, the group managed intensively were about half as likely to suffer cardiovascular problems. Now, 13 years after the study, the intensive therapy group still benefit from fewer cardiovascular events, and the death rate in this group is much reduced.

What does this mean?

The Steno-2 study reinforced the view that holistic management of Type 2 diabetes is the key and finally steered clinicians away from a view of the condition centering only on controlling sugar. It proved that treating to target is not just the preserve of randomized trials of new drugs, and that by adopting an aggressive approach to multiple targets, real benefits can be achieved.

37

Research and new developments

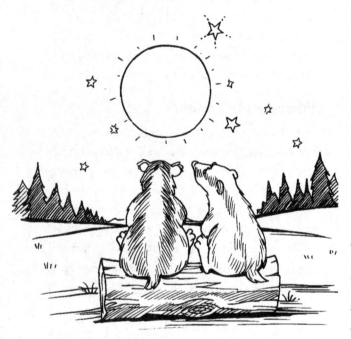

Huge efforts are put into diabetes research around the world, and more than 10,000 scientific studies are published every year. A large proportion of this is basic research, trying to throw light upon the causes of diabetes and the effects it may have on the body over the years. If you hear of a new treatment for diabetes from newspapers, television or the internet, you must be aware that many of these reports are not based on scientific fact. In any case, it takes several years before a new exciting treatment becomes widely available. Unfortunately, many new 'wonder drugs' never become established treatments.

No new drugs

A number of new drugs to help treat diabetes have been launched over the past 10 years and sadly there is now a gap with nothing new over the horizon for treating Type 2 diabetes.

Now the SGLT-2 inhibitors are available, there are no new drugs in the pipeline to treat diabetes. However, a great deal of research is in progress to work out how best to use the available drugs.

Very strict food restriction cures diabetes

An important research project was published in 2011 which showed that, by restricting food intake to 600 calories over the course of eight weeks, people with established diabetes could render their blood sugars normal. Over the 8 weeks of food restriction, participants lost an average of 13 kg (= 2 stones) and as a result their blood glucose results were normal. So far there has been no published information about how these people fared over the next 12 months.

Other research

Research into Type 2 diabetes is mainly focused on the following areas:
- Investigating the detailed mechanisms in the brain that control our eating and make us stop eating when we feel full.

- Looking into the mechanisms that cause racial and social differences in diabetes risk.

- Working out how best to screen populations for prediabetes and determining the most effective ways of preventing the condition from developing by education, lifestyle change and drugs.

- The new problem of Type 2 diabetes in young people and how best to help them through education.

Looking ahead

When your diabetes was diagnosed and while you were settling into a treatment pattern, it may have been difficult to view the future with optimism. Reading this book, you must be aware of a wide range of treatment that is available, and there is a promise of more effective methods of care in the future. In time, we can be sure that more effective and convenient forms of treatment will be developed.

Glossary

Terms in *italics* in these definitions refer to other terms in the glossary.

Acarbose A drug that slows the digestion and absorption of complex carbohydrates.

Acesulfame-K A low-calorie intense sweetener.

acetone One of the chemicals called ketones formed when the body uses up fat for energy. The presence of acetone in the urine usually means that more insulin is needed.

adrenaline A hormone produced by the adrenal glands, which prepares the body for action (the 'flight or fight' reaction) and also increases the level of blood glucose. Produced by the body in response to many stimuli, including a low blood glucose.

AGE Abbreviation for advanced glycation end products, the name given to glucose bound to fat which causes damage to certain cells in the body.

albumin A protein present in most animal tissues. The presence of albumin in the urine may denote kidney damage or be simply due to a urinary infection.

alpha cell The cell that produces glucagon – found in the *islets of Langerhans* in the pancreas.

alpha-glucosidase inhibitor A tablet that slows the digestion of carbohydrates in the intestine (acarbose).

analogue insulin Insulin that has the molecular structure changed to alter its action.

angiography A special type of X-ray where dye is injected into an artery to detect narrowing.

angioplasty A technique which uses an inflatable balloon to widen narrowed arteries.

antigens Proteins, which the body recognizes as 'foreign' and which trigger an immune response.

arteriosclerosis or **arterial sclerosis** or **arterial disease** Hardening of the arteries. Loss of elasticity in the walls of the arteries from thickening and calcification. Occurs with advancing years in those with or without diabetes. May affect the heart (causing thrombosis), the brain (a stroke) or the circulation to the legs and feet.

aspartame A low-calorie intense sweetener. Brand name NutraSweet.

autonomic neuropathy Damage to the system of nerves that regulate many automatic functions of the body such as stomach emptying, sexual function (potency) and blood pressure control.

bacterium (*pl.* bacteria) A type of germ.

balanitis Inflammation of the end of the penis, usually caused by yeast infections as a result of sugar in the urine.

beta-blockers   Drugs that block the effect of stress hormones on the cardiovascular system. Often used to treat angina and to lower blood pressure. May change the warning signs of *hypoglycaemia*.

beta cell   The cell that produces insulin – found in the *islets of Langerhans* in the pancreas.

biguanides   A group of anti-diabetes tablets that lower blood glucose levels. Their mode of action is not well understood, but they work in part by increasing the body's sensivity to insulin. Metformin is the only preparation in this group.

blood glucose monitoring   System of measuring blood glucose levels at home using a portable meter and reagent sticks.

bran   Indigestible husk of the wheat grain. A type of *dietary fibre*.

brittle diabetes   Refers to diabetes that is very unstable with swings from very low to very high blood glucose levels and often involves frequent admissions to hospital.

calories   Units in which energy or heat are measured. The energy value of food is measured in calories.

carbohydrates   A class of food that comprises starches and sugars and is most readily available to the body for energy. Found mainly in plant foods. Examples are rice, bread, potatoes, pasta, beans.

cataract   Opacity of the lens of the eye, which obscures vision. It may be removed surgically.

Charcot foot   Swelling of the foot, sometimes leading to deformity, as a result of lack of sensation (neuropathy).

clear insulin   This term used to refer to short-acting insulins. However, the two long-acting analogue *insulins* (Lantus and Levemir) are also clear so the term must be used with caution.

cloudy insulin   Longer-acting insulin with fine particles of insulin bound to protamine or zinc.

coma   A form of unconsciousness from which people can only be roused with difficulty. If caused by diabetes, may be a *diabetic coma* or an *insulin coma*.

complications   Long-term consequences of imperfectly controlled diabetes. For details, see Chapters 30, 31 and 32.

control   Usually refers to blood glucose control. The aim of good control is to achieve normal blood glucose levels (4– 10 mmol/L) and HbA_{1c} less than 7%.

coronary heart disease   Disease of the blood vessels supplying the heart.

cystitis   Inflammation of the bladder, which usually causes frequent passing of urine, accompanied by a burning pain.

DESMOND   Diabetes Education and Self Management for Ongoing and Newly Diagnosed. An education programme for people with Type 2 diabetes.

detemir   A new insulin analogue designed to last for 24 hours and act as basal insulin. Also called Levemir.

diabetes insipidus   A disorder of the pituitary gland accompanied by excessive urination and thirst. Nothing to do with diabetes mellitus.

diabetes mellitus   A disorder of the pancreas characterized by a high blood glucose level. This book is about *diabetes mellitus*.

diabetic amyotrophy   Rare condition causing pain in and/or weakness of the legs from the damage to certain nerves.

diabetic coma   Extreme form of *hyperglycaemia*, usually with ketoacidosis, causing unconsciousness.

diabetic diarrhoea   A form of diabetic *autonomic neuropathy* leading to diarrhoea.

diabetic foods   Food products targeted at people with diabetes, in which ordinary sugar (sucrose) is replaced with substitutes such as *fructose* or *sorbitol*. These foods are not recommended as part of your food plan.

diabetic nephropathy   Type of kidney damage that may occur in diabetes. See Chapter 31.

diabetic neuropathy   Type of nerve damage that may occur in diabetes. See Chapters 31 and 32.

diabetic retinopathy   Type of eye disease that may occur in diabetes. See Chapter 31.

dietary fibre   Part of the plant material that resists digestion and gives bulk to the diet. Also called fibre or roughage.

diuretics   Agents that increase the flow of urine, commonly known as water tablets.

DPP-4 inhibitors   New generation of agents to treat Type 2 diabetes. DPP-4 inhibitors (gliptins) can be taken in tablet form and work by slowing the breakdown of *GLP-1* (see below). Sitagliptin is now available and may be joined soon by vildagliptin.

erectile dysfunction   Inability to achieve or maintain an erection (*impotence*).

fibre   Another name for *dietary fibre*.

fructosamine   Measurement of diabetes control that reflects the average blood glucose level over the previous 2–3 weeks. Similar to *haemoglobin A_{1c}* which averages the blood glucose over the longer period

of 2–3 months.

fructose   Type of sugar found naturally in fruit and honey. Since it does not require insulin for its metabolism, it is often used as a sweetener in diabetic foods.

gangrene   Death of a part of the body due to a very poor blood supply. A combination of *neuropathy* and *arteriosclerosis* may result in infection of unrecognized injuries to the feet. If neglected, this infection may spread, causing further destruction.

gastroparesis   Delayed emptying of the stomach as a result of *autonomic neuropathy*. Can lead to erratic food absorption and vomiting.

gestational diabetes   Diabetes which is diagnosed during pregnancy.

glargine   A new insulin analogue designed to last for 24 hours to act as basal (background) insulin. Also called Lantus.

glaucoma   Disease of the eye causing increased pressure inside the eyeball.

glitazones   A group of drugs that reduce insulin resistance – see *thiazolidinedione*.

GLP-1   Glucagon-like peptide-1 – a hormone which increases the production of insulin in response to food and reduces the production of glucagon. Two GLP-1 agents (exenatide and liraglutide) are soon to arrive in the UK.

glucagon   A *hormone* produced by the *alpha cells* in the pancreas which causes a rise in blood glucose by freeing glycogen from the liver. Available in injection form for use in treating a severe *hypo*.

glucose   Form of sugar made by digestion of *carbohydrates*. Absorbed into the bloodstream where it circulates and is used as a source of energy.

glucose tolerance test   Test used in the diagnosis of *diabetes mellitus*. The glucose in the blood is measured at intervals before and after the person has drunk a large amount of glucose while fasting.

glycaemic index (GI)   A way of describing how a *carbohydrate*-containing food affects blood glucose levels.

glycogen   The form in which *carbohydrate* is stored in the liver and muscles. It is often known as animal starch.

glycosuria   Presence of *glucose* in the urine.

glycosylated haemoglobin   Another name for *haemoglobin A$_{1c}$*.

haemoglobin A$_{1c}$ The part of the haemoglobin or colouring matter of the red blood cell which has *glucose* attached to it. A test of diabetes control. The amount of haemoglobin A$_{1c}$ in the blood depends on the average blood glucose level over the previous 2–3 months.

HbA$_{1c}$ See *haemoglobin A$_{1c}$*.

hormone   Substance generated in one gland or organ which is carried by the blood to another part of the body to control another organ. *Insulin* and *glucagon* are both hormones.

human insulin   Insulin that has been manufactured to be identical to that produced in the human pancreas. Differs slightly from older insulins, which were extracted from cows or pigs.

hydramnios   An excessive amount of amniotic fluid, i.e. the fluid surrounding the baby before birth.

hyperglycaemia   High blood glucose (above 10 mmol/L).

hypo   Abbreviation for *hypoglycaemia*.

hypoglycaemia   (also known as a *hypo* or an insulin reaction) Low blood glucose (below 3.5 mmol/L).

impotence   Failure of erection of the penis.

Injector   Device to aid injections.

Innolet   A simple injector for insulin designed for people with poor vision or problems with their hands such as arthritis.

insulin   A *hormone* produced by the *beta cells* of the *pancreas* and responsible for control of blood glucose. Insulin can only be given by injection because digestive juices destroy its action if it is taken by mouth.

insulin coma   Extreme form of *hypoglycaemia* associated with unconsciousness and sometimes convulsions.

insulin-dependent diabetes (abbreviation **ID D**) Former name for *Type 1 diabetes*.

insulin pen   Device that resembles a large fountain pen that takes a cartridge of insulin. The injection of insulin is given after dialling the dose and pressing a button that releases the insulin.

insulin reaction   Another name for *hypoglycaemia* or a hypo. In America it is called an insulin shock.

insulin resistance   A condition where the normal amount of insulin is not able to keep the blood glucose level down to normal. Seen particularly in patients with Type 2 diabetes. Such people need large doses of insulin to control their diabetes. The glitazone group of tablets is designed to reduce insulin resistance.

intermediate-acting insulin   Insulin preparations with an action lasting 12–18 hours.

intradermal   Meaning 'into the skin'. Usually refers to injection given into the most superficial layer of the skin. *Insulin* must not be given in this way as it is painful and will not be absorbed properly.

intramuscular   A deep injection into the muscle.

islets of Langerhans   Specialized cells within the pancreas that produce insulin and glucagon.

isophane   A form of *intermediate-acting insulin* that has protamine added to slow its absorption.

joule   Unit of work or energy used in the metric system. There are about 4.18 joules in each calorie. Some dietitians calculate food energy in joules.

juvenile onset diabetes   Outdated name for *Type 1 diabetes*, so called because most patients receiving insulin develop diabetes under the age of 40. The term is no longer used because Type 1 diabetes can occur at any age, although it is more common in young people.

ketoacidosis   A serious condition due to lack of insulin which results in body fat being used up to form *ketones* and acids. Characterized by high blood glucose levels, ketones in the urine, vomiting, drowsiness, heavy laboured breathing and a smell of *acetone* on the breath.

ketones   Acid substances (including *acetone*) formed when body fat is used up to provide energy.

ketonuria   The presence of acetone and other ketones in the urine. Detected by testing with a special testing stick (Ketostix, Ketur Test). Presence of ketones in the urine is due to lack of

insulin or periods of starvation.

laser treatment   Process in which laser beams are used to treat a damaged retina (back of the eye). Used in *photocoagulation*.

lente insulin   A form of *intermediate-acting insulin* that has zinc added to slow its absorption.

lipoatrophy   Loss of fat from injection sites. It used to occur before the use of highly purified insulins.

lipohypertrophy   Fatty swelling usually caused by repeated injections of insulin into the same site.

maturity onset diabetes   Another term for *Type 2 diabetes*, most commonly occurring in people who are middle-aged and overweight.

metabolic rate   Rate of oxygen consumption by the body; the rate at which you 'burn up' the food you eat.

metabolism   Process by which the body turns food into energy.

metformin   A *biguanide* tablet that works by reducing the release of *glucose* from the liver and increasing the uptake of glucose into the muscle.

microalbuminuria   Small amounts of protein in the urine, not detectable by dipstick for albumin (*proteinuria*). Raised levels indicate early kidney damage.

microaneurysms   Small red dots on the retina at the back of the eye which are one of the earliest signs of diabetic *retinopathy*. Represent areas of weakness of the very small blood vessels in the eye. Microaneurysms do not affect the eyesight in any way.

micromole   One thousandth (1/1000) of a millimole.

millimole   Unit for measuring the concentration of glucose and other substances in the blood. Blood glucose is measured in millimoles per litre (mmol/L). It has replaced milligrammes per decilitre (mg/dl or mg%) as a unit of measurement, although this is still used in some other countries; 1 mmol/L = 18 mg/dl.

MODY   Maturity onset diabetes of the young: a form of Type 2 diabetes that affects young people and runs in families. See Chapter 22.

nateglinide   A prandial glucose regulator. nephropathy Kidney damage. In the first instance, this makes the kidney more leaky so that albumin appears in the urine. At a later stage, it may affect the function of the kidney, and in severe cases, it leads to kidney failure.

neuropathy   Damage to the nerves, which may be *peripheral neuropathy* or *autonomic neuropathy*. It can occur with diabetes especially when poorly controlled, but also has other causes.

NICE   National Institute for Health and Care Excellence. An independent organization to provide national guidance to promote good health. It provides guidelines for the use of new and existing drugs in the NHS.

non-insulin dependent diabetes (abbreviation **NIDD**)   Former name for *Type 2 diabetes*.

orlistat   A tablet that blocks the digestion of fat. Brand name Xenical. Used to help people lose weight, which in turn may improve control of diabetes.

pancreas   Gland lying behind the stomach, which as well as secreting a digestive fluid (pancreatic juice) also produces the *hormones insulin* and

glucagon. Contains the *islets of Langerhans*.

peripheral neuropathy   Damage to the nerves supplying the muscles and skin. This can result in diminished sensation, particularly in the feet and legs, and in muscle weakness. May also cause pain in the feet or legs.

phimosis   Inflammation and narrowing of the foreskin of the penis.

photocoagulation   Process of treating diabetic *retinopathy* with light beams, either laser beams or a xenon arc. This technique focuses a beam of light on a very tiny area of the *retina*. This beam is so intense that it causes a very small burn, which may close off a leaking blood vessel or destroy weak blood vessels that are at risk of bleeding.

pioglitazone   A glitazone tablet that targets insulin resistance. Trade name Actos.

PKC inhibitors (protein kinase C inhibitors)   Developed to try and reverse the changes in small blood vessels which cause diabetic eye disease (*retinopathy*). Though they seem to help in isolated cases, the overall results have been disappointing.

polydipsia   Being excessively thirsty and drinking too much. It is a symptom of untreated diabetes.

polyuria   The passing of large quantities of urine due to excess *glucose* in the bloodstream. It is a symptom of untreated diabetes.

pork insulin   Insulin extracted from the *pancreas* of pigs.

prandial glucose regulators   Tablets taken before meals that stimulate the release of insulin from the pancreas (repaglinide and nateglinide). Only used in Type 2 diabetes.

pre-eclampsia   A condition which occurs towards the end of pregnancy and leads to high blood pressure, protein in the urine and, in severe cases, convulsions. Pre-eclampsia normally resolves soon after delivery.

protein   One of the classes of food that is necessary for the growth and repair of tissues. Found in fish, meat, eggs, milk and pulses. Can also refer to *albumin* when found in the urine.

proteinuria   *Protein* or *albumin* in the urine.

pruritus vulvae   Irritation of the vulva (the genital area in women). Caused by an infection that occurs because of an excess of sugar in the urine and is often an early sign of diabetes in the older person. It clears up when the blood glucose levels return to normal and the sugar disappears from the insulin.

pyelonephritis   Inflammation and infection of the kidney.

renal threshold   The level of *glucose* in the blood above which it will begin to spill into the urine. The usual renal threshold for glucose in the blood is about 10 mmol/L; i.e. when the blood glucose rises above 10 mmol/L, glucose appears in the urine.

repaglinide   A *prandial glucose regulator*.

retina   Light-sensitive coat at the back of the eye.

retinal screening   Photograph of the *retina* to identify changes due to diabetes at a stage at which they can be treated to prevent loss of vision. Usually carried out once a year.

retinopathy   Damage to the *retina*.

rimonabant   New drug designed to help obese patients by reducing appetite. May also help people give up smoking, though it is not licensed for this. It is not yet available in the NHS and is being evaluated by *NICE*. Also named Acomplia.

roughage   Another name for *dietary fibre*.

saccharin   A synthetic sweetener that is calorie free.

short-acting insulin   Insulin preparations with an action lasting 6–8 hours.

sitaglitpin (Januvia)   A DPP-4 inhibitor tablet that increases levels of GLP-1, now available in the US and Europe.

Snellen chart   Chart showing rows of letters in decreasing sizes. Used for measuring *visual acuity*.

sorbitol   A chemical related to sugar and alcohol that is used as a sweetening agent in foods as a substitute for ordinary sugar. It has no significant effect upon the blood glucose level but has the same number of *calories* as ordinary sugar so should not be used by those who need to lose weight. Poorly absorbed and may have a laxative effect.

steroids   *Hormones* produced by the adrenal glands, testes and ovaries. Also available in synthetic form. Tend to increase the blood *glucose* level and make diabetes worse.

subcutaneous injection   An injection beneath the skin into the layer of fat that lies between the skin and muscle. The normal way of giving *insulin*.

sucrose   A sugar (containing *glucose* and *fructose* in combination) derived from sugar cane or sugar beet (i.e. ordinary table sugar). It is a pure *carbohydrate*.

sulphonylureas   Anti-diabetes tablets that lower the blood *glucose* by stimulating the *pancreas* to produce more insulin. Commonly used sulphonylureas are gliclazide and glibenclamide.

thiazolidinedione Generic name for the group of tablets that target *insulin resistance* and improve diabetes in *Type 2 diabetes*. A commonly used thiazolidinedione is pioglitazone. Brand name Actos.

thrombosis Clot forming in a blood vessel.

tissue markers *Proteins* on the outside of cells in the body that are genetically determined.

toxaemia Poisoning of the blood by the absorption of toxins. Usually refers to the toxaemia of pregnancy, which is characterized by high blood pressure, *proteinuria* and ankle swelling.

Type 1 diabetes Name for insulin-dependent diabetes which cannot be treated by diet and tablets alone. Age of onset is usually below the age of 40 years.

Type 2 diabetes Name for non-insulin-dependent diabetes. Age of onset is usually above the age of 40 years, often in people who are overweight, which contributes to insulin resistance. These people do not need insulin treatment immediately; their diabetes can usually be successfully controlled with diet alone or diet and tablets for a period of time. Formerly known as maturity onset diabetes.

U-40 insulin The old weaker strength of *insulin*, no longer available in the UK. It is still available in Eastern Europe and in some countries in the Far East, such as Vietnam and Indonesia.

U-100 insulin The standard strength of *insulin* in the UK, USA, Canada, Australia, New Zealand, South Africa, the Middle East and the Far East.

U-500 insulin A stronger strength of insulin used for patients who are particularly insulin resistant.

urine testing The detection of abnormal amounts of *glucose, ketones, protein* or blood in the urine, usually by means of urine testing sticks.

vildagliptin (trade name Galvus) A DPP-4 inhibitor tablet that is likely to be available soon.

virus A very small organism capable of causing disease.

viscous fibre A type of *dietary fibre* found in pulses (peas, beans and lentils) and some fruit and vegetables.

visual acuity Acuteness of vision. Measured by reading letters on a sight testing chart (a *Snellen chart*).

water tablets The common name for *diuretics*.

Xenical The brand name for *orlistat*.

Finding our more

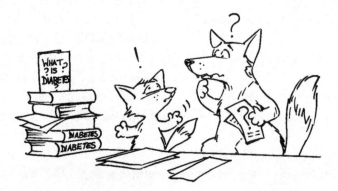

Dr Charles Fox and Dr Anne Kilvert have written another book, *Type 2 Diabetes: Answers at Your Fingertips* (now in its 7th edition), which contains over 400 questions from other patients together with answers. The book is published by Class Health and is available from www.class.co.uk

You are also advised to visit the diabetes UK website – www.diabetes.org.uk – for recommended books and leaflets which can be downloaded.

Index

allowances 198

alpha cells 21, 28, 29, 266g

alpha-glucosidase inhibitors 96–7, 266g

alternative therapies 13–14

Alva, Maria de 21

American Diabetes Association 82, 133, 171, 173

Amiel, Stephanie A. 143

amitriptyline 227

amphetamines 181

amputation 233

amylase 39, 48, 49

amylopectin 48, 49

anaemia 95, 226

Andersson, A.H., Asp, N-G. and Hallmans, G. 42

angina 184, 185

angiogram 233

angioplasty 234

angiotensin II receptor blockers (ARBs) (sartans) 219, 225, 226, 229, 260

angiotensin-converting (ACE) inhibitors 172, 192, 219, 225, 226, 229, 260

Anglo-Scandinavian Cardiac Outcomes Trial (ASCOT) 260–1

antibiotics 208

antibodies 113, 140

antidepressants 176

anxiety 30, 159, 212, 213–14

Apidra 105, 106, 108, 109, 110, 115, 122

appetite 136–7

'apple-shaped' body 56

apps 38, 133

Aqua Care 208

aqueous humour 36

ARBs (angiotensin II receptor blockers) (sartans) 219, 225, 226, 229, 260

Armed Forces 201

arteriosclerosis 47, 266g

ASCOT (the Anglo-Scandinavian Cardiac Outcomes Trial) 260–1

aspartame (E951) 53, 54

aspirin treatment 221, 243

associations, support 254

asthma 165

atherosclerosis 236

Atkins diet 46, 47, 60

atorvastatin 219, 261, 262

Attendance Allowance 253

Australia 40

autoimmunity 15, 236

autonomic nervous system 24diag, 142, 144, 147, 155, 181, 222, 227–8

autonomic neuropathy 230, 266g

'autonomic' or 'adrenergic' symptoms 142, 143, 144

autosomal dominant inheritance 172

azithromycin 208

background retinopathy 223

Balance 248

balanitis 32, 266g

bariatric surgery 62

B-D Safe Clip 124

bedtime injection, taking wrong type insulin 114, 115

benefits, claiming 252–3

benzodiazepines 181–2

beta cells, pancreas 16, 21, 22, 25, 27, 89, 98diag, 267g

biguanides (metformin) 16, 87–9, 267g
  and alcohol 88
  breastfeeding 88
  and cardiovascular disease 220
  combination with gliptins 93
  combination with glitazones 93, 94
  evidence for use 89
  and insulin 128, 137
  and monitoring 71
  older people 241
  PCOS 58, 237
  in pregnancy 88, 191, 193

Have you found **Type 2 Diabetes in Adults of all Ages** *useful and practical?*
If so, you may be interested in these other books from Class Publishing.

Type 2 Diabetes: Answers at Your Fingertips.

Dr Charles Fox and Dr Anne Kilvert   ISBN 9781859593233

This latest edition of our practical question-and-answer format handbook makes it easy for you to learn more about Type 2 diabetes. The authors comprehensively answer over 400 questions about every aspect of living with the condition, and their constructive approach will give you all the knowledge you need to deal confidently with your diabetes.

Type 2 Diabetes: Answers at your fingertips gives you:

- Up-to-date information on all the available – and forthcoming – medical treatments, including the current situation with Avandia (rosaglitizone)
- Advice on how to achieve the best possible control of your diabetes, working around your daily routine
- Answers to dozens of practical questions about lifestyle, work and holidays
- Guidance on healthy eating, exercise and complementary therapies

Type 2 Diabetes: Essentials

Dr Charles Fox and Dr Anne Kilvert   ISBN 9781859594872

This Essentials book answers all the key questions asked about Type 2 diabetes in succinct, accessible and up-to-date form. Type 2 diabetes tends to occur in people who are over thirty and above average weight (although there are exceptions). The onset tends to be gradual and the initial treatment is through diet and tablets. If your diabetes has been treated this way, this book is for you. This introductory guide answers 50 key questions asked by people with Type 2 diabetes and their families. It provides a summary of symptoms and treatments, and offers practical advice on living life with Type 2 diabetes.

Dump your Toxic Waist!, Lose Inches, Beat Diabetes and Stop that Heart Attack.

Dr Derrick Cutting   ISBN 9781859591918

The easy drug-free and medically accurate way to lose inches, beat diabetes and stop that heart attack. Excess fat round your belly is not just dead weight; it's a living liability. It's a fact. We are getting fatter and risking our health in the process. This is the only book you need to reverse the metabolic syndrome – the root cause of obesity, diabetes and heart disease.

"Highly recommended." - ***Michael Livingston, Director, H.E.A.R.T UK***

High Blood Pressure: Answers at Your Fingertips

Professor Tom Fahey, Professor Deirdre Murphy, Dr Julian Tudor Hart
ISBN 9781859590904

High blood pressure is the most common continuing medical condition seen by family doctors. Yet whilst lots of people have it, very few understand what is going on and why it is important to lower your blood pressure to a normal level and maintain it there.

In this practical guide, the expert medical authors use their experience to answer all your questions, giving you the information you need to bring your blood pressure down – and keep it down. Clear explanations of the causes and symptoms of high blood pressure and helpful advice will enable you to take positive steps towards managing your BP.

Heart Health: Answers at Your Fingertips

Graham Jackson   ISBN 9781859591574

Expert cardiologist Dr Graham Jackson takes the reader on a voyage of discovery and explanation in his clearly written and good-humoured text, which should allay fear through awareness of what heart disease is all about. This book answers over 420 real questions on all aspects of heart health – from coronary heart disease to angina, from palpitations to vascular disease. Heart Health also includes advice on healthy living, giving up smoking, HRT, sex & relationships and much more.

"Busy doctors or dissatisfied heart patients, could do better than invest in Dr Jackson's latest book...devoted to questions that patients ask and answers the doctor wishes he had given if only he'd had the time." – Dr Thomas Stuttaford, The Times

Type 1 Diabetes in Children, Adolescents and Young Adults

Dr Ragnar Hanas   ISBN 9781859593509
Highly Commended in the Popular Medicine Category of the BMA Medical Book Awards 2013

The number of children with Type 1 diabetes is steadily increasing. Medical research has conclusively proved that looking after your own diabetes - and keeping your blood glucose level down – is the key to avoiding the pitfalls and long-term risks.

In this practical, easy-to-read book Dr Ragnar Hanas shows you step-by-step how to become an expert in your own diabetes. By understanding your Type 1 diabetes and how to manage it, you can live a full, healthy and happy life.

The *Class Health* Feedback Form

We hope that you found this *Class Health* book helpful. We always appreciate readers' opinions and would be grateful if you could take a few minutes to complete this form for us.

1. **How did you acquire your copy of this book?**
   - [ ] From my local library
   - [ ] Read an article in a newspaper/magazine
   - [ ] Found it by chance
   - [ ] Recommended by a friend
   - [ ] Recommended by a patient organisation/charity
   - [ ] Recommended by a doctor/nurse/advisor
   - [ ] Saw an advertisement

2. **How much of the book have you read?**
   - [ ] All of it
   - [ ] More than half of it
   - [ ] Less than half of it

3. **Which copies/chapters have been most helpful?**

   ....

   ....

   ....

4. **Overall, how useful to you was this *Class Health* book?**
   - [ ] Extremely useful
   - [ ] Very useful
   - [ ] Useful

5. **What did you find most helpful?**

   ....

   ....

   ....

6. **What did you find least helpful?**

....

....

....

7. **Have you read any other health books?**

☐ Yes

☐ No

If yes, which subjects did they cover?

....

....

....

How did this _Class Health_ book compare?

☐ Much better

☐ Better

☐ About the same

☐ Not as good

8. **Would you recommend this book to a friend?**

☐ Yes

☐ No

Thank you for your help. Please send your completed form to:

FREEPOST
Class Learning

(No postcode required. No stamp needed if posted in the UK)

Title Prof/Dr/Mr/Mrs/Ms ....

Surname .... First name...............................

Address...

....

Town.. Postcode ....

Country ....

☐ Please add my name and address to receive details of related books.
(Please note, we will not pass on your details to any other company).